Atrial Fibrillation in Clinical Practice

Atrial Fibrillation in Clinical Practice

Gregory Y H Lip MD FRCP(Edin, Glasg) DFM FESC FACC
Consultant Cardiologist and Reader in Medicine
Haemostatis, Thrombosis and Vascular Biology Unit
University Department of Medicine
City Hospital
Birmingham, UK

MARTIN DUNITZ

First published in the United Kingdom in 2001 by
Martin Dunitz Ltd
The Livery House
7–9 Pratt Street
London NW1 0AE

Tel: +44-(0)20-7482-2202
Fax: +44-(0)20-7267-0159
E-mail: info@mdunitz.globalnet.co.uk
Website: http://www.dunitz.co.uk

A CIP catalogue record for this book is available from the British Library

ISBN 1-85317-895-0

Distributed in the United States by:
Blackwell Science Inc.
Commerce Place, 350 Main Street
Malden MA 02148, USA
Tel: +1-800-215-1000

Distributed in Canada by:
Login Brothers Book Company
324 Salteaux Crescent
Winnipeg, Manitoba R3J 3T2
Canada
Tel: +1-204-224-4068

Distributed in Brazil by:
Ernesto Reichmann Distribuidora de Livros, Ltda
Rua Coronel Marques 335, Tatuape 03440-000
Sao Paulo,
Brazil

Composition by Wearset, Boldon, Tyne and Wear
Printed and bound in Spain by Grafos S.A. Arte sobre papel

To Peck Lin, Philomena and Aloysius

Contents

Preface

Atrial fibrillation (AF) is the most common sustained cardiac rhythm disorder, with an increasing prevalence in an increasingly elderly population. The great interest in AF relates to the substantial mortality and morbidity associated with it, with an increased risk of stroke and thromboembolism, in addition to heart failure and decreased exercise tolerance. Indeed, we are not dealing with a benign condition, but neither are we dealing with a new or uncommon problem.

Indeed, there is also more to AF management than digoxin, and things have moved far beyond the days of *digitalis purpurea* use by William Withering of Birmingham. Nevertheless the management of patients with AF today is still often suboptimal, with marked disparity in treatment between cardiologists and non-cardiologists. We recognise however that pharmacological therapy for AF has significant limitations, with arrhythmia suppression (and not abolition) but at the expense of drug adverse effects. The cynical view that 'all antiarrhythmics are poisonous' and the increasing viability of new non-pharmacological techniques to improve quality of life and symptomology in short-term studies of patients with AF opens new management possibilities for the future. The value of thromboprophylaxis in AF is also well-established but despite the compelling evidence of the benefits of stroke reduction in AF, antithrombotic therapy continues to be under-utilised. Indeed, the challenge ahead is to find the 'magic bullet' that substantially reduces stroke and thromboembolism, but with minimal bleeding risk.

Atrial Fibrillation in Clinical Practice aims to set out in a logical fashion where we are today with AF, and to highlight the clinical epidemiology, pathophysiology, clinical features and management of this condition, in a practical, clinically-orientated and up-to-date manner. This book will therefore be of use to all clinicians and health care professionals dealing with this common cardiac arrhythmia.

Gregory Y H Lip
Consultant Cardiologist and
Reader in Medicine
University Department of Medicine
City Hospital
Birmingham

Acknowledgements

Many colleagues and patients have perpetuated my interest in atrial fibrillation, and I am grateful to them for their advice and intellectual stimulation over many years. Dr Denis Krikler very kindly enlightened me on the historical aspects of atrial fibrillation. I also thank Alan Burgess and Dan Edwards from Martin Dunitz for their patience.

Gregory YH Lip

I
Epidemiology and Importance

1

History of atrial fibrillation

Introduction

Atrial fibrillation (AF) is the most common sustained cardiac rhythm disorder, with an increasing prevalence in an increasingly elderly population. The presence of AF confers significant mortality and morbidity, with an increased risk of stroke and thromboembolism, in addition to important haemodynamic effects, resulting in decreased exercise tolerance and heart failure. The symptoms of AF can occasionally be quite disabling, and the disorder often requires important therapeutic considerations as regards the need for anti-arrhythmic and antithrombotic therapy.

The diverse clinical presentations of AF makes the development of generalised management strategies difficult. AF is commonly associated with heart disease, but a significant proportion of patients (about one third) have no detectable heart disease. Patients with paroxysmal AF also represent a problem: these patients tend to be younger than those in sustained AF, about 50% have "lone" AF, and many will have asymptomatic paroxysms. Investigation and management should thus be tailored and individualised to the specific clinical scenario associated with AF.

As more is understood about the epidemiology, pathophysiology, and electrophysiology of this disorder, many controversies regarding the appropriate management of AF are becoming apparent. In the past decade, significant advances have been made in the management of AF, which reflect not only technological advances but, perhaps more importantly, a deeper understanding of the consequences of this arrhythmia and prevention strategies.

A brief history of atrial fibrillation

The presence of an irregular pulse was known to many ancient physicians. Nevertheless, the earliest description of AF is perhaps to be found in *The Yellow Emperor's Classic of Internal Medicine* (Huang Ti Nei Ching Su Wên). The legendary Emperor Physician is believed to have ruled China between 2598 and 1696 BC, and his textbook took the form of a dialogue between the emperor and his assistants about various medical ailments and disorders (Figure 1.1).

> "... When the pulse is irregular and tremulous and the beats occur at intervals, then the impulse of life fades; when the pulse is slender [smaller than feeble, but still perceptible, thin like a thread], then the impulse of life is small ..."
>
> Huang Ti Nei Ching Su Wên
>
> *The Yellow Emperor's Classic of Internal Medicine*

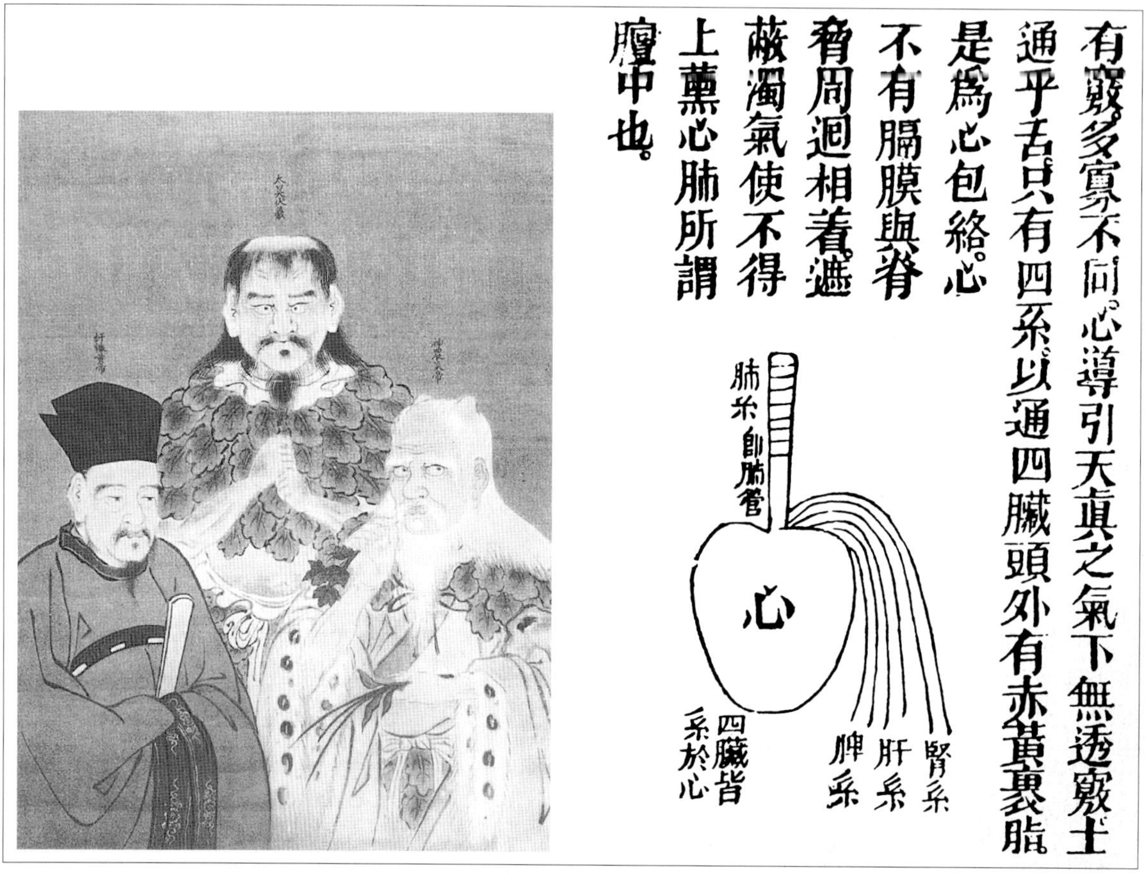

Figure 1.1
Huang Ti Nei Ching Su Wên and the heart. The thin lines pointing below indicate the connection of the heart with (from right to left) the kidneys, the liver, and the spleen. The tube leading into the heart from above forms the connection with the lungs and the trachea.

The poor prognosis associated with chaotic irregularity of the pulse was clearly appreciated by most of the ancient physicians, but in recorded history, William Harvey in 1628 was probably first to describe "fibrillation of the auricles" in animals. In *De Motu Cordis*, Harvey reported that "... when the auricle was ceasing to beat and appeared on the point of death, an obscure movement, undulation/palpation clearly continued ..." in the heart. Vulpian also visually observed AF in vivo and wrote in 1874 on "mouvement fibrillaire", with his observations of the chaotic rhythm of the atria during experiments in the intact dog heart.

In clinical practice, and with the aid of Laénnec's recently invented stethoscope, in 1827 Robert Adams of Dublin reported the association of irregular pulses with mitral stenosis, and in 1863, Etienne Marey published a pulse tracing from such a patient. Other early descriptions of AF and its significance were published in the early years of the 20th century, by Sir James Mackenzie and Heinrich Hering.

Digitalis

The discovery of the therapeutic properties of digitalis leaf (*Digitalis purpurea*) in 1785 by William Withering (Figure 1.2) of Birmingham brought some relief to patients with gross heart failure. Withering practised as a physician at the Birmingham General Hospital, and was aware of a herbal recipe used by an old woman from Shropshire for the treatment of "dropsy", which we now recognise to be heart failure. The recipe contained, amongst other things, leaves from the purple foxglove *Digitalis purpurea* (Figure 1.3). The latter contained a range of cardiac glycosides, most notable of which was digitoxin. Withering stressed the importance of digitalis as a diuretic, stating that "it has a power over the motion of the heart, to a degree yet unobserved in any other medicine, and that this power may be converted to salutary ends". It is also interesting that Withering recorded a patient who had a weak irregular pulse which became "more full and more regular" after five draughts containing *Fol Digital Purp oz iv*.

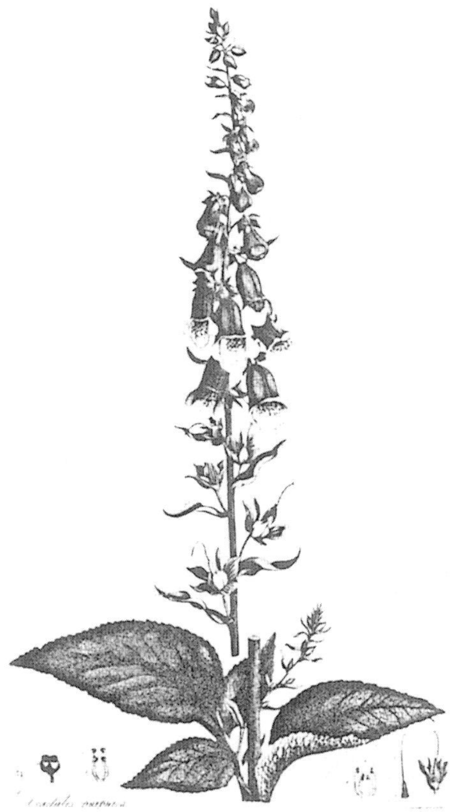

Figure 1.3
Digitalis purpurea.

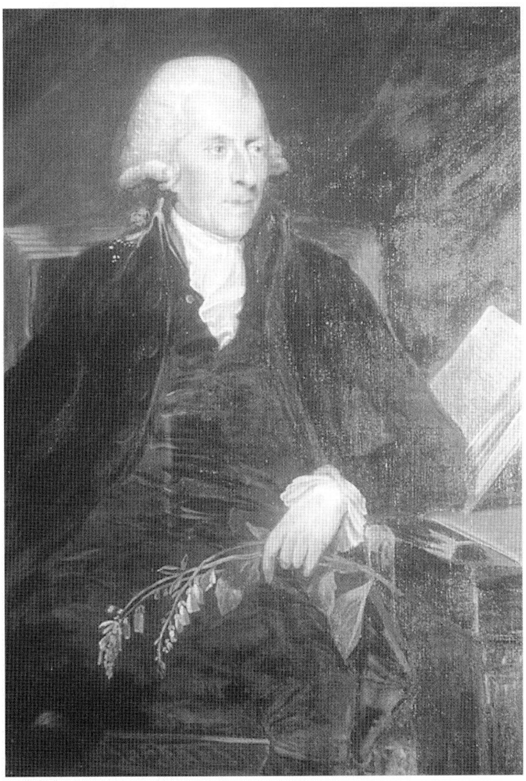

Figure 1.2
William Withering.

In 1799, Ferriar published an essay of the medical properties of *Digitalis purpurea* or foxglove and noted "... the power of reducing the pulse is its true characteristic". In

1935, Jean Baptiste Bouillaud said that he considered digitalis to be "*cette sorte d'opium du coeur*". He observed that digitalis reduced the heart rate dramatically even though irregularity of pulse still persisted. Most commercial digoxin is now obtained from the white foxglove (*Digitalis lanata*).

The ECG

The main diagnostic breakthrough was clearly the invention of the electrocardiograph (ECG) by Waller in 1887, and its modern form by Einthoven (Figure 1.4a) in 1900. Experimentally, Cushny described AF in the dog in 1899. The first electrocardiographic recordings of AF in man were made by Rothberger and Winterberg in 1909. In Britain, a close friend of Einthoven, Sir Thomas Lewis (Figure 1.4b) at University College Hospital, London, was the first to use an ECG in a patient with AF; this description came about 2 months after the description by Rothberger and Winterberg, and Lewis was totally unaware of their work.

(a)

(b)

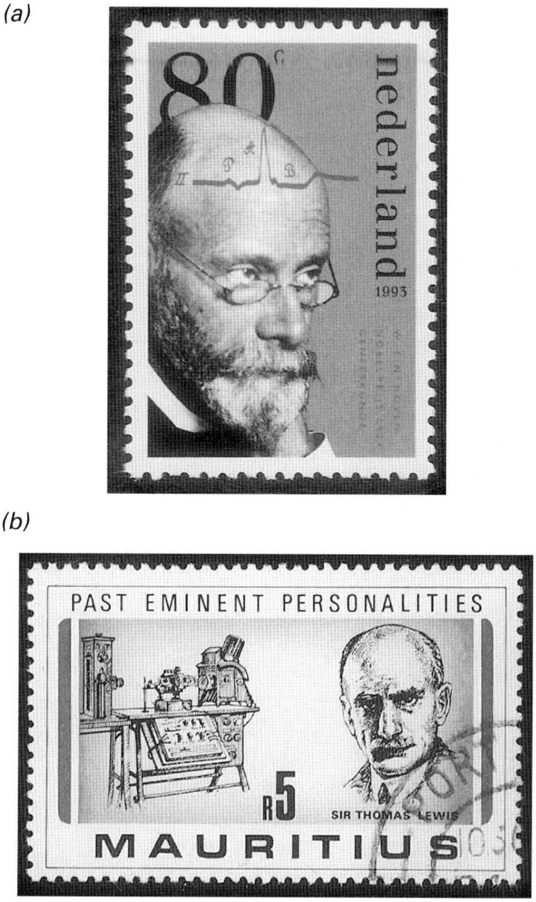

Figure 1.4
(a) William Einthoven; (b) Thomas Lewis.

Mechanism and significance of AF

The exact mechanisms and significance of AF remained controversial. In 1894, Engelmann hypothesised that AF was caused by multiple foci within the atria. Also in 1894, Sir James MacKenzie published observations on AF based on his work with the polygraph. Mackenzie had also noted that when AF was present the jugular vein lost its atrial contraction wave, and the presystolic murmur of mitral stenosis disappeared. Thus, AF was described as a "functional paralysis of the atria". However, he was wrong that the irregularity of the pulse in AF was due to a nodal rhythm, with the atrioventricular node taking over the functions of the sinoatrial node.

Sir Thomas Lewis described AF in human beings in 1909, which he described as "a common clinical condition", and additionally hypothesised that digitalis controlled the ventricular rate in AF by increasing the atrioventricular block.

> *About digitalis in atrial fibrillation:* "Although it is usually possible to control the rate ... at rest or quietly exercising, it is rarely possible to control the rates adequately in conditions of freer exercise."
>
> *Sir Thomas Lewis, 1934*

He disagreed with Mackenzie's viewpoint that digitalis reduced the ventricular rate in AF through the vagus nerve. Lewis and Mackenzie soon fell out over this point, which was exacerbated by the rejection of Mackenzie's manuscript for publication in *Heart* by Lewis, who was the journal's editor at that time. Eventually, Mackenzie was proved to be right. In 1911, Lewis published a classic visual description of AF in a horse.

> "The symptomology consisted of very irregular and tumultuous action of the heart, marked breathlessness, epistaxis, faltering and occasionally falling, upon moderate exertion ... The heart was absolutely irregular, long pauses of 2 seconds were frequent and short runs of rapid beats were noted from time to time ... The heart beats were more numerous than the arterial pulsations."
>
> *Sir Thomas Lewis, 1911*

After the horse had been shot and the chest opened, he noted that "close inspection of the musculature [of the atria] revealed the presence of fibrillatory movements ... the ventricle continued its active coordinate but irregular movements". Well before Moe's work in the 1960s, Lewis had already postulated circus movement as the cause of AF.

In 1970, Bootsma and colleagues, with the aid of computers, concluded that the totally irregular response of the ventricles was due to the effect of "randomly spaced atrial impulses of random strength reaching the atrioventricular node from random directions". Further development of the mechanisms of AF includes the work by Moe (1962), in which AF is thought to be due to multiple coexisting re-entrant wavefronts of activation within the atria, whilst Allesie's model from the 1970s considered that AF was due to multiple wavelets continuously sweeping around the atria in irregular, shifting patterns, repeatedly encountering excitable myocardium, and requiring a critical surface area. Meijler and Fisch worked on the question of atrioventricular node conduction during AF. Indeed, several anatomical and functional aspects of atrioventricular conduction systems in mammals of all sizes showed that the "delaying role" of the atrioventricular conduction system, which allows synchronisation of atrial and ventricular contractions by a varying delay, diminishes as the size of the mammal increases; whereas the "protective role" of the atrioventricular node, which protects the ventricles from rapid atrial arrhythmias, probably increases. In humans, the function of the atrioventricular node was intermediate between that of the small and large mammals.

Improvements in cardiac electrophysiology have provided further insights into the mechanisms of AF over the last decade, and have provided possible therapeutic options.

The epidemiological significance of AF as an important precursor of cardiac and cerebrovascular death was investigated in detail in the Framingham study by William Kannel and colleagues in 1982. Over the past 10 years, there has been increasing awareness of the hazards of sustained non-rheumatic AF, and of the benefits of thromboprophylaxis in preventing stroke and thromboembolism. Indeed, further developments have included the exploration of new antithrombotic strategies and improvements in risk stratification for identifying patients with AF who are at highest risk for stroke and who could be targeted for anticoagulation. Advances in elucidating the mechanisms for the high risk of thrombogenesis in AF have included improved cardiac imaging (for example, transoesophageal echocardiography) and work into abnormalities of haemostasis, platelets, and endothelial dysfunction, suggesting that AF may confer a hypercoagulable state *per se*, independent of underlying structural heart disease or aetiology. The increasing public-health profile of AF and the issue of thromboprophylaxis have also led to developments in the delivery of anticoagulation services, such as near patient testing and domicillary anticoagulation services. Finally, the past decade has seen developments in electrophysiologial techniques and non-pharmacological strategies for the management of AF, including atrioventricular node modification, atrial defibrillators, multi-site pacing, and internal cardioversion.

Author	*Year*	*Comments*
Adams	1827	Probably the first to recognise AF clinically but as "a sign of mitral stenosis"
Bouilland	1835	Digitalis reduced the rate dramatically even though irregularity of pulse persisted
Marey	1863	Publication of a pulse tracing of AF from a patient with mitral stenosis
Vulpian	1874	Observation of AF in vivo (dog) "mouvement fibrillaire"
Engelman	1894	AF caused by multiple foci in the atria
Einthoven	1900	Invention of the ECG
Lewis	1909	AF recording on ECG; work on mechanisms of AF
Rothenberger and Winterberg	1909	"arrhythmia perpetua"; "fibrillation of the auricles"
Lown	1969	Cardioversion of AF

Reproduced with permission from Acierno LJ, 1994.

Table 1.1
History of atrial fibrillation.

The future

AF has been described as "the final frontier" for cardiac arrhythmia management. The progress in our understanding of the condition and the many developments in the management of AF suggests that very soon it will be highly likely that we will boldly go where no man (or cardiologist?) has gone before!

References

Acierno LJ. *The history of cardiology*. New York. Parthenon Publishing Group. 1994.

Flegel KM. From delerium cordis to atrial fibrillation: historical development of a disease concept. *Ann Intern Med* 1995; **122**: 867–73.

Kannell WE, Abbott RD, Savage DD, McNamara PM. Epidemiological features of chronic atrial fibrillation. The Framingham Study. *N Engl J Med* 1982; **306**: 1018–22.

Krikler DM. The foxglove, "The Old Woman from Shropshire" and William Withering. *J Am Coll Cardiol* 1985; **5**: 3A–9A.

Krikler DM. Historical aspects of electrocardiography. *Cardiol Clin* 1987; **5**: 349–55.

Lewis T. Auricular fibrillation: a common clinical condition. *BMJ* 1909; **2**: 1528.

Lown B. Electrical reversion of cardiac arrhythmias. *Br Heart J* 1967; **29**: 469–89.

Mackenzie J. The venous and liver pulses, and the arrhythmic contraction of the cardiac cavities. *J Pathol Bacteriol* 1894; **2**: 84–154.

McMichael J. Sir James Mackenzie and atrial fibrillation: a new perspective. *J R Coll Gen Pract* 1981; **31**: 402–6.

Meijler FL, Fisch C. Does the atrioventricular node conduct? *Br Heart J* 1989; **61**: 309–15.

Meijler FL. Comparative aspects of the dual role of the human atrioventricular node. *Br Heart J* 1986; **55**: 286–90.

Withering W. *An account of the foxglove, and some of its medical uses: with practical remarks on dropsy and other diseases*. London. GGJ and J Robinson. 1785.

2

Epidemiology of atrial fibrillation

Introduction

Estimates of the prevalence of atrial fibrillation (AF) vary widely around the world and depend upon the population studied. Much of the clinical epidemiology of AF is also based on data from predominantly white populations, and information on AF in non-white populations is scarce (Table 2.1).

Age and sex

The risk of AF is well recognised to increase with age and with underlying heart disease (Feinberg et al, 1995). The prevalence of AF roughly doubles with each advancing decade of age, from 0.5% at age 50–59 years to almost 9% at age 80–90 years (Kannel et al, 1982, 1998). AF is also becoming significantly more prevalent in men aged 65–84 years (3.2% in 1968–70, 9.1% in 1987–89), which is not explained by an increase in age, valve disease, or myocardial infarction.

The incidence of new onset of AF also doubles with each decade of age, independent of the increasing prevalence of known predisposing conditions. The incidence of new cases of AF also in people over the age of 65 is about 1% per annum. Based on 38-year follow-up data from the Framingham study, men have a 1.5-fold greater risk of developing AF than women, after adjustment for age and predisposing conditions.

Indeed, AF is very uncommon in infants and children, unless concomitant structural or congenital heart disease is present. Healthy young adults are also at low risk of developing AF. For example, one early report suggested that only five of 122 043 routinely evaluated, healthy Air Force personnel had AF (Hess and Lamb, 1962). Thus, AF is primarily a disease of older people. This is particularly important as the general population (at least in the UK) is getting older.

Predisposing factors

The prevalence of common predisposing factors to AF, such as hypertension and ischaemic heart disease, will also influence the prevalence of AF in a population. Epidemiological studies have shown that many of the risk factors for AF can be subject to control (for example, systolic blood pressure, blood glucose, and valvular heart disease). For example, treatment of hypertension might prevent the development of left ventricular hypertrophy and left atrial enlargement, and thereby prevent AF.

Of cardiovascular risk factors, only hypertension and diabetes were significant independent predictors of AF, adjusting for age and other predisposing conditions in the Framingham study. Cigarette smoking was a significant risk factor in women, adjusting only for age (odds ratio = 1.4), but was just short of significance on adjustment for other risk

Study/ author	*Study period*	*Patients (n)*	*Age (yr)*	*Prevalence (%)*	*Comment*
US Air Force	1957–1962	122,043	15–50	0.004	US Air Force cadets and personnel: electrocardiograms on all fliers and trainees
Tecumseh (male/female)	1959–1960	5,129 (52%/48%)	≥16	0.4 0.52/0.33	Community survey: 85% of individuals 16 yr old or older had electrocardiograms
		480	>60	3.3	
Whitehall	1967–1969	19,018	40–69	0.4	Screening of male civil servants, all employment grades
			40–49	0.16	
			60–64	1.13	
Reykjavik (male/female)	1967–1970	9,067 (48%/52%)	32–64	0.28	Population sample
CASS		18,343		0.6	Multicenter registry: patients with angiographically proven coronary artery disease
			18–39	0.02	
			40–59	0.04	
			≥60	1.4	
Hill	1983–1985	819	>65	3.7	"Symptomless patients" from UK general practice
Edinburgh (male/female)	1972–1977	487 (56%/44%)	62–90	5.0	Random sample from 27,000 older people living in defined area of city
Campbell (male/female)	1970–1973	2,254 (39%/61%)	≥65	2.0	Electrocardiographic survey of majority of elderly people at home in Scottish community
			≥75	5.0	
Australia (male/female)	1966–1981	1,770 (52%/48%)	>60		Triennial population survey
			60–64	1.7	
			65–69	3.0	
			70–74	7.0	
			≥75	11.6	

CASS, Coronary Artery Surgery Study.
Reproduced with permission from Cairns and Connolly, 1991.

Table 2.1
Prevalence of atrial fibrillation.

factors. Neither obesity nor alcohol intake was associated with AF incidence in either sex in the Framingham study (Kannel et al, 1998). For men and women, respectively, diabetes conferred a 1.4- and 1.6-fold risk of AF, and hypertension a 1.5- and 1.4-fold risk of AF, after adjusting for other associated conditions. Because of its high prevalence in the population, hypertension caused more AF in the population (14%) than any other risk factor.

Intrinsic overt cardiac conditions will confer a substantially higher risk of developing AF. For example, heart failure is associated with AF in about one-third of cases; however, adjusting for other relevant conditions, heart failure is associated with a 4.5- and 5.9-fold risk of AF, and valvular heart disease a 1.8- and 3.4-fold risk of AF, in men and women, respectively. Whilst uncomplicated coronary artery disease is a rare cause of AF, the presence of myocardial infarction significantly increases the risk factor-adjusted likelihood of AF by 40%, but in men only.

Structural heart disease detected by echocardiography has been related to the risk of AF. For example, echocardiographic predictors of non-rheumatic AF include left atrial enlargement (39% increase in risk per 5 mm increment), left ventricular fractional shortening (34% per 5% decrement), and left ventricular wall thickness (28% per 4 mm increment). Electrocardiographic left ventricular hypertrophy increases the risk of AF 3- to 4-fold after adjusting only for age, but this risk ratio is decreased to 1.4 after adjustment for the other associated conditions.

Nevertheless, up to one third of patients with AF may have idiopathic or "lone" atrial fibrillation, where no precipitating cause can be identified, and there is no evidence of organic heart disease (Kopeckly et al, 1987); nevertheless, the true prevalence of lone AF depends on the definition and criteria for diagnosis. The subject of lone AF is discussed in detail in Chapter 6.

Prognostic implications

The chief hazard of AF is stroke and thromboembolism, the risk of which is increased 4 to 5-fold. Because of its high prevalence in advanced age, AF assumes great importance as a risk factor for stroke and by the ninth decade becomes a dominant factor (Wolf et al, 1998) (Table 2.2). The attributable risk for stroke associated with AF increases steeply from 1.5% at age 50–59 years to 23.5% at age 80–89 years. AF is associated with a doubling of mortality in both sexes, which is decreased to 1.5 to 1.9-fold after adjusting for associated cardiovascular conditions. Decreased survival associated with AF occurs across a wide range of ages (Wolf et al, 1998) (Figure 2.1).

Population studies

North America

The prevalence of AF in the USA rises from about 2–3% at age 60 to 65 to 8–10% at age 80; about 70% of all affected patients are at least 65 years old (Feinberg et al, 1995; Psalty et al, 1997). The Cardiovascular Health Study was a population-based, longitudinal study of risk factors for coronary artery disease and stroke in 5201 American men and women aged over 65 years, which included a proportion of subjects undergoing 24 h ambulatory electrocardiographic monitoring; that study reported a prevalence of AF of about 9.1% in men and women with clinical cardiovascular disease, 4.6% in patients with evidence of subclinical but no clinical cardiovascular disease, and only 1.6% in subjects with neither clinical nor subclinical cardiovascular disease (Furberg et al, 1994; Manolio et al, 1984). A history of

Age (yr) and Sex	*Relative Mortality Risk (95% Confidence Interval)*	
Men		
65–74	1.21*	(1.00–1.46)
75–84	1.07	(0.96–1.19)
85–89	1.10*	(1.04–1.16)
Women		
65–74	1.20	(1.00–1.45)
75–84	1.20*	(1.09–1.32)
85–89	1.22*	(1.14–1.29)

Age (yr) and Sex	*Relative Stroke Risk (95% Confidence Interval)*	
Men		
65–74	1.20	(0.99–1.45)
75–84	1.05	(0.94–1.16)
85–89	1.08*	(1.02–1.14)
Women		
65–74	1.23*	(1.02–1.48)
75–84	1.25*	(1.14–1.37)
85–89	1.22*	(1.15–1.30)

* Odds ratio differs from unity at $p < .05$. Adjusted for primary diagnoses of acute myocardial infarction, unstable angina, stable angina, and congestive heart failure: and secondary diagnoses of hypertension, diabetes, valvular disease, stroke, and chronic obstructive pulmonary disease. Patients were eliminated at death from the stroke regression analysis.
Reproduced with permission from Wolf et al (1998).

Table 2.2
Adjusted mortality and stroke risk associated with atrial fibrillation following hospital admission by age and sex.

congestive heart failure, valve disease and stroke, dilated left atria on echocardiography, abnormal mitral or aortic valve function, treated systemic hypertension, and advanced age were independently associated with the prevalence of AF.

The Framingham study reported that the incidence of AF in subjects over 22 years' follow-up was 2%, being slightly more common in men (2.2%) than in women (1.7%); the prevalence ranged from 0.5% for subjects in the age range 50–59 years to 8.8% in subjects aged 80–89 years (Benjamin et al, 1994; Wolf et al, 1991) (Figure 2.2) (Table 2.3).

The most recent analysis from the Framingham study examined the mortality of subjects 55–94 years of age who developed AF during 40 years of follow-up from the original Framingham Heart study cohort (Benjamin et al, 1998) (Figures 2.3a and 2.3b). Of the original 5209 subjects, 296 men and 325 women developed AF, and those who did so were more likely to have hypertension, smoking, left ventricular hypertrophy on ECG, myo-

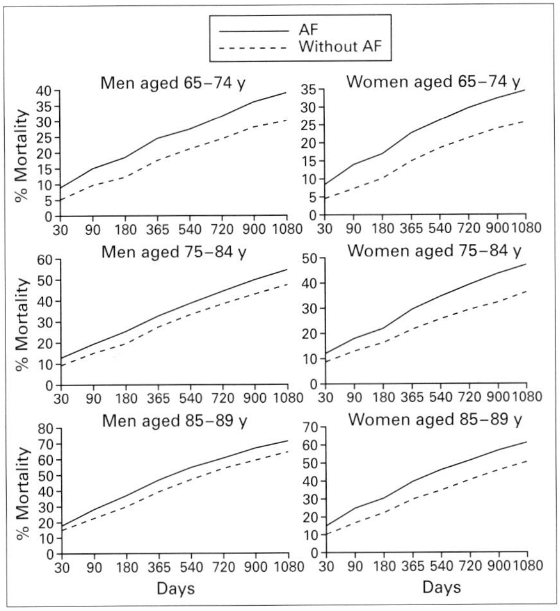

Figure 2.1
Cumulative mortality following index admission by age and sex. Sample of Medicare patients hospitalized in 1989 with a diagnosis of cardiovascular disease with and without atrial fibrillation. Reproduced with permission from Wolf et al (1998).

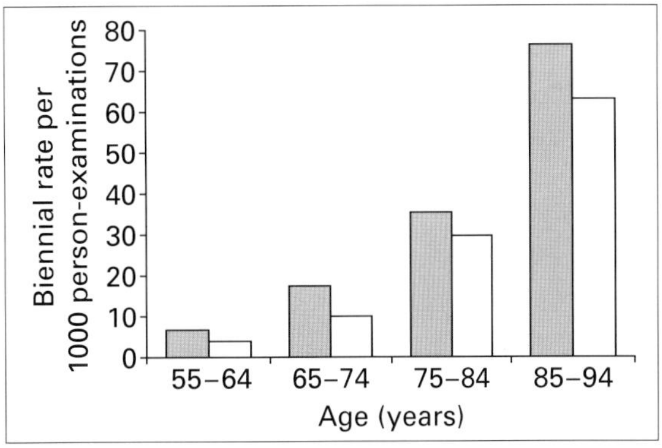

Figure 2.2
Incidence of atrial fibrillation. Framingham Heart Study 38-year follow-up. ▨, men; □, women.

cardial infarction, congestive heart failure, valvular heart disease, and cerebrovascular disease at baseline. The striking feature, however, was that AF was associated with an odds ratio for death of 1.5 for men and 1.9 in women, which did not vary by age, but most of the excess of mortality attributed to AF occurred early after diagnosis of AF. There was also a significant interaction between AF and sex with respect to mortality (Benjamin et al, 1998) (Figure 2.3). The reasons for this early mortality are, however, uncertain, although causes of death were related to cardiovascular or cerebrovascular disease.

In the Manitoba Follow-up Study, a longitudinal study of 3983 male air-crew recruits for 44 years, with nearly 154 131 person-years of observation, about 7.5% developed AF (Krahn et al, 1995). The risk in this cohort increased with advancing age, rising from 0.5 per 1000 person-years before age 50 to 9.7 per 1000 person years after age 70. The risk of developing AF varied with aetiology: ischaemic heart disease had amongst the highest relative risks for AF (3.62 for myocardial infarction, 2.84 for angina) using a multivariate Cox model, compared with a lower relative risk from hypertension of 1.42.

United Kingdom

In the UK, there have been few studies of the prevalence of AF in the community (Hill et al, 1987; Rose et al, 1978; Camm et al, 1980; Kennedy and Caird 1972; Campbell et al, 1974; Kitchin and Milne 1977), and these have been criticised for being too small and involving small numbers of elderly patients from unrepresented populations (Sudlow et al, 1997). For example, Hill et al (1987) screened 819 general practice patients, and found 30 patients (3.7%) with AF. Kennedy and Caird (1972) studied the electrocardiograms of 400

	Men†			Women‡		
Variable	*AF*	*No AF*	*Odds Ratio (95% CI)*	*AF*	*No AF*	*Odds Ratio (95% CI)*
Age (mean), y	72	65	...	75	66	...
Cigarette smoking, %	34.8	33.7	1.0 (0.8–1.4)	28.5	23.4	1.4§ (1.0–2.0)
Diabetes, %	16.3	10.2	1.7‖ (1.2–2.3)	15.5	7.5	2.1¶ (1.5–2.8)
ECG LV hypertrophy, %	10.7	4.4	3.0¶ (1.9–4.8)	13.6	3.8	3.8¶ (2.6–5.6)
Hypertension, %	44.1	30.9	1.8¶ (1.4–2.3)	51.7	40.7	1.7¶ (1.3–2.2)
Myocardial infarction, %	25.5	13.0	2.2‖ (1.6–2.8)	13.0	4.6	2.4‖ (1.7–3.4)
Congestive heart failure, %	20.6	3.2	6.1¶ (4.5–8.4)	26.0	2.9	8.1¶ (6.1–10.7)
Valve disease, %	16.7	6.7	2.2¶ (1.6–3.1)	29.5	8.7	3.6¶ (2.8–4.6)
Body mass index (mean)	26.2	26.0	1.03 (0.99–1.06)	26.0	25.7	1.02 (1.00–1.05)
Ethanol, oz/wk	5.4	5.1	1.01 (0.99–1.03)	1.5	1.8	0.95 (0.89–1.02)

* Variables are expressed as age-adjusted % (categorical data) and means (continuous data); odds ratios are age-adjusted from 2-year pooled logistic regression, subjects with compared with those without AF. CI indicates confidence interval; ECG, electrocardiographic; and LV, left ventricular.
† There were 264 incident cases of AF among men in 18 245 follow-up person-examinations.
‡ There were 298 incident cases of AF among women in 26 277 follow-up person-examinations.
§ $P \leq .05$.
‖ $P \leq .01$.
¶ $P \leq .0001$.
Reproduced with permission from Benjamin et al (1994)

Table 2.3
Risk factors for developing incident atrial fibrillation (AF).*

Figure 2.3
(a) Kaplan-Meier mortality curves for subjects 55–74 years of age. Vertical axis shows percent of subjects dead at follow-up (0–80%); horizontal axis, up to 10 years follow-up. Subjects included men with AF (n = 159), men without AF (n = 318), women with AF (n = 133), and women without AF (n = 266). Both men and women with AF had significantly higher mortality than age-, sex-, and calendar year-matched non-AF subjects. Log rank test for men gave $\chi^2 = 42.90$ ($p < 0.0001$); for women, $\chi^2 = 70.93$ ($p < 0.0001$). (b) Kaplan-Meier mortality curves for subjects 75–94 years of age. Vertical axis shows percent of subjects dead at follow-up (0–80%); horizontal axis, up to 5 years of follow-up. Subjects included men with AF (n = 137), men without AF (n = 274), women with AF (n = 192), and women without AF (n = 384). Both men and women with AF had significantly higher mortality than age-, sex-, and calendar year-matched non-AF subjects. Log rank test for men gave $\chi^2 = 51.44$ ($p < 0.0001$); for women, $\chi^2 = 101.51$ ($p < 0.0001$). Reproduced with permission from Benjamin et al (1998).

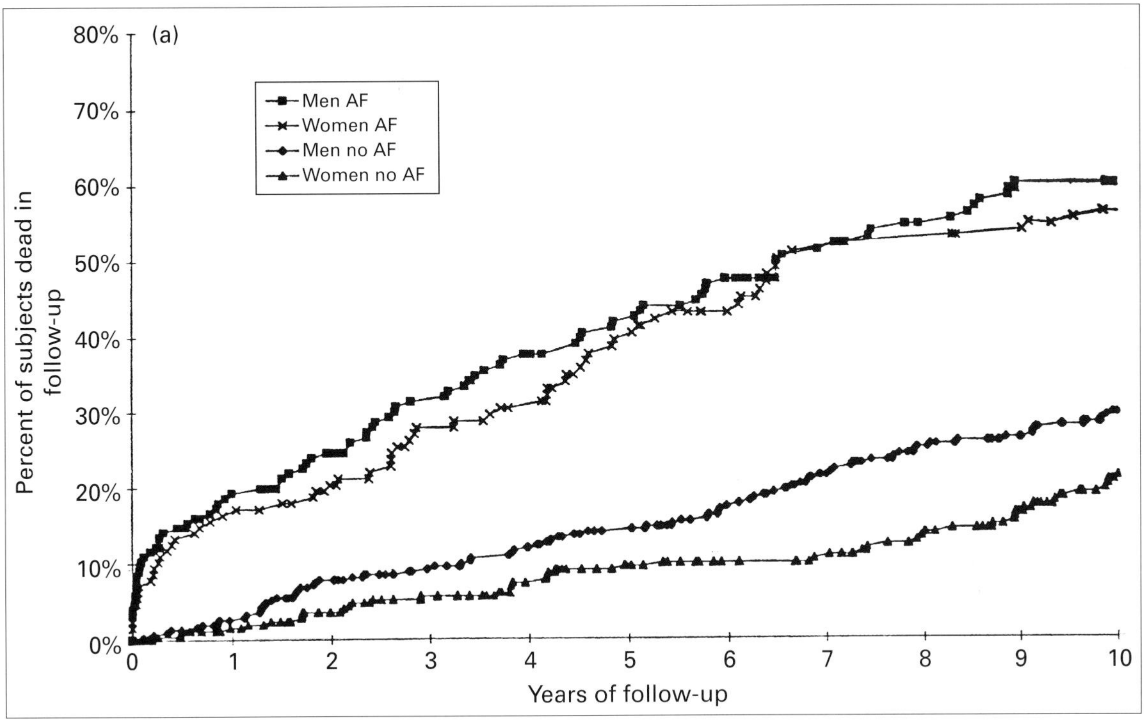
(a)
Men AF
Women AF
Men no AF
Women no AF
Percent of subjects dead in follow-up
80%
70%
60%
50%
40%
30%
20%
10%
0%
0
1
2
3
4
5
6
7
8
9
10
Years of follow-up

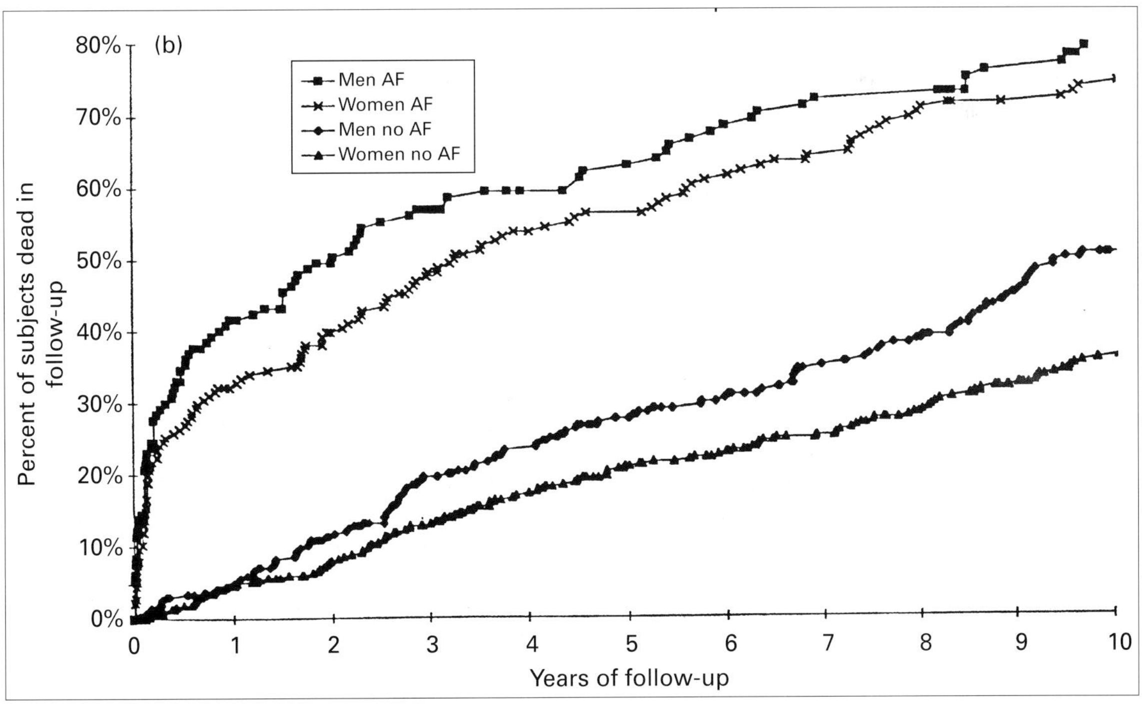
(b)
Men AF
Women AF
Men no AF
Women no AF
Percent of subjects dead in follow-up
80%
70%
60%
50%
40%
30%
20%
10%
0%
0
1
2
3
4
5
6
7
8
9
10
Years of follow-up

elderly people over 65 years, and found that only 11 patients had AF. Sudlow et al (1995) estimated that AF may in fact be more prevalent in the UK than in the USA or Australia, and suggested that "between 160 000 and 644 000 patients aged over 65 years in Great Britain would have atrial fibrillation".

In the West Birmingham Atrial Fibrillation project, the prevalence of AF was 2.4% in two general practices, where the commonest aetiological causes were hypertension (37%) and ischaemic heart disease (29%); interestingly, however, only a third of patients in the survey had ever presented to hospital (Lip et al, 1997) (Figure 2.4). In that survey, cardiac failure was associated with AF in a third of patients, and cerebrovascular events had occurred in 18%. Further extension of this project showed that the prevalence of AF in Indo-Asians aged more than 50 years in the general practice population was 0.6% (Lip et al, 1998).

The Echocardiographic Heart of England Screening (EcHoES) study was a population survey of patients with left ventricular dysfunction in the west Midlands. The study showed a prevalence of AF amongst patients aged over 65 years of 3.8% (95% CI 2.5–5.1; Davis et al, 1999). In the overall population sample aged 45 years or more, the prevalence was 1.7%, but amongst high risk subgroups (heart failure, previous myocardial infarction, hypertension, angina, diabetes) the prevalence was 11.6%. Echocardiographic abnormalities were found in 67%, and only 21% were actually on warfarin. The investigators concluded that screening may be most cost-effective if targeted at patients at high risk of AF.

The recently published Newcastle survey screened 4843 people aged 65 years or more in general practices and found a prevalence of AF of 4.7% (Sudlow et al, 1998). This survey also provided interesting data on the eligibility for anticoagulation in this community study.

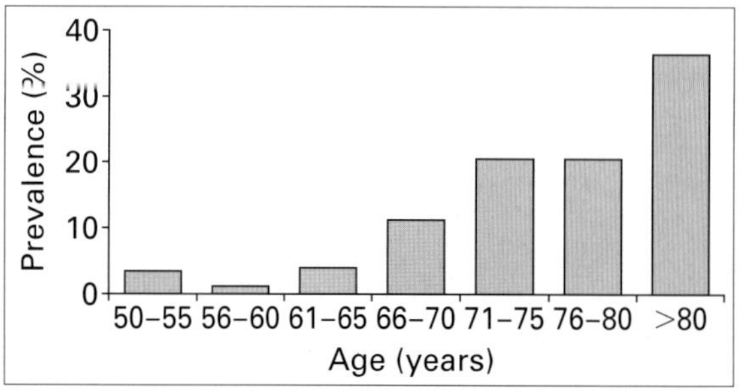

Figure 2.4
Age distribution of patients with atrial fibrillation in general practice. Reproduced with permission from Lip et al (1997).

The same research group compared screening methods for AF ("feeling the pulse", case note search, ECG screening) and reported specificity and sensitivity rates for these methods (Sudlow et al, 1998).

Australia

A study from the Busselton community in Western Australia reported a prevalence of AF that increased from 1.7% at age 60–64 years to 11.6% in those aged over 75 years (Lake et al, 1989) (Table 2.4). In that study of 1770 people aged over 60 years, 2.3% were found to be in AF at their first survey and a further 2.7% developed AF or atrial flutter during follow-up; 9% of those with AF had paroxysmal AF. The average cumulative incidence of new AF was 15 per 1000 people. The predominant aetiological factors in men and women from this survey are summarized in Table 2.4. The relative mortality in those with AF compared with those without AF was 1.92 for all causes, 1.82 for cardiovascular causes (excluding stroke), and 3.78 for deaths from stroke.

France

The recent ALFA study (Levy et al, 1999) characterised various clinical presentations

	No AF (%)	AF (%)	p value
Angina	14.4	24.1	$p = 0.023$
Previous myocardial infarction	10.6	18.3	$p = 0.048$
ECG-Left bundle branch block	2.4	18.4	$p < 0.001$
ST depression	4.8	5.7	$p = 0.90$
Left ventricular hypertrophy	0.9	2.3	$p = 0.44$
Hypertension	15.3	11.5	$p = 0.41$
History of rheumatic fever	1.0	2.3	$p = 0.48$
Current smoker	37.4	28	$p = 0.26$
Alcohol consumers			
All	59.1	43.1	$p = 0.016$
Males	63.0	42.1	$p = 0.016$
Females	54.5	44.4	$p = 0.41$

Reproduced with permission from Lake et al (1989).

Table 2.4
Busselton Study: associations with AF.

and underlying conditions of 756 patients (19–95 years old) with AF, in general practice in France. In this cohort, 670 (88.6%) patients were symptomatic. The relative prevalences of paroxysmal (<7 days), chronic (last episode >1 month), and recent onset AF (persistent >7 days and <1 month) were 22.1%, 51.4%, and 26.4%, respectively. Cardiac disorders were present in 534 (70.6%) patients, and included hypertension (39.4%), coronary artery disease (16.6%), and myocardial disorders (15.3%). Rheumatic valvular disease was common in women (25.0%) but not in men (8.0%). As expected, the paroxysmal group differed by a high percentage of palpitations (79.0%) and a low percentage of underlying heart disease (53.9%). With a mean follow-up of nearly 9 months, 28 (3.7%) patients died, including six fatal cerebrovascular accidents. Among the 728 patients who survived, congestive heart failure occurred in 30 (4.1%) patients, and embolic complications occurred in 13 (1.8%) patients. In the paroxysmal AF group, 13 (8.0%) patients developed chronic AF and 51 (31.3%) had AF recurrences. At the time of follow-up, 53 (14.3%) patients from the chronic AF group and 108 (55.7%) patients from the recent onset AF group were in sinus rhythm.

Hospital studies

One measure of the problem of AF is a review of studies based on hospital practice. However, this may give a biased view of the clinical epidemiology of AF, since only one-third of patients with AF may actually have been admitted to hospital (Lip et al, 1997). In one preliminary study from North America, AF accounted for over a one-third of hospital admissions due to cardiac arrhythmias (Bialy et al, 1992) (Figure 2.5).

In a survey of AF amongst acute medical admissions to a district general hospital in Glasgow, UK, Lip et al (1994) reported a prevalence of 6.3%, with the predominant associated medical conditions being ischaemic heart disease, hypertension, and valve disease. The presenting symptoms was typically cardiorespiratory, with dysponea in 52%, chest pain in 34%, palpitations in 26%, and dizziness/syncope in 19%.

A similar hospital survey in the west of Birmingham, UK, in a multi-ethnic population showed a lower prevalence of AF (2.3%) but associated medical conditions and presenting symptoms were broadly similar to the Glasgow study (Zarifis et al, 1997).

Nevertheless, some of these surveys were undertaken before publication of some of the more recent trials on the value of antithrombotic therapy. However, Stewart et al (1999) recently reported the prevalence of AF in patients admitted acutely to the general medical service at Auckland Hospital over a 12-week period: they found 147 patients (52% male) who were admitted 165 times out of the 1637 admissions over the study period (a prevalence of 10.4%, 95% CI 8.6–11.5%). The main causes of admission were heart failure (23%), pneumonia or sepsis (17%), cerebrovascular events (14%), and ischaemic heart disease (11%). Past medical history included hypertension (46%), ischaemic heart disease (39%), congestive heart failure (58%), valvular heart disease (12%), chronic obstructive airways disease (24%), cerebrovascular or thromboembolic event (24%), and diabetes (17%). Thyroid function tests were done in 50% of patients, and echocardiograms in 38%. Only 28% were discharged on warfarin, 33% on aspirin, and one patient on both; nevertheless, 52% had contraindications to warfarin therapy. Thus the general picture still remained the same in this study.

In the hospital surveys there was generally a suboptimal application of standard investigations for AF, and only a limited use of anticoagulation and consideration for cardioversion.

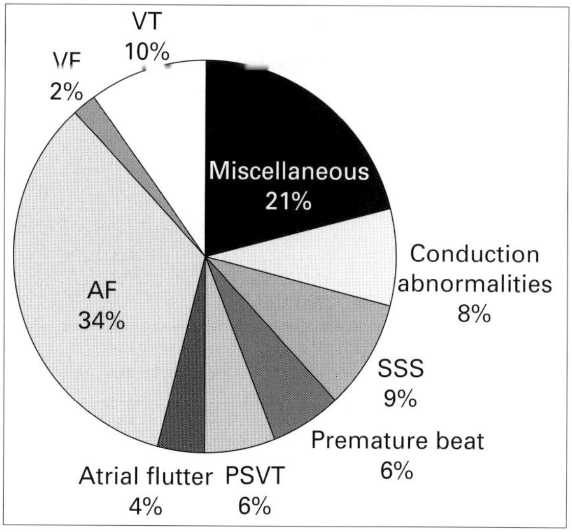

Figure 2.5
US hospital admissions for arrhythmias.
VT = ventricular tachycardia; VF = ventricular fibrillation; SSS = sick sinus syndrome; PSVT = paroxysmal supraventricular tachycardia. Adapted from Bialy et al (1992).

The low prevalence of anticoagulation despite the absence of contraindications was also illustrated by reports from London (Bath et al, 1993) and Glasgow (Hendry et al, 1994), which are based on hospital case-note review. For example, in the study by Hendry et al (1994), 53% of patients with AF, who were mainly elderly (mean age 79 years, range 53–95) and without contraindications, were discharged without antithrombotic therapy.

Ethnicity and AF

Much of the clinical epidemiology of AF from the Framingham study, from the UK and other countries including Australia, has been derived from predominantly white populations. Whilst there are recognised ethnic differences in cardiovascular disease and stroke, with a high prevalence of ischaemic heart disease in the Indo-Asian population and hypertension (and its related problems, such as stroke) in Afro-Caribbean populations (Balarajan, 1991), the world literature on the clinical epidemiology of AF in non-white groups is limited. We are only aware of small surveys on the prevalence of AF in non-white groups from Africa (Maru, 1997), Japan (Kitamuru et al, 1991; Takahashi et al, 1981) and Hong Kong (Lok and Lau, 1995) in addition to our own work in a multi-ethnic city centre population in Birmingham, UK (Lip et al, 1998; Zarifis et al, 1997).

For example, Maru (1997) reported a survey of 136 Ethiopian cardiac outpatients with AF in whom the mean age was 41 years and the commonest aetiological causes of AF were rheumatic heart disease (66%), hypertension (10%), cardiomyopathy (9%), and ischaemic heart disease (7%). In a review of 291 predominantly Chinese patients with AF attending a regional hospital in Hong Kong, the mean age was 73 years and the commonest aetiological factors were hypertension (29%), vascular disease (25%), and rheumatic heart disease (18%; Lok and Lau, 1995). Takahashi et al (1981) reported 94 Japanese patients with paroxysmal AF, of whom 54% had hypertension and/or coronary artery disease, whilst 3.2% had rheumatic valve disease, 2% had hyperthyroidism, and 25% had lone AF. A Japanese report of secular trends in the prevalence and incidence of AF amongst a rural population aged 40-69 years found an association of AF with hypertension, but over 80% did not have any clinical evidence of

	White (n = 213)	*Black (n = 10)*	*Asian (n = 22)*
Age			
Years mean (s.d.)	*75.3 (11.0)*	*73.1 (12.1)*	*62.4 (15.5)*
Past medical history			
None	19	1	2
Ischaemic heart disease	53 (24.9%)	1	10 (45.5%)
Valvular heart disease	11	0	2
Ischaemic and valvular heart disease	5	0	0
Thyroid disease	16 (7.5%)	0	0
Cardiomyopathy	0	0	2
Heart failure	39	3	4
Hypertension	45 (21.1%)	5 (50%)	1
Cerebrovascular disease	29 (13.6%)	0	2
Diabetes mellitus	22	0	2
Other	8	0	2

Reproduced with permission from Zarifis et al (1997).

Table 2.5
Ethnic differences in atrial fibrillation.

heart disease or thyroid disease (Kitamuru et al, 1991).

In a survey of acute medical admissions with AF to our city centre hospital in Birmingham, England, serving a multi-ethnic population of 300 000 (64% white, 11% black/Afro-Caribbean, 25% Indo-Asian), we reported that 87% of the patients with AF were white, 4% black/Afro-Caribbean, and 9% Indo-Asian (Zarifis et al, 1997) (Table 2.5). Indo-Asian patients with AF in our study were generally younger, with a mean age of 62 years, compared with Afro-Caribbeans and whites (mean age 73 and 75 years, respectively). This age difference may account for the relatively lower prevalence of AF in Indo-Asians, since they are generally first-generation migrants to the UK, who may be relatively younger than the white population. The predominant aetiological factor associated with AF in our Afro-Caribbean patients was hypertension, whilst in Indo-Asians the main aetiological factor was ischaemic heart disease.

In the West Birmingham Atrial Fibrillation project, our survey of six general practices with a combined population of 25 051 (with 65% Indo-Asians) only identified 12 Indo-Asian patients (mean age 67 years) with known AF, suggesting a prevalence of AF in Indo-Asians aged above 50 years of 0.6% (Lip et al, 1998). The common associated medical conditions were ischaemic heart disease, heart failure, hypertension, and valve disease. The lower prevalence of AF amongst Indo-Asian patients in general practice compared with our hospital survey may be a reflection of a higher relative proportion of Indo-Asians with AF who required hospital admission, perhaps due to concurrent ischaemic heart disease (or its complications) that could make such patients more unwell. Nevertheless, the relatively small numbers of subjects identified in most of these studies of AF in non-white groups may limit any meaningful analysis of aetiology or outcome in non-whites with AF.

References

Balarajan R. Ethnic differences in mortality from ischaemic heart disease and cerebrovascular disease in England and Wales. *BMJ* 1991; **302:** 560–4.

Bath PMW, Prasad A, Brown MM, MacGregor GA. Survey of use of anticoagulation in atrial fibrillation. *BMJ* 1993; **307:** 1045.

Benjamin EJ, Levy D, Varizi SM et al. Independent risk factors for atrial fibrillation in a population based cohort: the Framingham Heart Study. *JAMA* 1994; **271:** 840–4.

Benjamin EJ, Wolf PA, D'Agostino et al. Impact of atrial fibrillation on the risk of death. *Circulation* 1998; **98:** 946–52.

Bialy D, Lehman MH, Schumacher DN, Steinman RT, Meissner MD. Hospitalisation for arrythmias in the United States: importance of atrial fibrillation. *J Am Coll Cardiol* 1992; **19:** 14A.

Cairns JA, Connolly SJ. Nonrheumatic Atrial Fibrillation: risk of smoke and role of antithrombotic therapy. *Circulation* 1991; **81:** 470.

Camm JC, Evans KE, Ward DE, Martin A. The rhythm of the heart in active elderly subjects. *Am Heart J* 1980; **99:** 598–603.

Campbell A, Caird FI, Jackson TFM. Prevalence of abnormalities of electrocardiogram in old people. *Br Heart J* 1974; **36:** 1005–11.

Davis RC, Hobbs R, Kenkre J et al. Atrial fibrillation prevalence in the general population and in high risk groups. *J Am Coll Cardiol* 1999; **33(suppl A):** 265A.

Feinberg WM, Blackshear JL, Laupacis A et al. Prevalence, age distribution, and gender of patients with atrial fibrillation. Analysis and implications. *Arch Intern Med* 1995; **155:** 469.

Furberg CD, Psaty BM, Manolio TA et al. Prevalence of atrial fibrillation in elderly subjects. The Cardiovascular Health Study. *Am J Cardiol* 1994; **74:** 236–41.

Hendry A, Campbell AM, Campbell G et al. Antithrombotic therapy prescribed for patients with non-rheumatic atrial fibrillation. *Scott Med J* 1994; **39:** 110–11.

Hess RG, Lamb LE. Electrocardiographic findings in 122,043 individuals. *Circulation* 1962; **25:** 947.

Hill JD, Mottram EM, Killeen PD. Study of the prevalence of atrial fibrillation in general practice patients over 65 years of age. *J R Coll Gen Pract* 1987; **37:** 172–3.

Kannel WB, Wolf PA, Benjamin EJ, Levy D. Prevalence, incidence, prognosis, and predisposing conditions for atrial fibrillation: population-based estimates. *Am J Cardiol* 1998; **82:** 2N–9N.

Kannel WB, Abbot RD, Savage DD, McNamara PM. Epidemiological features of chronic atrial fibrillation. The Framingham Study. *N Engl J Med* 1982; **306:** 1018–22.

Kennedy RD, Caird FI. The application of the Minnesota code to population studies of the electrocardiogram in the elderly. *Gerontol Clinic* 1972; **14:** 5–16.

Kitamuru A, Shimamoto T, Doi M et al. Secular trends in prevalence and incidence of atrial fibrillation and associated factors in a Japanese rural population. *Nippon Koshu Eisei Zasshi* 1991; **38:** 95–105.

Kitchin AH, Milne JS. Longitudinal survey of ischaemic heart disease in randomly selected sample of older population. *Br Heart J* 1977; **39:** 889–93.

Kopecky SL, Gersh BJ, McGoon MD et al. The natural history of lone atrial fibrillation. A population-based study over three decades. *N Engl J Med* 1987; **317:** 669–74.

Krahn AD, Manfreda J, Tate RB et al. The natural history of atrial fibrillation: Incidence, risk factors, and prognosis in the Manitoba Follow-up Study. *Am J Med* 1995; **98:** 476.

Lake FR, Cullen KJ, de Klerk NH et al. Atrial fibrillation and mortality in an elderly population. *Aust N Z J Med* 1989; **19:** 321–6.

Levy S, Maarek M, Coumel P et al. Characterization of different subsets of atrial fibrillation in general practice in France: the ALFA study. *Circulation* 1999; **99:** 3028–35.

Lip GYH, Bawden L, Hodson R. Atrial fibrillation

amongst the Indo-Asian general practice population. The West Birmingham Atrial Fibrillation Project. *Int J Cardiol* 1998; **65:** 187–92.

Lip GYH, Golding DJ, Nazir M et al. A survey of atrial fibrillation in general practice: The West Birmingham Atrial Fibrillation Project. *Br J Gen Pract* 1997; **47:** 285–9.

Lip GYH, Tean KN, Dunn FG. Treatment of atrial fibrillation in a district general hospital. *Br Heart J* 1994; **71:** 92–5.

Lok NS, Lau CP. Presentation and management of patients admitted with atrial fibrillation: a review of 291 cases in a regional hospital. *Int J Cardiol* 1995; **48:** 271–8.

Manolio TA, Furberg CD, Rautaharju PM et al. Cardiac arrhythmias on 24 hour ambulatory electrocardiography in older women and men. The Cardiovascular Health Study. *J Am Coll Cardiol* 1984; **23:** 916–25.

Maru M. Atrial fibrillation and embolic complications. *East Afr Med J* 1997; **74:** 3–5.

Psalty BM, Manolio TA, Kuller LH et al. Incidence of and risk factors for atrial fibrillation in older adults. *Circulation* 1997; **96:** 2455.

Rose G, Baxter PJ, Reid DD, McCartney P. Prevalence and prognosis of electrocardiography findings in middle-aged men. *Br Heart J* 1978; **40:** 636–43.

Stewart FM, Singh Y, Persson S et al. Atrial fibrillation: prevalence and management in an acute general medical unit. *Aust N Z J Med* 1999; **29:** 51–8.

Sudlow CM, Rodgers H, Kenny RA, Thomson RG. Service provision and use of anticoagulants in atrial fibrillation. *BMJ* 1995; **311:** 558–61.

Sudlow M, Rodgers H, Kenny RA et al. Population based study of use of anticoagulants among patients with atrial fibrillation in the community. *BMJ* 1997; **314:** 1529–30.

Sudlow M, Thomson R, Thwaites B et al. Prevalence of atrial fibrillation and eligibility for anticoagulants in the community. *Lancet* 1998; **352:** 1167–71.

Takahashi N, Seki A, Imataka K, Fujii J. Clinical features of paroxysmal atrial fibrillation. An observation of 94 patients. *Jpn Heart J* 1981; **22:** 143–9.

Wolf PA, Mitchell JB, Baker MPP et al. Impact of atrial fibrillation on mortality, stroke and medical costs. *Arch Intern Med* 1998; **158:** 229–34.

Zarifis J, Beevers DG, Lip GYH. Acute admissions with atrial fibrillation in a British multiracial hospital population. *Br J Clin Pract* 1997; **51:** 91–6.

3

Clinical implications and importance

Introduction

Since the prevalence of atrial fibrillation (AF) increases with ageing, this common arrhythmia is a frequent problem not only for hospital physicians but also for primary-care physicians (Figure 3.1). Most of AF appears to be managed by the general practitioner, and in fact, only one third of patients with AF have been admitted to hospital for AF (Lip et al, 1997).

AF in the community

Initial detection and management

In the UK, with an ageing population, which is increasing at twice the rate of growth of the general population, the proportion of those over 70 years old will constitute 20–25% of the total population by the turn of the century. AF will therefore be an increasingly common cause of stroke, thromboembolism, and heart failure, and is therefore an important public-health problem.

The general practitioner is likely to remain as the "front line" for the initial detection, assessment, and management of patients with AF (Table 3.1). A high index of suspicion is necessary when reviewing high-risk individuals, such as those with hypertension, heart failure, thyroid disease, or ischaemic heart disease. For example, AF is present in about a third of patients with heart failure, and subclinical hyperthyroidism is common in the elderly who may not show overt symptoms. Indeed, recent onset symptoms of palpitations or reduced exercise tolerance, especially in the presence of an irregular pulse, will require further investigation with an ECG. It is therefore important to know when to "screen" for AF amongst the patients attending for a general practice consultation.

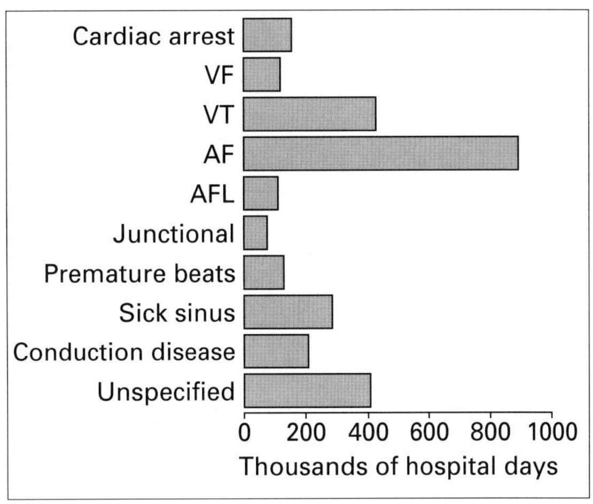

Figure 3.1
Estimated number of hospital days with arrhythmia as the principal diagnosis.

- Identification of patients with new onset AF.
- Assessment of thromboembolic risk and the early initiation of antithrombotic therapy — warfarin will be required for most patients, whilst aspirin may be suitable for young patients (age <65 years) with no cardiac risk factors or structural heart disease.
- Assistance with monitoring of anticoagulant therapy.
- Referral of appropriate patients to a cardiologist for further assessment (including ECG) and consideration of cardioversion.
- Awareness of potential drug interactions and toxicity with antiarrhythmic drugs and anticoagulants.

Table 3.1
Role of the general practitioner.

Drug use for AF and the general practitioner

Many patients with AF will also be taking antiarrhythmic drugs and anticoagulants. Since many patients are elderly, and have other medical conditions, side-effects and drug interactions will become increasingly common clinical problems. For example, hypokalaemia secondary to the use of high doses of loop diuretics may result in dangerous proarrhythmia in patients taking antiarrhythmic drug therapy or digoxin. Indeed, class I and III antiarrhythmic agents can cause QT prolongation and thus interact with electrolyte abnormalities (hypokalaemia, hypomagnesaemia), "over-the-counter" drugs (antihistamines) and other commonly prescribed drugs (tricyclic antidepressants, macrolide antibiotics such as erythromycin), leading to polymorphic ventricular tachycardia (*torsades des pointes*). Furthermore, many drugs have potentially serious interactions with warfarin. For example, cimetidine may inhibit the metabolism of warfarin, resulting in overanticoagulation.

The frequent use of drugs such as amiodarone may result in drug interactions with warfarin and digoxin, with consequent toxicity. Such possibilities emphasise the need for full recording of information on concurrent drug therapy and the need for a high index of suspicion. Non-compliance with therapy, owing to inadequate understanding or supervision, may also be dangerous, and careful monitoring of requests for repeat prescriptions is therefore essential. Finally, it is crucial to recognise when referral of a patient with AF to a cardiologist should be made (Table 3.2).

Anticoagulation and the general practitioner

The increasing prevalence of AF results in an increase in the numbers of patients on anticoagulant therapy. In our experience, a high proportion of patients in general practice would have risk factors for thromboembolism, which would require long-term anticoagulant therapy. This presents two problems: inconvenience and safety.

Despite the compelling evidence of the benefits of stroke reduction in patients with AF,

- Young patient with AF.
- AF resistant to "usual" drugs for rate control.
- Patient suitable for cardioversion.
- Further assessment required (e.g. valvular heart disease, preexcitatiom syndrome).
- Patient with moderate to severe heart failure, or resistant heart failure.
- Frequent attacks of paroxysmal AF.
- Syncopal attacks due to AF.

Table 3.2
When to refer a patient with AF to a cardiologist.

antithrombotic therapy is still under-used, ranging from 11% to 44% use in those eligible for oral anticoagulants (Sudlow et al, 1995). This is particularly so in elderly patients (over 75 years old) even though the benefits of antithrombotic therapy might be expected to be greatest in those patients. Clinician surveys have consistently cited patients age as a deterrent to warfarin usage (McCroy et al, 1995). Other risk factors such as poor compliance, recurrent falls, cognitive impairment, and the risk of interaction with multiple drug therapies should be considered, especially in the elderly (Kutner et al, 1991).

Many health authorities and general-practitioner groups have attempted to address this issue by providing guidelines for the use of anticoagulation in AF. The availability of various guidelines for AF may in fact add to the disparity, and it has been estimated that if various guidelines were applied to a population of patients with AF, the rate of anticoagulation would range from 13% to 100% (Thompson et al, 1998).

One suggested option to improve anticoagulation management of these patients with AF may be to increase involvement by general practitioners. Although regular monitoring of anticoagulation intensity and adjustment of dosage is often done at hospital-based or satellite-community-based anticoagulant clinics, this task is now undertaken by some general practitioners. Indeed, many general practitioners do feel they can take on this role (Rogers et al, 1997). If better, safer, and increasing use of anticoagulation in patients with AF is intended, increasing provision of general practitioner-based anticoagulation monitoring aided by computerised support systems and near patient testing may become a necessary step (Fitzmaurice et al, 1998). Indeed, anticoagulant monitoring by general practitioners has been found much better than that in hospital clinics (Pell et al, 1993), and many patients prefer to attend their local general practitioner. However, general practitioners do vary in their willingness to undertake anticoagulation monitoring, and much will depend on local enthusiasm and specialist support.

Screening for AF

With the potentially increasing importance of AF as a cause of mortality or morbidity, the question arises as to whether screening programmes will be cost-effective? All general practitioners should at least have easy access to a reliable ECG machine to confirm AF.

Currently, 5% of total UK National Health Service (NHS) expenditure can be attributed to stroke, and thus there would be expected to be about 1000 new cases of stroke per annum in a typical health authority serving a population of half a million people. Therefore, any screening programme that might lead to an important reduction in stroke incidence needs

- Patients complaining of palpitations or syncope.
- Patients with stroke or transient ischaemic attacks.
- Patients with heart failure.
- Patients on regular diuretic or digoxin therapy.

Table 3.3
"Screening" for AF in general practice.

serious consideration, because of the potential for health gain and the potential for reduced overall NHS expenditure. Since AF is an important risk factor for stroke in population terms (associated with 15% of all strokes) and since anticoagulation is a highly effective treatment to reduce this risk, screening for AF might be one such programme. Indeed, the optimal treatment of AF in the population might reduce the overall incidence of stroke by 10%. The incidence of new cases of AF in people over the age of 65 is about 1% per annum. However, any formal screening in general practice would have considerable implications in terms of manpower and costs.

However, before implementing a screening programme for AF, unresolved questions must be answered over how the screening should be conducted:

- What is the appropriate target population for the screening programme?
- What is the most appropriate screening test for AF? Whilst the 12-lead ECG is recognised as the gold standard, this test is relatively time-consuming as a formal screening tool. Therefore, it is important to consider simpler tests such as taking the pulse and simpler ECGs.
- Does the ECG need to be read by a cardiologist? Cardiologists will offer the most accurate readings of ECGs, but satisfactory interpretations can occasionally be obtained by the general practitioner, the practice nurse, or computerised diagnostic software.
- Once somebody has been identified as having AF, should they also receive an echocardiogram to assess their risk of stroke, or is clinical assessment of risk adequate?

The simplest screening strategy for AF is one of an "opportunistic case finding" programme, in which a general practitioner will take the opportunity to feel a patient's pulse during a consultation (Table 3.3). If the general practitioner notes it to be irregular, they might make a clinical diagnosis of AF, or request an ECG as a confirmatory test. However, opportunistic case finding is likely to miss a significant proportion of people who would otherwise have benefited from treatment, especially those AF patients in the community who may be symptom-free, or those with paroxysmal AF who happen to be in sinus rhythm at the time of pulse checking.

Another possible approach is to screen patients who are at higher risk of AF — a "targeted screening" programme. Heart failure, myocardial infarction, diabetes, hypertension, and rheumatic heart disease are important precursors of AF. AF is also more common in people with a history of hyperthyroidism, stroke, or transient ischaemic attack than people without these disorders. A targeted screening programme could use computerised general practice disease registers to identify such high-risk patients, or use prescribing information on the computerised records.

A third possible approach is to screen everyone over the age of 65 years for AF — a "whole population" screening programme. This would have substantial implications for resources and costs.

Screening for AF would result in an increasing referral rate for specialist advice and cardiological investigations (such as ECG). The cost-benefit ratio of such an exercise would need to be addressed. It has been estimated that a screening programme for AF in general practice would require 625 ECG examinations in each district general hospital serving a population of 250 000; this programme might prevent 19 strokes in each year. However, open access to general practitioners for ECG in local hospitals for patients with heart failure has been tried successfully in some centres, and there is a good case for extending this facility to the management of AF.

As with other chronic diseases, the adequate treatment of AF needs an effective channel of communication between hospital and general practice. Decisions on the advantages and disadvantages of anticoagulant therapy need to involve the physician, the general practitioner and, of course, the individual patient.

AF in hospital practice

As with general practice, the future increasing prevalence of AF will mean there will be more patients at increased risk of stroke and heart failure, with significant mortality and morbidity.

The increasing incidence of AF has important implications for the provision of cardiological investigations such as ECG. Most cardiologists would use this investigation for their patients with AF. In patients presenting with syncope, 24-h Holter monitoring is advisable. Since syncope is a common symptom in patients with AF, the question therefore arises whether we can afford to investigate all patients with AF with so many detailed and expensive investigations?

A recent survey of hospital consultant physicians in the UK has also identified significant differences in management approaches, with more cardiologists than non-cardiologists considering anticoagulation and cardioversion (Lip et al, 1996). Similarly, one US study identified significant variations from the recommended guidelines for anticoagulation in relation to cardioversion of AF (Schlicht et al, 1996).

Indications for hospital admission

Another important issue is whether the patient with the acute onset of AF requires hospital admission. Indeed, AF is a common reason for hospital admission because of cardiac arrhythmia.

One frequent reason for admission to the hospital is to “rule out” an acute myocardial infarction, although AF is rarely the manifestation of a symptom-free acute ischaemic event or myocardial infarction (MI). Thus, there is no real reason to admit the patient to a coronary care unit (CCU) with AF for this indication unless there are other reasons for doing so, such as classic ischaemic anginal pain or an ECG that shows an acute infarct or ischaemia. In these instances, it is generally not clear whether the MI precipitated the AF, or AF and the rapid ventricular rates caused cardiac ischaemia and an MI. In the study by Friedman and colleagues (1987) of 245 patients with AF admitted to a coronary care unit, only five had raised cardiac enzymes indicative of an acute MI. All five had at least two of the following clinical features: LVH on the ECG, an old MI on the ECG, typical angina pectoris, and duration of symptoms of less than 4 h. In another study of 97 patients with new onset AF, only one had an acute MI that was clearly identified by ECG changes (Shlofmitz et al, 1986).

However, hospital admission may be

required in some patients with AF, if an associated medical problem, which may be the reason for the arrhythmia, requires treatment, such as a chest infection. Elderly patients may be occasionally more safely treated in hospital, especially those with significant underlying heart disease who have haemodynamic consequences from the AF or those who are at risk of a complication resulting from treatment of the AF.

Implications for more anticoagulant clinics

The increasing use of warfarin as thromboprophylaxis requires regular anticoagulant clinic attendances for monitoring of the International Normalised Ratio (INR). Patients would also need well-designed instructions phrased in non-technical prose to inform them of what to do in the event of unusual symptoms or signs of bleeding. If such patients are reliant on expensive hospital-provided transport, this adds to the overall costs of treating them, and one option is to run domicillary anticoagulant checks, which minimise this expense.

Dedicated hospital outpatient clinics have been reported as less than satisfactory, with less than 50% of the results falling within the therapeutic range, and nearly one-third of patients being classed as "poorly controlled". This finding may be due to the high workload and inadequate time available to communicate with the patient. Patients may also have to travel long distances to the nearest clinic and may therefore default in attendance. As discussed above, more involvement and provision of anticoagulation-therapy monitoring by the general practitioner may be needed.

Effect of AF on mortality, stroke, and medical costs

We can generally assume that the effect of AF on mortality, stroke, and medical costs is considerable (Tables 3.4 and 3.5). However there are few studies that specifically address this issue. A recent prospective cohort study of hospitalised Medicare patients with AF showed that mortality rates were high in patients with AF and cardiovascular disease, ranging from 19.0% to 52.1% in the first year (Wolf et al, 1998). Adjusted relative mortality risk was about 20% higher in patients with AF in all age-sex strata during each of the 3 years studied; the incidence of stroke was highest in those with cardiovascular disease with and without AF (range 6.2–15.4% in 1 year), and was at least 5-fold higher than in individuals without cardiovascular disease. In those with cardiovascular disease, stroke rates were about 25% higher in women with AF ($p < 0.05$) but only 10% higher in men. Adjusted total Medicare spending in 1 year was 8.6 to 22.6-fold greater in men, and 9.8 to 11.2-fold greater in women with AF.

The cost-effectiveness of thromboprophylaxis is an important issue: balance is needed between the reduction in ischaemic stroke or thromboembolism and inconvenience associated with regular anticoagulation monitoring and the risks associated with bleeding whilst on anticoagulation (Cleland et al, 1996). Gustafsson and colleagues (1992) reported that primary prophylaxis with anticoagulant therapy in AF was cost-effective if the rate of intracranial bleeding during such therapy was only 0.3%, as in the major published trials. However if this rate increased to 2% or more per year, anticoagulation therapy was no longer cost effective. It should be appreciated that this "cost" has to be balanced against the reduction of the annual risk of stroke and the

Study	Study Period	Follow-up (yr)	Patients (n) (n with AF)	Age (yr)	Mortality (%) AF	Mortality (%) No AF	Mortality (%) RR	Study architecture
Framingham (male/female)	1948–1952	24	5,191 (98) (45%/55%)	30–62	*All cause*			Population sample, incident cases of chronic AF, age- and sex-matched controls, biennial follow-up
					Male 59.2	34.3	1.7	
					Female 44.9	25.3	1.8	
					Cardiovascular			
					Male 42.9	21.2	2.0	
					Female 40.8	15.1	2.7	
Reykjavik (male/female)	1967–1970	14	9,067 (25) (48%/52%)	32–64	*All cause*			Population sample, prevalent cases of chronic AF, age- and sex-matched controls, follow-up at 14 yr
					32	20	1.9	
					Vascular			
					20	6	6.1	
					Cerebrovascular			
					20	2	12.3	
Whitehall (male)	1967–1969	18	19,018 (63) (100%)	40–69			2.6	Screening of male civil servants, prevalent cases of chronic nonrheumatic AF, age-matched controls
British Regional Heart (male)	1979–1980		7,727 (48) (100%)	40–59				General practice sample, prevalent cases of chronic nonrheumatic AF, age-matched controls
					All cause			
Edinburgh (male/female)	1972–1977	5	487 (44%/56%)	62–90	67	27.3	2.3	Population sample of older people, prevalent cases of AF, age-matched controls
					Ischemic heart disease			
							7.3	
Australia (male/female)	1966–1981	2–17	1,770 (87) (48%/52%)	>60	*All cause*			Triennial population survey, prevalent and incident cases of paroxysmal and chronic AF, adjusted for age, sex, and other risk factors
					42.5		1.9	
					Cardiovascular (nonstroke)		1.8	
					Stroke		3.8	
Framingham	1948–1952	24	1,037 (71)	30–62	*Male*			Population sample, incident cases of chronic and paroxysmal AF in patients with coronary heart disease, age- and sex-matched controls, biennial follow-up
					Chronic AF		2.7	
					Transient AF		0.7	
					Female			
					Chronic AF		1.0	
					Transient AF		1.9	
CASS		7	18,343 (116)	All ages; 67%, 40–59	62	20	2.0	Multicenter registry, patients with angiographically proven coronary artery disease, prevalent cases of AF compared with those with NSR

AF, atrial fibrillation; RR, relative risk; CASS, Coronary Artery Surgery Study; NSR, normal sinus rhythm.
Reproduced with permission from Cairns and Connolly (1991).

Table 3.4
Prognosis of atrial fibrillation — mortality.

Study	Date of cohort assembly	Follow-up (yr)	Patients (n) (n with AF)	Age (yr)	Stroke (%/yr) AF	No AF	RR	Study architecture
Framingham	1948–1952	24	5,184 (98)	30–60	4.1 (nonrheumatic) 4.5 (rheumatic)	0.29 0.29	5.6 17.6	Population sample: incident cases of chronic AF, age- and sex-matched controls, includes TIA; biennial follow-up
Framingham	1948–1952	30	5,184 (303)	30–62	3.8 (nonrheumatic)	0.31	4	As above but nonrheumatic AF only
Reykjavik	1967–1970	14	9,067 (25)	32–64	4.43		7.1	Population sample: prevalent cases of chronic AF, age- and sex-matched controls; follow-up at 14 yr
Whitehall	1967–1969	18	19,018 (63)	40–69	1.8		6.9	Screening of male civil servants: prevalent cases of chronic nonrheumatic AF, age-matched controls, not TIA
British Regional Heart	1979–1980	5	7,727 (48)	40–59	0.3		2.3	General practice sample: prevalent cases of chronic nonrheumatic AF, age-matched controls, not TIA
Montreal (male/female)	1979–1983	3.3 (mean)	(254) (48%/52%)	18–86	5.5			Retrospective chart review: all patients had chronic or paroxysmal AF, includes TIA, nonanticoagulated cohort
AFASAK (male/female)	1985–1988	2	(336) (54%/46%)	38–91 74.6 (mean)	4.9			Outpatient chronic AF, nonrheumatic AF only, not TIA, placebo group
SPAF (male/female)	1987–1989	1.13 (mean)	(528) (71%/29%)	66.9 (mean)	5.7			Inpatient or outpatient chronic or paroxysmal AF, nonrheumatic AF only, not TIA, placebo group

AF, atrial fibrillation; RR, relative risk; TIA, transient ischemic attack; AFASAK, Copenhagen Atrial Fibrillation Trial; SPAF, Stroke Prevention in Atrial Fibrillation. Reproduced with permission from Cairns and Connolly (1991).

Table 3.5
Prognosis of atrial fibrillation — stroke.

associated morbidity and mortality "costs", which are likely to be substantial.

Postoperative AF is also a health-care problem that leads to an increase in stroke, thromboembolism, and heart failure, and prolonged hospital stay and costs. AF after cardiac surgery can occur in about one third of patients, is associated with an increase in adverse events in all measurable outcomes of care, and increases the use of hospital resources and, therefore, the cost of care. Strategies to reduce the incidence of AF after cardiac surgery should favourably affect surgical outcomes and reduce resource use, and

- To relieve symptoms of congestive heart failure, hypotension or angina that can be directly attributed to a rapid heart rate.
- To improve overall cardiac function.
- To improve exercise tolerance.
- To reduce the risk of thromboembolism and stroke.

Table 3.6
Importance of treating atrial fibrillation.

thus lower the cost of care. “High risk” patients can be identified and appropriate antiarrhythmic prophylaxis initiated. For example, in the study by Almassi and colleagues (1997) the prevalence of postoperative AF was 29.6%, which was predicted by the following: advancing age (odds ratio [OR] 1.61), chronic obstructive pulmonary disease (OR 1.37), use of digoxin within 2 weeks before surgery (OR 1.37), low resting pulse rate of less than 80 beats per min (OR 1.26), high resting systolic blood pressure of more than 120 mmHg (OR 1.19), mitral valve repair (OR 2.86) and replacement (OR 2.33), and prolonged use of inotropic agents (OR 1.36). Morbid events, hospital mortality, and 6-month mortality were significantly higher in AF patients.

In the elderly, the effect of AF may be a particular problem. In the population-based study by Kaarisalo and colleagues (1997a) amongst elderly (aged over 75 years) mortality was higher in the AF group at 28 days (33.9% *vs* 28.1%) and at 1 year after first ischaemic stroke (52.7% *vs* 43.0%). The age-adjusted and sex-adjusted relative risk of death was 1.25 in the AF group (95% CI 1.04–1.50) at 28 days, and 1.41 (1.18–1.67) at 1 year. The strongest risk factor predicting 1-year mortality was recent myocardial infarction (relative risk 1.90 [95% CI 1.49–2.42]). Although estimates of relative risk attributable to AF are of the same magnitude in older and in middle-aged stroke patients, the much higher prevalence of AF in the older patients emphasizes its absolute effect on the mortality and recurrence after the first ischaemic stroke in that age group.

Stroke patients with AF are at particularly high risk of death both at the acute phase of stroke and during the year after the first acute stroke event. In the study by Kaarisalo and colleagues (1997b), mortality was higher in the AF group both at 28 days (19.5% *vs* 14.4%) and at 1 year after the attack (30.5% *vs* 21.8%). In the proportional hazards model, AF was still a significant independent risk factor for 1-year mortality, with a hazard ratio of 1.26 (95% CI 1.09–1.46). Nevertheless the analysis by Stevenson and colleagues (1996) suggested that the prognosis of patients with advanced heart failure and AF may actually be improving. Their findings support the practice of avoiding class I antiarrhythmic drugs in this group, and may reflect recent beneficial changes in heart failure therapy.

Thus, the prevention of AF and treatment of patients with AF and associated cardiovascular disease are likely to yield benefits in terms of reduced mortality and stroke, as well as reducing health-care costs. The treatment of coexisting cardiac disease also has the potential to prevent deaths and recurrent stroke events, especially in older people in whom the impact of AF is likely to be the greatest (Table 3.6).

References

Almassi GH, Schowalter T, Nicolosi AC et al. Atrial fibrillation after cardiac surgery: a major morbid event? *Ann Surg* 1997; **226:** 501–10; discussion 511–3.

Cairns JA and Connolly SJ. Nonrheumatic atrial fibrillation. Risk of stroke and role of antithrombotic therapy. *Circulation* 1991; **84:** 469–74.

Cleland JGF, Cowburn PJ, Falk RH. Should all patients with atrial fibrillation receive warfarin? *European Heart Journal* 1996; **17:** 674–81.

Fitzmaurice DA, Hobbs FD, Murray ET. Primary care anticoagulant clinic management using computerized decision support and near patient International Normalized Ratio (INR) testing: routine data from a practice nurse-led clinic. *Fam Pract* 1998; **15:** 144–6.

Friedman HZ, Weber-Bornstein N, Deboe SF et al. CCU admission criteria for suspected acute myocardial infarction in new onset atrial fibrillation. *Am J Cardiol* 1987; **59:** 866.

Gustafsson C, Asplund K, Britton M et al. Cost-effectiveness of primary stroke prevention in atrial fibrillation: Swedish national perspective. *BMJ* 1992; **305:** 1457–60.

Kaarisalo MM, Immonen-Raiha P, Marttila RJ et al. Atrial fibrillation in older stroke patients: association with recurrence and mortality after first ischemic stroke. *J Am Geriatr Soc* 1997(a); **45:** 1297–301.

Kaarisalo MM, Immonen-Raiha P, Marttila RJ et al. Atrial fibrillation and stroke. Mortality and causes of death after the first acute ischemic stroke. *Stroke* 1997(b); **28:** 311–15.

Kutner M, Nixon G, Silverstone F. Physicians' attitudes towards oral anticoagulants and antiplatelet agents for stroke prevention in elderly patients with atrial fibrillation. *Arch Intern Med* 1991; **151:** 1950–3.

Lip GYH, Golding DJ, Nazir M et al. A survey of atrial fibrillation in general practice: the West Birmingham Atrial Fibrillation Project. *Br J Gen Pract* 1997; **47:** 285–9.

Lip GYH, Zarifis J, Watson RD, Beevers DG. Physician variation in the management of patients with atrial fibrillation. *Heart* 1996; **7:** 200–5.

McCrory DC, Matchar DB, Smasa G et al. Physician attitudes about anticoagulation for nonvalvular atrial fibrillation in the elderly. *Arch Intern Med* 1995; **155:** 277–81.

Pell JP, McIver B, Stuart P et al. Comparison of anticoagulant control among patients attending general practice and a hospital anticoagulant clinic. *Br J Gen Prac* 1993; **43:** 152–4.

Rogers H, Sudlow M, Dobson R et al. Warfarin anticoagulation in primary care: a regional survey of present practice and clinicians' views. *Br J Gen Pract* 1997; **47:** 309–10.

Schlicht JR, Davis RC, Naqi K et al. Physician practices regarding anticoagulaion and cardioversion of atrial fibrillation. *Arch Intern Med* 1996; **156:** 290–4.

Shlofmitz RA, Hirsch BE, Meyer BR. New-onset atrial fibrillation. Is there a need for emergent hospitalization? *J Gen Intern Med* 1986; **1:** 139.

Stevenson WG, Stevenson LW, Middlekauff HR et al. Improving survival for patients with atrial fibrillation and advanced heart failure. *J Am Coll Cardiol* 1996; **28:** 1458–63.

Sudlow CM, Rodgers H, Kenny RA, Thomson RG. Service provision and use of anticoagulants in atrial fibrillation. *BMJ* 1995; **315:** 558–61.

Taylor F, Ramsay M, Voke J, Cohen H. Anticoagulation in patients with atrial fibrillation: GPs not prepared for monitoring anticoagulation. *BMJ* 1993; **307:** 1493.

Thomson R, McElroy H, Sudlow M. Guidelines on anticoagulant treatment in atrial fibrillation in Great Britain: variation in content and implications for treatment. *BMJ* 1998; **316:** 509–13.

Wolf PA, Mitchell JB, Baker CS et al. Impact of atrial fibrillation on mortality, stroke, and medical costs. *Arch Intern Med* 1998; **158:** 229–34.

II
Aetiology

4

Common causes of atrial fibrillation

Introduction

Atrial fibrillation (AF) may be paroxysmal or chronic, and is commonly associated with the common cardiovascular disorders. The latter are often associated with atrial enlargement, an elevation in atrial pressure, or even infiltration or inflammation of the atria. In the Framingham study, for example, the development of AF was associated with increasing age (odds ratio [OR] 2.1 for men and 2.2 for women, $p < 0.0001$), diabetes (OR 1.4 for men and 1.6 for women), hypertension (OR 1.5 for men and 1.4 for women), valve disease (OR 1.8 for men and 3.4 for women), (Benjamin et al, 1994). Myocardial infarction was significantly associated with the development of AF in men, whilst women were more likely to have valve disease as a risk factor for AF. AF is also commonly associated with, and complicated by, congestive heart failure and strokes.

The coexistence of cardiovascular disease and chronic AF significantly worsens the patient's prognosis. As discussed later, in chapter 16, the presence of cardiovascular risk factors such as hypertension, diabetes, or heart failure, and prior cerebrovascular events significantly increases the risk of further stroke and thromboembolism (AF Investigators 1994). In the Framingham study, the association between AF and cardiovascular disease may even double the cardiovascular mortality (Kannel et al, 1982). By comparison, patients under the age of 60 who have AF but no apparent heart disease are considered to have lone AF, and to be a group with a much better prognosis. However, a 30-year follow up from the Framingham study did report that patients with lone AF had a 5-fold increase in mortality, but this population was older and had a higher prevalence of hypertension (Brand et al, 1985).

Causes of AF

The causes of AF can be cardiac (Table 4.1) and non-cardiac (Table 4.2). In about 80% of

Common
- Ischaemic heart disease
- Rheumatic heart disease
- Hypertension
- Sick sinus syndrome
- Pre-excitation syndromes (e.g. Wolff-Parkinson-White)

Less commonly
- Cardiomyopathy or heart muscle disease
- Pericardial disease, including effusion, constrictive pericarditis
- Atrial septal defect
- Atrial myxoma

Table 4.1
Cardiac causes of atrial fibrillation.

- Acute infections, especially pneumonia
- Lung carcinoma
- Other intrathoracic pathology e.g. pleural effusion
- Alcohol excess
- Postoperative, especially after thoracotomy or coronary artery bypass surgery
- Pulmonary thromboembolism
- Thyrotoxicosis

Unknown
- Idiopathic or "lone" atrial fibrillation

Table 4.2
Non cardiac causes of AF.

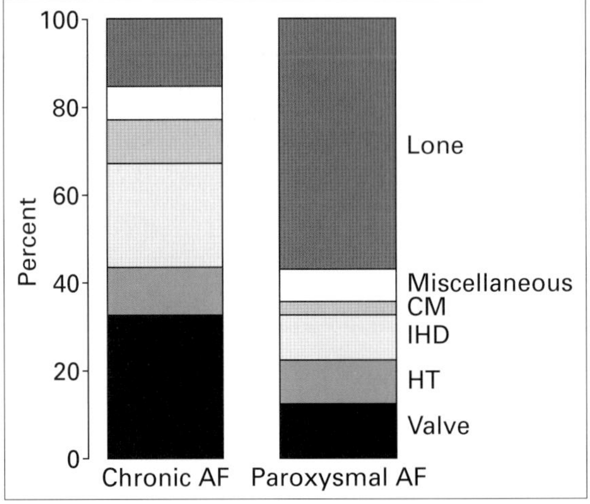

Figure 4.1
Aetiology of AF in 246 patients undergoing DC conversion for chronic AF and 161 patients with paroxysmal AF. Miscellaneous includes sinus node disease. CM = cardiomyopathy; IHD = ischaemic heart disease; HT = hypertension; valve = valvular heart disease, including rheumatic and significant mitral valve prolapse. reproduced with permission from Murgatroyd et al (1993).

cases, AF is associated with organic heart disease, including coronary heart disease, hypertension (especially if LVH is present), valvular heart disease (mostly mitral disease), hypertrophic or dilated cardiomyopathy, or congenital heart disease. Other possible aetiologies include restrictive cardiomyopathy (including infiltrations such as amyloidosis, haemochromatosis, and endomyocardial fibrosis), and constrictive paricarditis. When patients with chronic AF are compared with those with paroxysmal AF, the latter group tends to be younger and nearly half do not have underlying heart disease (Figure 4.1).

Nevertheless, AF may also occur in the absence of detectable organic heart disease, but underlying heart disease may still appear as time progresses especially in the elderly. Non-cardiac causes would include any pyrexial illness or infection, thyroid disease, chronic obstructive lung disease, alcohol, and the postoperative state.

Hypertension

In developed countries, hypertensive heart disease is now the most common underlying disorder in patients with AF. In the Framingham study, for example, hypertension was considered to be the most common cause of AF, being present in over 50% of patients (Kannel et al, 1982). In fact, hypertension was associated with a relative risk of 1.9 for developing AF in the Framingham study. In the Manitoba follow-up study, hypertension was also common (53% cases) and was associated with a relative risk of 1.42 (Krahn et al, 1995). In that study, either hypertension or ischaemic heart disease preceded AF in 65% of cases, suggesting that both hypertension and ischaemic heart disease accounted for a large proportion of cases of AF.

The picture seems different, however, in

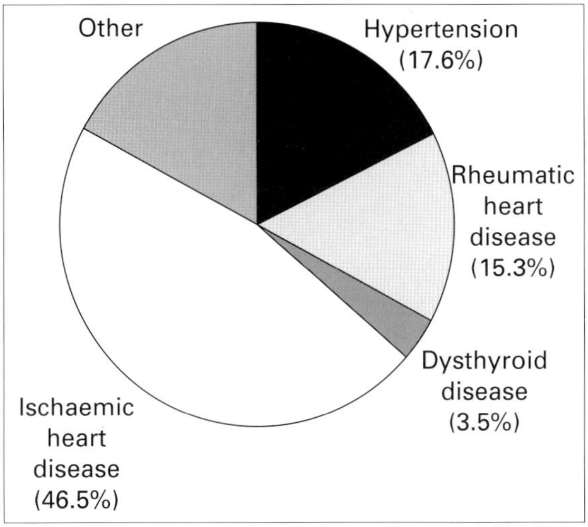

Figure 4.2
Aetiology of atrial fibrillation amongst acute admissions to a Scottish district general hospital. Reproduced with permission from Lip (1994).

some studies from the UK. For example, in a study of acute hospital admissions with AF from Glasgow (Lip et al, 1994) and Birmingham (Zarifis et al, 1997), ischaemic heart disease was the most common associated factor, followed closely by hypertension (Figure 4.2). In particular, hypertension was the most common underlying medical condition in black or Afro-Caribbean patients, whilst in South Asians the most common cause was ischaemic heart disease. In our survey of AF in general practice, hypertension was the most common underlying medical problem, being present in over a third of patients (Lip et al, 1997); this may be a reflection of the differences between community and hospital-based populations. In a study of AF amongst Hong Kong Chinese (Lok and Lau, 1995), AF was frequently associated with hypertension (29%), compared with atherosclerotic vascular disease (25%) and rheumatic heart disease (18%).

It is well recognised that patients with chronic hypertension, particularly those with associated left ventricular hypertrophy, develop left atrial dilatation. The latter alters the electrophysiological properties of the atrium, resulting in the propensity to develop AF. Excess alcohol intake may also contribute to hypertension and to AF. Patients with hypertension can develop significant diastolic dysfunction and the concomitant increase in left atrial pressure is another predisposing factor. Importantly, patients with hypertension are more prone to develop coronary artery disease, which is another important risk for developing AF. In the Stroke Prevention in Atrial Fibrillation (SPAF) study, the echocardiographic substudy suggested that left ventricular hypertrophy was an added risk for stroke and AF on univariate analysis, but on multivariate analysis only the presence of left atrial dilatation and left ventricular dysfunction emerged as independent risk factors (SPAF Investigators, 1992b). A previous history of hypertension in patients with AF also merits consideration for anticoagulation, since such patients are at high risk of stroke and thromboembolism (SPAF, 1992a).

However, patients with uncontrolled hypertension require control of blood pressure before initiation of anticoagulation, to avoid the risk of cerebral haemorrhage, since there is an association between uncontrolled blood pressure and this adverse effect of warfarin therapy.

Coronary artery disease

There is a high prevalence of coronary disease in the population, and thus coronary artery disease (CAD) is a common cause of AF. AF is however not commonly associated with isolated CAD per se, unless complicated by acute MI or congestive heart failure.

AF occurs transiently in about 20% of patients with an acute MI, presumably due to atrial ischaemia or atrial stretching secondary to heart failure; these patients tend to have larger infarcts and a poor prognosis (Sugiura et al, 1985; Goldberg et al, 1990; Sakata et al, 1997). If AF occurs in the setting of an acute MI, it usually occurs in the first 24 h and is usually self-limiting.

The time of onset of AF may, however, be useful to assess cardiac status and prognosis for these patients. In the study by Sakata and colleagues (1997), amongst 1039 patients with acute MI 9.6% developed AF; 45% did so within 24 h of MI onset (Group I), 41% developed AF over 24 h after MI onset (Group II), whilst 14% developed AF before the onset of MI (Group III) (Figure 4.3). Complications such as heart failure, cardiogenic shock, and in-hospital mortality were higher for patients with AF than for patients who were in sinus rhythm. AF was also an independent predictor of cardiac death in patients developing AF within 24 h (odds ratio 2.5% [95% CI 1.2–5.0]) and those developing AF over 24 h (odds ratio 3.7 [95% CI 1.8–7.5]).

The GISSI-2 trial evaluated over 11 000 patients treated with thrombolytic therapy for acute MI, and when compared with those without AF, patients with AF had a higher mortality rate both in-hospital (18% *vs* 8.6%) and at 6 months (8.2% *vs* 3.1%, Ledda et al, 1994).

Nevertheless, the development of AF may simply reflect co-morbidity. In the study by Goldberg and colleagues (1990) of 4108 patients with an acute MI the overall incidence of new AF was 9.7%, and this was associated with a 1.7-fold increase in mortality. On multivariate analysis, AF was not an independent risk factor for mortality, but was associated with older age and a higher prevalence of heart failure, shock, or ventricular arrhythmias — all factors associated with an increased mortality.

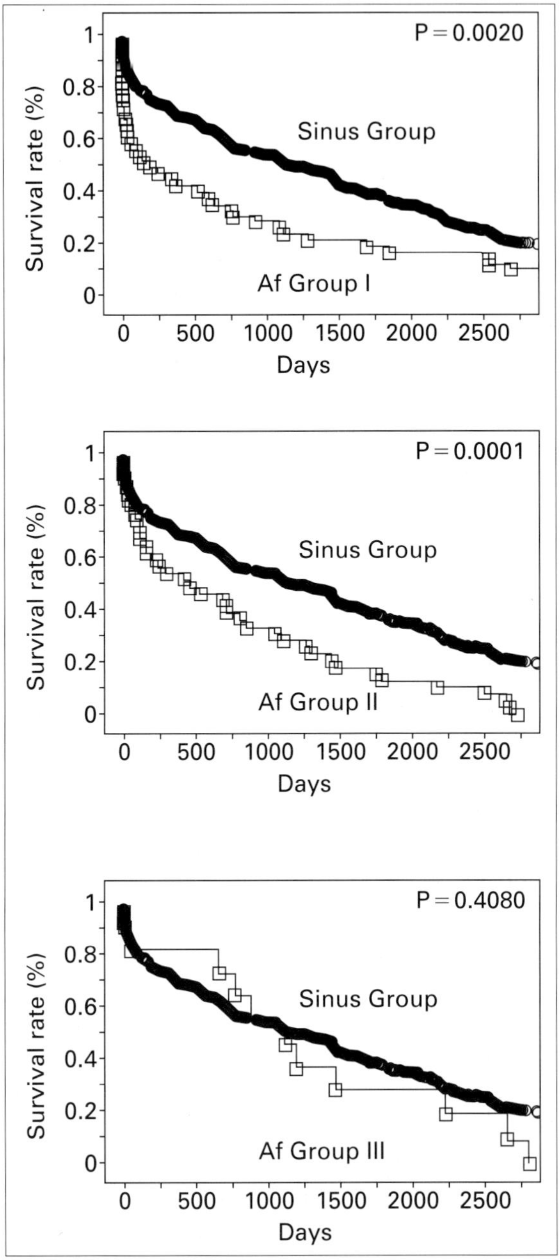

Figure 4.3
Kaplan-Meier analysis of cumulative survival rates for patients with myocardial infarction during 8-year follow-up. Survival rates are stratified by presence or absence of AF. Reproduced from Sakata et al (1997), with permission from Excerpta Medica Inc.

In patients with chronic stable CAD the incidence of AF is much lower. For example, Kramer and colleagues (1982) reported that only 0.8% of patients with high-grade coronary lesions at angiography are in AF, which was considered to be a marker of left ventricular dysfunction. In the Coronary Artery Surgical Study (CASS), the prevalence of chronic AF was 0.6%, which was associated with age over 60 years, male sex, mitral regurgitation, and congestive heart failure, but not with the number of coronary arteries involved (Cameron et al, 1988). Nevertheless the presence of AF is an independent predictor or increased mortality with a 7-year survival of 38%, compared with 80% for those without AF (relative risk 1.98, Cameron et al, 1988).

Heart failure

AF occurs frequently in association with heart failure. Nevertheless, as AF can predispose to heart failure by fast ventricular rates and rate-related ischaemia; and congestive heart failure can lead to AF due to high intracardiac pressures, this leads to a "chicken or egg" scenario. In addition, both AF and heart failure are closely related to heart disease and hypertension. Alcohol can also precipitate AF and result in heart failure due to alcoholic cardiomyopathy.

The prognostic significance of AF in patients with heart failure remains controversial. There is evidence that the presence of heart failure or impaired left ventricular function on ECG substantially adds to the increased risk of stroke and thromboembolism in AF (see chapter 16). Furthermore, a retrospective analysis from the SOLVD registry found that the presence of AF was significantly associated with an increase in all-cause mortality, progressive pump failure, and risk of death or rehospitalisation (Dries et al, 1998).

Valve disease

Rheumatic heart disease is now less frequent in developed countries. For example, valve disease was present only in the minority in our general-practice survey (Lip et al, 1997). Nevertheless valve disease is, however, associated with a high prevalence of AF, and worldwide, rheumatic valve disease is still a very important cause of AF.

In a study of the predictors for AF in about 1100 patients with rheumatic heart disease, the highest frequency of AF (70%) was found in those with mitral stenosis, mitral regurgitation, and tricuspid regurgitation, whilst AF occurred in 29% with isolated mitral stenosis, 16% with isolated mitral regurgitation, and 52% with both conditions (Diker et al, 1996). However, when concurrent mitral valve disease is absent, AF is relatively infrequent in patients with aortic stenosis (about 1%) unless heart failure is present (Diker et al, 1996).

Valve disease is particularly important since its presence increases the thromboembolic risk of patients with chronic AF by about 18-fold. Up to 20% of patients with mitral stenosis and AF develop embolic events, and these most commonly (60–75%) affect the cerebral circulation. This risk of stroke and thromboembolism for patients in AF is 3 to 7 times that of patients with mitral stenosis in sinus rhythm.

Thyroid disease

AF occurs in about 20 to 25% of older patients with thyrotoxicosis, but is less common under the age of 30. However, it may also be underdiagnosed, since thyroid-function tests are often neglected, particular in the elderly in whom classical signs of thyrotoxicosis may not be obvious. One clinical clue may be the failure of digoxin to control the ventricular rate without the addition of beta-blockers.

Increased beta-adrenergic tone may be in part responsible for the development of AF, and may also contribute to the rapid ventricular response in this disorder. Attempted electric or pharmacological cardioversion should not therefore be attempted whilst the patient remains thyrotoxic, as AF usually recurs. Nevertheless, spontaneous reversion to sinus rhythm often occurs within 6 weeks in younger patients who are rendered euthyroid; whilst older patients show less spontaneous reversion which is age-related. There is a risk of thromboembolism and anticoagulation would be prudent.

The risk of AF is increased up to 3-fold in patients with subclinical hyperthyroidism (Sawin et al, 1994; Krahn et al, 1996). Sawin and colleagues (1994) assessed the frequency of hyperthyroidism in 726 patients with recent onset AF and found low Thyroid Stimulating Hormone (TSH) values in 5.4%. Nevertheless, thyroid function tests are infrequently checked (Lip et al, 1994) and only a small proportion are subsequently cardioverted.

Alcohol

Cardiac arrhythmias, especially supraventricular arrhythmias, seem to occur much more commonly in heavy drinkers, particularly after weekend or holiday-related bouts of heavy consumption. Such observations have led to the term "holiday heart syndrome", referring to acute disturbances of cardiac rhythm with heavy alcohol consumption in people with "normal hearts" (Ettinger et al, 1978; Lowenstein et al, 1983; Thornton, 1984).

The study by Ettinger and colleagues described 32 episodes of atrial arrhythmias in 24 chronic heavy users of alcohol, which mainly occurred during the holiday season. Lowenstein and colleagues reported that in younger patients (aged <65 years) with new onset AF, alcohol caused or contributed to the arrhythmia in 63% of cases. In our survey of two general practices in the west of Birmingham, however, alcohol-related AF was found in only 5.4% of cases (Lip et al, 1997). Interestingly, there was actually a lower consumption of alcohol amongst patients with AF compared with those without AF (43% *vs* 59%) in the Busselton study (Lake et al, 1989).

The mechanisms for alcohol-related AF may be related to increases in levels of catecholamines, the direct toxic effect of alcohol exerted by acetaldehyde on the myocardium, and changes in conduction and refractory times (Table 4.3). Alcohol may also cause arrhythmogenic changes in serum electrolyte concentrations. Acute alcohol ingestion can influence the parasympathetic system, especially with vomiting; such vagal stimulation can provoke atrial arrhythmias. Furthermore, alcohol use is related to hypertension, which is an important cause of AF, and alcohol may result in a dilated cardiomyopathy, resulting in

Mechanisms
- Alcohol ingestion results in release of cathecholamines.
- Plasma acetaldehyde, the main metabolite of ethanol, raises cathecholamine concentrations.
- Direct effect of alcohol (or its metabolites) on the heart, with prolongation of PR, QRS and QT times, facilitating atrial arrhythmias.
- Alcohol withdrawal increases cathecholamine release.

Table 4.3
Alcohol and AF.

high intra-atrial pressures and the development of AF.

Congenital heart disease

AF can be associated with congenital heart disease. In particular, AF is found in 19% of adults with an atrial septal defect (Tikoff et al, 1968). AF also occurs in other forms of congenital heart disease that affect the atria, including Ebstein's anomaly and patent ductus arteriosus, and after surgical correction of some other abnormalities, including ventricular septal defect, Tetralogy of Fallot, pulmonic stenosis, and transposition of the great vessels. Since many such patients are now surviving to adulthood because of improving surgical techniques, the development of AF may result in clinical deterioration or cardiac decompensation, and increase the need for antithrombotic therapy.

Cardiomyopathy

Cardiomyopathies can predispose to the development of AF. The prognostic importance of AF in these patients is nevertheless unclear.

For example, AF is present in up to 28% of patients with hypertrophic cardiomyopathy. This may confer a worse prognosis, with sudden cardiac death in 16% and a reduced 15-year survival (76% *vs* 97% in those without AF) (Cecchi et al, 1995). Some patients with hypertrophic cardiomyopathy have significant diastolic dysfunction, and the rhythm change from sinus rhythm to AF may result in clinical deterioration and diastolic heart failure. Nevertheless, one other study found no increase in mortality risk with AF, but some symptomatic deterioration did occur in 89%, which was generally reversable with cardioversion or heart rate control (Robinson et al, 1990).

AF is present in up to 20% of patients with dilated cardiomyopathy, but prognosis is dependent upon the severity of myocardial dysfunction. In mild to moderate heart failure, AF does not increase morbidity or mortality, but total and sudden death mortality is increased in patients with significantly advanced heart failure (Carson et al, 1993; Middlekauff et al, 1991; Mahoney et al, 1999).

Chest disease

Any thoracic pathology can contribute to AF — this can range from a simple pyrexial infection to lung carcinoma, pericardial disease, infections, and pleural disease. Up to 10% of patients with documented pulmonary thromboembolism have AF, although the commonest ECG abnormality in that disorder is still sinus tachycardia (Weber et al, 1966) (Figure 4.4).

Familial

Brugada and colleagues (1997) described a family of 26 members, of whom ten had familial AF, segregating as an autosomal dominant disease. Genetic linkage analysis has localised the gene responsible to chromosome 10q in the region of 10q22-q24, which may contribute to the substrate for the development of AF.

Drug-induced AF

Some medications can cause or contribute to the development of AF. Theophylline or caffeine are examples. In addition, increased vagal tone induces AF experimentally, and drugs that increase vagal tone, such as digitalis, may share this effect.

Other causes of AF

AF is common in the postoperative period, especially after cardiothoracic surgery. This

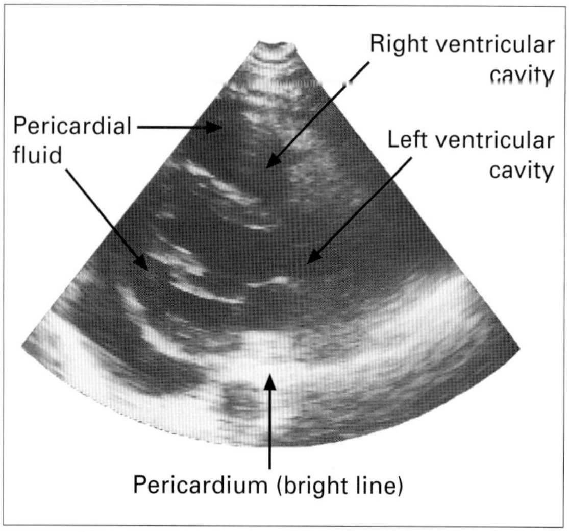

Figure 4.4
Two-dimensional echocardiogram showing large pericardial effusion.

important area is discussed further in chapter 5. Less common causes of AF include peripartum cardiomyopathy, lupus myocarditis, the cardiomyopathy associated with severe obesity, and both idiopathic and uraemic pericarditis.

AF is common in individuals with paroxysmal supraventricular tachycardia (PSVT). As an example, AF occurs in up to a third of individuals with the Wolff-Parkinson-White syndrome (Campbell et al, 1977), and ablation of the accessory pathways usually leads to a reduction in subsequent AF.

In one study of 169 patients who presented with PSVT and were followed by clinic visits and transtelephonic ECG monitoring during symptomatic episodes, 19% had an episode of AF during a mean follow-up of 31 months; 6% of episodes had occurred within 1 month, 9% within 4 months, and 12% within 1 year (Hamer et al, 1995). The time to occurrence of AF was not influenced by either the mechanism or the rate of the PSVT.

References

Atrial Fibrillation Investigators. Risk factors for stroke and efficacy of antithrombotic therapy in atrial fibrillation. *Arch Intern Med* 1994; **154:** 1449–57.

Benjamin EJ, Levy D, Varizi SM et al. Independent risk factors for atrial fibrillation in a population based cohort: the Framingham Heart Study. *JAMA* 1994; **271:** 840–4.

Brand FN, Abbott RD, Kannel WB, Wolf PA. Characteristics and prognosis of lone atrial fibrillation: 30 year follow up in the Framingham study. *JAMA* 1985; **254:** 3449.

Brugada R, Tapscott T, Czernuszewicz G et al. Identification of a genetic locus for familial atrial fibrillation. *N Engl J Med* 1997; **336:** 905.

Cameron A, Schwartz MJ, Kronmal RA et al. Prevalence and significance of atrial fibrillation in coronary artery disease (CASS Registry). *Am J Cardiol* 1988; **61:** 714.

Campbell RWF, Smith RA, Gallagher JJ et al. Atrial fibrillation in the preexcitation syndrome. *Am J Cardiol* 1977; **40:** 514.

Carson PE, Johnson GR, Dunkman B et al for the V-HeFT VA Cooperative Studies Group. The influence of atrial fibrillation on prognosis in mild-moderate heart failure. The V-HeFT Studies. *Circulation* 1993; **87(suppl VI):** IV102.

Cecchi F, Olivotto I, Montereggi A et al. Hypertrophic cardiomyopathy in Tuscany: clinical course and outcome in an unselected regional population. *J Am Coll Cardiol* 1995; **26:** 1529.

Diker E, Aydogdu S, Ozdemir M et al. Prevalence and predictors of atria fibrillation in rheumatic heart disease. *Am J Cardiol* 1996; **77:** 96.

Dries DL, Exner DV, Gersh BJ et al. Atrial fibrillation is associated with an increased risk for mortality and heart failure progression in patients with asymptomatic and symptomatic left ventricular dysfunction: a retrospective analysis of the SOLVD trials. *J Am Coll Cardiol* 1998; **32:** 695–703.

Ettinger PO, Wu CF, DelaCruz C et al. Arrhythmias and the "holiday heart". Alcohol associated cardiac rhythm disorders. *Am Heart J* 1978; **95:** 555.

Goldberg RJ, Seeley D, Becker RC et al. Impact of atrial fibrillation on the in-hospital and long term survival of patients with an acute myocardial infarction: a community wide perspective. *Am Heart J* 1990; **119:** 991.

Hamer ME, Wilkinson WE, Clair WE et al. Incidence of symptomatic atrial fibrillation in patients with paroxysmal supraventricular tachycardia. *J Am Coll Cardiol* 1995; **25:** 984.

Kannel WB, Abbott RD, Savage DD, McNamara PM. Epidemiologic features of chronic atrial fibrillation. *N Engl J Med* 1982; **306:** 1018.

Krahn AD, Manfreda J, Tate RB et al. The natural history of atrial fibrillation: incidence, risk factors and prognosis in the Manitoba Follow-Up study. *Am J Med* 1995; **98:** 476–84.

Krahn AD, Klein GJ, Kerr CR. How useful is thyroid function testing in patients with recent-onset atrial fibrillation? *Arch Intern Med* 1996; **156:** 2221.

Kramer RJ, Zeldis SM, Hamby RI. Atrial fibrillation, a marker for abnormal left ventricular function in coronary heart disease. *Br Heart J* 1982; **47:** 606.

Lake FR, Cullen KJ, de Klerk NH et al. Atrial fibrillation and mortality in an elderly population. *Aust N Z J Med* 1989; **19:** 321–6.

Ledda A, Maggioni AP, Franzosi MG et al. Incidence and prognostic value of paroxysmal atrial fibrillation in 11,493 patients with confirmed acute myocardial infarction treated with thrombolytic agents. *J Am Coll Cardiol* 1994; **23:** 313A.

Lip GYH, Golding DJ, Nazir M et al. A survey of atrial fibrillation in general practice: the west Birmingham Atrial Fibrillation Project. *Br J Gen Pract* 1997; **47:** 285–9.

Lip GYH, Tean KN, Dunn FG. Treatment of atrial fibrillation in a district general hospital. *Br Heart J* 1994; **71:** 92–5.

Lok NS, Lau CP. Presentation and management of patients admitted with atrial fibrillation: a review of 291 cases in a regional hospital. *Int J Cardiol* 1995; **48:** 271–8.

Lowenstein SR, Gabow PA, Cramer J et al. The role of alcohol in new-onset atrial fibrillation. *Arch Intern Med* 1983, **113:** 1882–5.

Mahoney P, Kimmel S, DeNofrio D et al. Prognostic significance of atrial fibrillation in patients at a tertiary medical center referred for heart transplantation because of severe heart failure. *Am J Cardiol* 1999; **83:** 1544–7.

Middlekauff HR, Stevenson WG, Stevenson LW. Prognostic significance of atrial fibrillation in advanced heart failure: a study of 390 patients. *Circulation* 1991; **84:** 40.

Murgatroyd FD, Camm AJ. Atrial arrhythmias. *Lancet* 1993; **341:** 1317–22.

Robinson K, Frenneaux MP, Stockins B et al. Atrial fibrillation in hypertrophic cardiomyopathy: a longitudinal study. *J Am Coll Cardiol* 1990; **15:** 1279.

Sakata K, Kurihara H, Iwamori K et al. Clinical and prognostic significance of atrial fibrillation in acute myocardial infarction. *Am J Cardiol* 1997; **80:** 1522–7.

Sawin CT, Geller A, Wolf PA et al. Low serum thyrotropin concentrations as a risk factor for atrial fibrillation in older persons. *N Engl J Med* 1994; **331:** 1249.

Stroke Prevention in Atrial Fibrillation Investigators. Predictors of thromboembolism in atrial fibrillation: I. Clinical features of patients at risk. *Ann Intern Med* 1992a; **116:** 1–5.

Stroke Prevention in Atrial Fibrillation Investigators. Predictors of thromboembolism in atrial fibrillation: II. Echocardiographic features of patients at risk. *Ann Intern Med* 1992b; **116:** 6–12.

Sugiura T, Iwasaka T, Ogawa A et al. Atrial fibrillation in acute myocardial infarction. *Am J Cardiol* 1985; **56:** 27.

Thornton JR. Atrial fibrillation in healthy non-alcoholic people after an alcoholic binge. *Lancet* 1984; **2:** 1013–5.

Tikoff G, Schmidt AM, Hecht HH. Atrial fibrillation in atrial septal defect. *Arch Intern Med* 1968; **121:** 402.

Weber DM, Phillips JH. A reevaluation of electrocardiographic changes accompanying acute pulmonary embolism. *Am J Med Sci* 1966; **251:** 381.

Zarifis J, Beevers DG, Lip GYH. Acute admissions with atrial fibrillation in a British multiracial hospital population. *Br J Clin Pract* 1997; **51:** 91–6.

5

Atrial fibrillation and surgery

Introduction

Atrial fibrillation (AF) is common after surgery, especially cardiothoracic operations. Overall, the presence of the AF after cardiac surgery not only results in prolongation of hospital stay but also increases risk of heart failure, stroke, or thromboembolism, and brings significant increases in hospital costs.

For example, the prevalence of supraventricular arrhythmias, predominantly AF, is between 17%–33% of patients who undergo coronary artery bypass graft surgery (CABG), and particularly after valvular heart surgery (Leitch et al, 1990; Polanczyk et al, 1998; Crosby et al, 1990). In the recent study by Almassi and colleagues (1997), the incidence of postoperative AF was 29.6%, with morbidity, hospital mortality, and 6-month mortality being significantly higher in the AF patients. Indeed, if AF occurs, the length of stay in hospital after CABG surgery can be extended by about 3 days, with additional costs of thousands of UK pounds per patient. AF can also occur after cardiac transplantation, commonly in the absence of significant rejection, but the occurrence of AF is associated with an increased risk of subsequent death (Pavri et al, 1995).

The size of the problem

Many studies consistently show the problem of AF and other supraventricular arrhythmias in relation to both cardiac and non-cardiac surgery. There is generally a wide range of incidence figures for surgery-related AF between different studies. One reason for this difference may be a reflection of the criteria for arrhythmia definition, when and where monitoring is done, and the intensity and duration of monitoring. Many series also group AF with atrial flutter and other supraventricular arrhythmias.

For example, one prospective series of 295 patients undergoing thoracic surgery for non-cardiac disease (mainly lung cancer) showed that 13% developed AF after surgery (Neilson et al, 1973). In a prospective cohort of 916 patients aged over 40 years who underwent major non-cardiac surgery, only 4% developed supraventricular arrrhythmias (mainly AF) after surgery (Goldman, 1978). Johnston (1989) reported a multicentre prospective study of patients undergoing non-ruptured abdominal aortic aneurysm repair and showed a 3.2% incidence rate of supraventricular arrhythmias.

Nevertheless, AF is particularly common after cardiothoracic surgery, especially mitral valve surgery. For example, one recent analysis of a cohort of 915 consecutive adult patients undergoing isolated valvular heart surgery with preoperative sinus rhythm showed that the incidence of postoperative AF

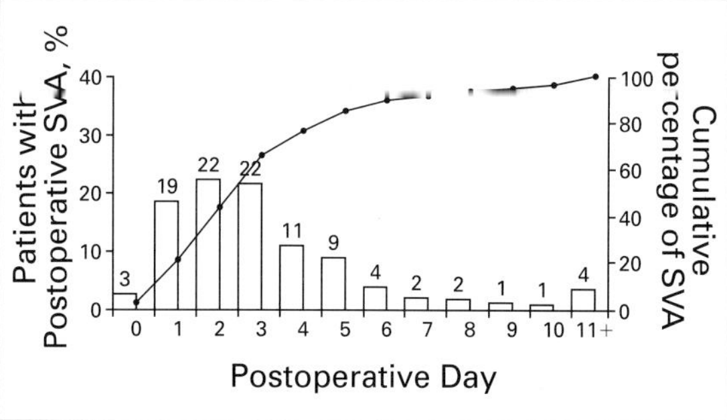

Figure 5.1
Distribution of supraventricular arrhythmias (SVA) according to the time of first occurrence among the 256 patients who developed arrhythmias after surgery. Reproduced with permission from Polanczyk et al (1998).

was 36.7% (Asher et al, 1998). In a review of data from 16 randomised prophylactic trials between 1974 and 1984, supraventricular arrhythmias after CABG occurred in between 11.4% and 100% of cases (mean 33%), (Vecht et al, 1986). However, AF after cardiac surgery for valvular heart disease occurs at rates that far exceed that of isolated CABG. In the study by Cresell and colleagues (1993) of 3983 patients undergoing cardiac surgery, atrial arrhythmias occurred in 31.9% of patients after CABG alone, 48.4% after CABG with aortic valve replacement, and 63.6% after CABG and mitral valve replacement.

After cardiac surgery, AF onset appears to peak on day 2 (Figure 5.1). For example, one analysis of 1166 patients after CABG showed a 4.7% incidence of supraventricular arrhythmias on the day of surgery, with a peak incidence of 43.1% on day 2, but decreasing to 0.4% at 9 or more days after surgery (Fuller et al, 1989). This peak of onset may reflect postoperative factors such as ischaemia and inotrope use, but (as discussed further below) the picture is likely to be more complex than this.

Pathogenesis

A wide variety of predisposing factors during surgery can lead to the development of AF, as summarised in table 5.1. These can include hypoxia or atrial ischaemic with cardioplegia during bypass, atrial trauma due to cannulation, atrial hypertension or infarction, acute atrial enlargement secondary to raised intra-atrial pressure, age-dependant atrial atrophic changes, and other electrophysiological properties. Electrolyte abnormalities such as hypomagnesaemia and hypokalaemia, inflammation due to pericarditis, and the withdrawal of preoperative beta-blockers may also predispose to postoperative development of AF.

Very commonly, multiple factors confound for one another. In the study by Asher and colleagues (1998), independent predictors of postoperative AF included the following: advanced age (odds ratio [OR] 1.51 per decade [95% CI 1.35–1.68); mitral stenosis (2.07 [1.21–3.52]); left atrial enlargement (1.47 [1.07–2.01]); use of systemic hypothermia (0.57 [0.42–0.78]); and a history of cardiac surgery (0.68 [0.47–0.98]). In a cohort of 189 patients who had undergone successful mitral valve reconstruction, predictors for recurrent AF were preoperative AF ($p = 0.0001$), preoperative antiarrhythmic drug treatment ($p = 0.005$), heart rate ($p = 0.01$), left ventricular ejection fraction ($p = 0.01$) and increased left ventricular posterior wall thickness ($p = 0.05$; Vogt et al, 1998). Older patients with a history of AF, antiarrhythmic treatment, or raised pulmonary artery pressure may also present with AF late after successful mitral valve repair. In a cohort of 436 patients undergoing isolated CABG surgery, in whom 23% developed AF (Borzack et al, 1998), AF patients were usually older and more likely to have obstructive lung dis-

	Risk of developing AF
Preoperative factors	
Older age	4
Valvular heart disease	3
Surface P-wave duration on ECG	2
Preoperative digoxin use	1
Preoperative beta-blocker use	1
Chronic obstructive lung disease	1
Right coronary artery stenosis	1
Intraoperative factors	
Internal mammary artery graft	2
Hypomagnesaemia	2
Type of cardioplegia	1
Prolonged aortic cross-clamp and bypass time	1
Matters of cannulation	1
Postoperative factors	
Postoperative beta-blocker usage (protective)	4
Postoperative beta-blocker withdrawal	1
Pericarditis or pericardia infusion	1

Key: 1 = some uncertainty; 2 = some evidence; 3 = moderate evidence; 4 = strong evidence.

Table 5.1
Risk factors for development of AF after cardiothoracic surgery.

ease than patients without AF; however, patients with and without AF had similar left ventricular function and extent of coronary disease. As expected, intensive care unit and hospital stays were longer in patients with AF. Borzack and colleagues (1998) suggest that although AF is strongly associated with advanced age, most of the prolonged hospital stay appears to be attributable to the rhythm itself and not to patients' characteristics. Thus, the development of AF leads to complications (such as heart failure) that need to be dealt with, the consideration of rate control or cardioversion, and anticoagulation therapy.

Some patients may be intrinsically vulnerable to development of postoperative AF. For example, there is a consistent association between advancing age and the development of postoperative AF. Suppression of sinoatrial node responsiveness after cessation of cardiopulmonary bypass has also been noted in patients who subsequently develop postoperative AF, which is independent of preoperative beta-blocker usage. Postoperative atrial distension, ischaemia, or infarction, or more direct cardiac injury related to surgery, added to pre-existing atrophic changes related to age, or perhaps some perioperative inflammation, can significantly affect atrial electrophysiological properties or conduction. These factors may serve to enhance vulnerability or serve as triggers for the development of postoperative AF.

Interestingly, the use of internal mammary artery conduits may increase the risk of postoperative AF. For example, the study by Salem and colleagues (1991) showed that in 80 patients, 31% of those receiving internal mammary artery grafts in addition to vein graphs developed postoperative AF, compared with 24% of those who received vein grafts alone.

Postoperative electrolyte abnormalities may contribute to the development of AF. For example, hypomagnesaemic patients are more likely to develop postoperative supraventricular cardiac arrhythmias in the intensive care unit, compared with those with normal magnesium levels (England et al, 1992). The recent report by Wahr and colleagues (1999) found that serum potassium level of less than 3.5 mmol/L was a predictor of serious perioperative arrhythmia (2.2 [95% CI 1.2–4.0]), intraoperative arrhythmia ([1.0–3.6]), and postoperative AF/flutter (1.7 [1.0–2.7]). Thus, perioperative arrhythmia (including AF) increased with electrolyte abnormalities, although the value of electrolyte supplementation or repletion in patients scheduled for cardiac surgery is still uncertain.

Although circulating catecholamines in the postoperative period are raised, no consistent correlations with the development of postoperative AF have been shown. Engleman and colleagues (1983) showed increased serum catecholamines in the early postoperative period after coronary bypass and valve procedures, but found no consistent relation with the development of AF, and, importantly, no significant protection from beta-blocker use. Nevertheless, discontinuation of preoperative beta-blocker usage after cardiac surgery may be a possible mechanism in pathogenesis of supraventricular arrhythmias after surgery, in keeping with a beta-blocker withdrawal phenomenon. In view of the possible involvement of the adrenergic system in the pathogenesis of AF, a change in guanine nucleotide-binding protein (G protein) expression has been postulated to play a part in the development of post-CABG AF (Tittelbach et al, 1999) — an increase of the G(s alpha)/G(i alpha) ratio in mononuclear leukocytes appears to be associated with the development of AF after CABG surgery.

Since postoperative AF is most common 2–3 days after surgery, one hypothesis is that an inflammatory mechanism may be implicated in its pathogenesis. Indeed, the presence of pericardial effusion after cardiac surgery (perhaps indicating pericarditis) appears to be a strong risk factor for the development of AF. Angelini and colleagues (1987) reported on a series of 114 patients after CABG and valve surgery who underwent echocardiography within 3–5 days after surgery. The patients with pericardial effusions had a significant increase in incidence of supraventricular arrhythmias compared with those who did not develop pericardial effusions (63% *vs* 11%).

Management

Although postoperative AF is usually transient and generally self-limiting, some patients have significant associated morbidity, such as haemodynamic compromise, heart failure, and thromboembolism, which would justify intervention. In particular, those patients who are actually haemodynamically unstable, or who develop cardiac ischaemia or heart failure consequent upon the fast irregular ventricular response, should undergo cardioversion to sinus rhythm with a 200 joule synchronised DC shock. Atrial overdrive pacing can perhaps be attempted if atrial flutter is the dominant rhythm, using temporary epicardial pacing leads.

In less-urgent situations, however, control of the ventricular rate may be more appropriate. The use of digoxin alone for rate control in the postoperative patient is often inadequate, due to the high postoperative catecholamine load. Nevertheless, beta-blockers and calcium antagonists may be effectively used. In a recent randomised comparison of intravenous diltiazem and digoxin for ventricular rate control in AF after CABG surgery, ventricular rate control was achieved more rapidly with intravenous diltiazem than digoxin (75% *vs* 35%, at 2 h), although 12-h and 24-h response rates, cardioversion rates (55% *vs* 65% at 24 h), and duration of postoperative hospital stay associated with the two drugs were similar (Tisdale et al, 1998). Another option is the use of short acting intravenous agents such as esmolol, which has a short half-life and short duration of action if the infusion is discontinued. In one recent trial, patients with postoperative supraventricular arrhythmias (mainly AF) who were randomized to receive esmolol were converted to sinus rhythm within 2 h of treatment in 59% of cases, compared with only 33% of patients randomised to receive diltiazem, although ventricular rates were similarly controlled in the two treatment groups (Balser et al, 1998).

In patients with persistent stable AF, chemical or electrical cardioversion can eventually be attempted. One recent report suggests that atrial defibrillation with temporary epicardial wire electrodes can be done safely and effectively, with low shock energy and often without anaesthesia in patients after cardiac operations (Liebold et al, 1998). Nevertheless, the recurrence rates of postoperative AF after conversion to sinus rhythm despite maintenance of antiarrhythmic agents have not been well established. The need for continuation of anticoagulation after DC cardioversion in the postoperative period has also not been firmly established, although current guidelines suggest that anticoagulation for at least 4 weeks after cardioversion would reduce stroke and thromboembolic events after cardioversion.

Prophylaxis

A great variety of pharmacological agents has been tested as prophylaxis against the development of postoperative AF. These agents have included digoxin, beta-blockers, and calcium antagonists, as well as other antiarrhythmic agents. Studies have assessed the role of pacing to prevent post-operative AF. Nevertheless, one recent study of post-CABG pacing found that it did not prevent AF, although there was a trend toward less AF in the paced groups treated with beta-blockade (Gerstenfeld et al, 1999). Similarly, a recent prospective randomized study to test the effect of biatrial synchronous pacing via epicardial electrodes on the incidence of AF after heart surgery compared with conventional therapy was prematurely aborted because postoperative deterioration of atrial sensing and its profibrillatory effect that resulted in a higher incidence of AF (Kurz et al, 1999).

In general, there appears to be little benefit of using digoxin in the prevention of supraventricular arrhythmia after CABG. This is based on relatively small studies, some of which have been non-randomised or conducted as open-label studies. Some of the trials of digoxin (and other antiarrhythmic agents) have been confounded by preoperative or postoperative use of beta-blockers and other antiarrhythmic agents. As will be discussed in later chapters, digoxin is ineffective for the cardioversion of AF and the maintenance of sinus rhythm after cardioversion, and may even make paroxysmal AF worse.

Based on two meta-analyses of prophylactic pharmacological agents in preventing post-CABG AF, beta-blockers are probably the most useful agents in preventing AF after surgery. For example, the overview by Kowey and colleagues (1992) of 2482 postoperative patients treated prophylactically with beta-blockers (seven trials), digoxin (five trials) and combination therapy with digoxin and beta-blockers (two trials) to prevent supraventricular arrhythmia early after coronary artery bypass grafting showed that beta-blockers alone reduced supraventricular arrhythmias from 20.2% in the controls to 9.8% in those taking beta-blockers ($p < 0.001$). The combination of beta-blockers and digoxin was more impressive (albeit with fewer patients and only two trials), with a reduction from 29.4% to 2.2% ($p < 0.001$). One reason for the possible synergy between digoxin and beta-blockers may be the vagomimetic effect of digoxin and the suppression of catecholamine excess with the beta-blockers.

The second meta-analyses by Andrews and colleagues (1991) of 22 randomised controlled trials (18 beta-blocker, five digoxin, three verapamil) similarly concluded that beta-blocker prophylaxis was effective for the prevention of supraventricular arrhythmias after coronary artery bypass surgery, irrespective of the type of agent used, the time of initiation, or the dose; there was an impressive reduction of supraventricular arrhythmias from 34.0% in controls to 8.7% in treated patients ($p < 0.0001$). In both meta-analyses, it was clear that digoxin alone and verapamil monotherapy did not provide adequate prophylaxis against supraventricular arrhythmias after CABG surgery.

Nevertheless, many clinicians still favour verapamil or diltiazem — even if it does not usually prevent AF after CABG. When AF does occur, the ventricular rate tends to be slower in the treated patients. Furthermore, in one study, intravenous diltiazem started intraoperatively and continued for 24 h reduced postoperative AF from 21 to 2%, but in that report the main effect of diltiazem may have been related to beneficial effects on cardiac ischaemia, as reduced ST segmental changes, myocardial infarction and maximal creatinine kinase release was seen in the diltiazem-treated patients (Seitlberger et al, 1992).

The use of sotalol, a class III antiarrhythmic agent, is also effective in reducing postoperative supraventricular arrhythmias, with no excess proarrhythmia. For example, the study by Nystrom and colleagues (1993), which randomised patients after coronary artery bypass surgery to sotalol 160 mg bd or controls (reduced dose or no beta-blocker), showed reduced AF in the sotalol group (29% *vs* 10%, $p = 0.028$). A selective approach — that is, treatment with sotalol of high-risk patients — only reduced the incidence of AF from 76% to 50% ($p = 0.0295$) compared with a reduction from 44% to 26% ($p = 0.0065$) when all patients were treated. More importantly, with the non-selective approach, all patients were exposed to the possible side-effects of sotalol and costs compared with 24% by the selective approach (Weber et al, 1998).

A few other studies have examined other antiarrhythmic agents with varying success. For example, Hohnloser and colleagues (1991) conducted a prospective placebo-controlled study using intravenous amiodarone in 77 patients post-CABG and reported a reduction in AF from 21% to 5%. A recent double-blind trial comparing oral amiodarone with placebo for the prevention of AF after CABG (Redle et al, 1999) showed a non-significant reduction (24.7% *vs* 32.8%) in average heart rates at onset of AF and shorter duration of AF with oral amiodarone. Nevertheless, Daoud et al (1997) did find some benefit from preoperative amiodarone on prophylaxis against AF after heart surgery (Figure 5.2).

Whilst there appears to be an increase in postoperative AF with hypomagnesaemia,

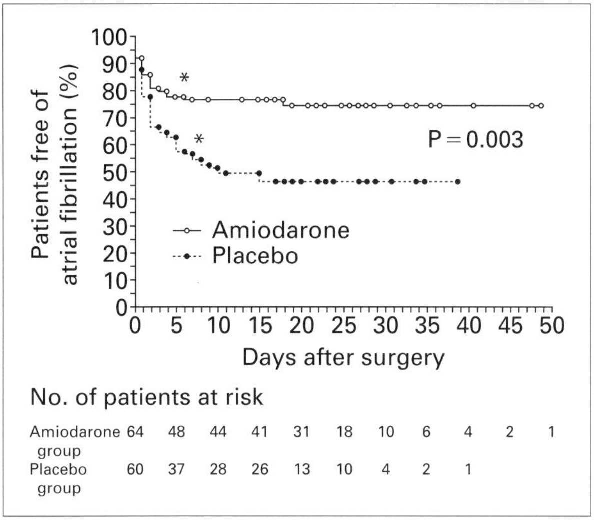

Figure 5.2
Kaplan-Meier analysis of the percentages of patients remaining free of atrial fibrillation after surgery in the amiodarone and placebo groups. The asterisks indicate the mean days of hospital discharge. Reproduced with permission from Daoud et al (1997).

studies on the efficacy of magnesium in the prevention of postoperative AF have been disappointing, showing rather inconsistent results. Apart from correction of electrolyte abnormalities (including hypomagnesaemia and hypokalaemia) there is no clearly defined role for the routine use of intravenous magnesium as prophylaxis against postoperative AF.

After mitral valve replacement or repair in some patients who had chronic AF preoperatively, it may be worthwhile attempting cardioversion to sinus rhythm. The main consideration appears to be the duration of previous AF and degree of structural heart disease. For example, the study by Flugelman and colleagues (1984) of 40 patients with pure mitral stenosis and chronic AF undergoing mitral valve replacement, who were cardioverted electrically and treated with quinidine or disopyramide, resulted in 60% of patients remaining in sinus rhythm for more than 3 months after cardioversion. Nevertheless, in patients with a preoperative left atrial size greater than 5.2 cm and symptoms for more than 3 years, the likelihood of successful cardioversion may be too low to justify any attempt at cardioversion.

Prognosis of AF following surgery

AF developing in relation to surgery may be related to outcomes. For example, in one recent cohort of 462 consecutive patients after noncardiothoracic surgery, patients with new onset atrial arrhythmias (10.2%, mainly AF) had a higher mortality rate (23.4%), longer intensive care unit stay, and extended hospital stay compared with patients without atrial arrhythmias (Brathwaite et al, 1998). In this cohort, 13% of patients had a past history of atrial arrhythmias, and also had a higher mortality rate (8.6%) and longer intensive care unit stays than controls. Patients admitted to a surgical intensive care unit after noncardiothoracic surgery, who had a history of or who developed new atrial arrhythmias, also had greater mortality and longer intensive care unit stays than patients without arrhythmias. However, the atrial arrhythmias were not the primary cause of death, but appeared to be markers of increased mortality and morbidity.

The incidence of stroke or transient ischaemic attack (TIA) after CABG ranges from 1–3%, and the development of postoperative AF significantly adds to this risk. Several studies have clearly shown an association between postoperative AF and cerebrovascular events. For example, in a study by Taylor and colleagues (1987), stroke or TIA occurred in 2.2% of 453 patients undergoing CABG, usually in the first 10 days after surgery; importantly, stroke or TIA occurred in 7% of patients with post-operative AF compared with only 1% of patients without postoperative AF. In general, there is about a 4-fold increase in the risk of stroke or TIA for patients with a carotid bruit, and a 3-fold increase associated with postoperative AF after CABG (Reed et al, 1988).

Haemodynamic instability associated with postoperative AF is uncommon, but may have implications for morbidity and mortality from heart failure or shock. The severity of the haemodynamic disturbance depends on the ventricular rate, the ventricular function, duration of arrhythmia, and dependence on atrial contraction. For example, a patient with fast AF would be particularly compromised with fast ventricular rates, if poor left ventricular function was present and diastolic abnormalities (such as left ventricular hypertrophy) required greater contribution from atrial transport. Persisting fast AF can also lead to a tachycardia-mediated cardiomyopathy, and a prolonged duration in AF reduces the chances of successful cardioversion to sinus rhythm.

Finally, AF can affect the length of hospital stay, costs, and resource use after CABG. On average, the length of the hospital stay increases by 2–3 days in patients developing AF after CABG. In the study by Redle and colleagues (1999), the development of AF was associated with an increased cost of US $7011 compared with those who remained in sinus rhythm. A recent analysis of 570 CABG patients also showed that the adjusted length of stay attributable to AF was 4–9 days, at the cost of over US $19,000 in hospital charges (Aranki et al, 1996).

Solomon and colleagues (1998) recently assessed an early discharge scheme of patients with new-onset AF after cardiovascular surgery: patients discharged in AF tended to be older, with higher Parsonnet risk scores and an increased incidence of valvular heart surgery. These patients had a shorter length of hospital stay, and decreased hospital costs and hospital charges compared with patients with postoperative AF discharged in sinus rhythm. In the patients discharged in AF, no repeat hospital admission, bleeding complications, or thromboembolic events occurred. This was a small study, suggesting that further evaluation is needed.

References

Almassi GH, Schowalter T, Nicolosi AC et al. Atrial fibrillation after cardiac surgery: a major morbid event? *Ann Surg* 1997; **226:** 501–11; discussion 511–3.

Andrews TC, Raimold SC, Berlin JA, Antman EM. Prevention of supraventricular arrhythmias after coronary artery bypass surgery: a meta-analyses of randomised controlled trials. *Circulation* 1991; **84:**(suppl III): III236–III244.

Angelini GD, Penny WJ, El-Ghamary F et al. The incidence and significance of early pericardial infusion after open heart surgery. *Eur J Cardiothoracic Surg* 1987; **1:** 165–8.

Aranki SF, Shaw DP, Adams DH et al. Predictors of atrial fibrillation after coronary artery surgery; current trends impact on hospital resources. *Circulation* 1996; **94:** 390–7.

Asher CR, Miller DP, Grimm RA et al. Analysis of risk factors for development of atrial fibrillation early after cardiac valvular surgery. *Am J Cardiol* 1998; **82:** 892–5.

Balser JR, Martinez EA, Winters BD et al. Beta-adrenergic blockade accelerates conversion of postoperative supraventricular tachyarrhythmias. *Anesthesiology* 1998; **89:** 1052–9.

Borzak S, Tisdale JE, Amin NB et al. Atrial fibrillation after bypass surgery: does the arrhythmia or the characteristics of the patients prolong hospital stay? *Chest* 1998; **113:** 1489–91.

Brathwaite D, Weissman C. The new onset of atrial arrhythmias following major noncardiothoracic surgery is associated with increased mortality. *Chest* 1998; **114:** 462–8.

Cresell LL, Schuesseler RB, Rosenbloom M, Cox JL. Hazards of post-operative atrial arrhythmias. *Ann Thoracic Surg* 1993; **56:** 539–49.

Crosby LH, Pifalo WB, Woll KR, Borkholder JA. Risk factors for atrial fibrillation after coronary artery bypass grafting. *Am J Cardiol* 1990; **66:** 150–2.

Daoud EG, Strickberger SA, Ching Man A et al. Preoperative amiodarone as prophylaxis against atrial fibrillation after heart surgery. *New Engl J Med* 1997; **337:** 1785.

Engelman RM, Haag B, Lemshow S et al. Mechanism of plasma catecholamines increases during coronary artery bypass and valve procedures. *J Thoracic Cardiovas Surg* 1983; **86:** 608–15.

England MR, Gordon G, Falem M, Chernow B. Magnesium administration and dysrhythmias after cardiac surgery: placebo-controlled, double-blind randomised trial. *JAMA* 1992; **268:** 2395–402.

Flugelman MY, Hasin Y, Katznelson N et al. Restoration and maintenance of sinus rhythm after mitravalve surgery for mitrostenosis. *Am J Cardiology* 1984; **54:** 617–9.

Fuller JA, Adams GG, Buxton B. Atrial fibrillation after coronary artery bypass grafting. Is it a disorder of the elderly? *J Thoracic Cardiovas Surg* 1989; **97:** 821–5.

Gerstenfeld EP, Hill MR, French SN et al. Evaluation of right atrial and biatrial temporary pacing for the prevention of atrial fibrillation after coronary artery bypass surgery. *J Am Coll Cardiol* 1999; **33:** 1981–8.

Goldman L. Supra-ventricular tachyarrhythmias in hospitalised adults after surgery. *Chest* 1978; **73:** 450–4.

Hohnloser SH, Meinertz T, Dammbacher T et al. Electrocardiographic and anti-arrhythmic effects of intravenous amiodarone; results of a prospective, placebo-controlled study. *Am Heart J* 1991; **121:** 89–95.

Johnston KW. Multicentre prospective study of non-ruptured abdominal aortic aneurysm. *J Vasc Surg* 1989; **9:** 437–47.

Kowey PR, Taylor JE, Rials SJ, Marinchak RA. Meta-analyses of the effectiveness of prophylactic drug therapy in preventing supraventricular arrhythmia early after coronary artery bypass grafting. *Am J Cardiol* 1992; **69:** 863–5.

Kurz DJ, Naegeli B, Kunz M et al. Epicardial, biatrial synchronous pacing for prevention of atrial fibrillation after cardiac surgery. *Pacing Clin Electrophysiol* 1999; **22:** 721–6.

Liebold A, Wahba A, Birnbaum DE. Low-energy cardioversion with epicardial wire: new treatment of atrial fibrillation after open heart surgery. *Circulation* 1998; **98:** 883–6.

Leitch JW, Thompson D, Baird DK, Harris PJ. The importance of age as a predictor of atrial fibrillation and flutter after coronary artery bypass grafting. *J Thoracic Cardiovas Surg* 1990; **100:** 338–42.

Neilson JB, Sorensen HR, Arstrup P. Atrial fibrillation following thoracotomy for non-cardiac diseases in particular cancer of the lung. *Acta Med Scand* 1973; **193:** 425–9.

Nystrom U, Edverdsson N, Berggren H et al. Oral sotalol reduces incidence of atrial fibrillation after coronary artery bypass surgery. *Thoracic Cardiovasc Surg* 1993; **41:** 34–7.

Pavri BB, O'Nunain SS, Newell JB et al. Prevalence and prognostic significance of atrial arrhythmias after orthotopic cardiac transplantation. *J Am Coll Cardiol* 1995; **25:** 1673.

Polanczyk PA, Goldman L, Marcantonio ER et al. Supraventricular arrhythmia in patients having noncardiac surgery: clinical correlates and effect of length of stay. *Ann Int Med* 1998; **129:** 279–85.

Redle JD, Khurana S, Marzan R et al. Prophylactic oral amiodarone compared with placebo for prevention of atrial, fibrillation after coronary artery bypass surgery. *Am Heart J* 1999; **138:** 144–50.

Reed GL, Singer DE, Picard EH, Desanctis RW. Stroke following coronary artery bypass surgery. *N Engl J Med* 1988; **319:** 1426–50.

Salem DI, Choudhry A, Hikal M et al. Sustained supraventricular tachyarrhythmias following coronary artery bypass surgery comparing mammary versus saphenous vein graphs. *Angiology* 1991; 441–6.

Seitlberger R, Hannes W, Schindler M et al. Anti-ischaemic and anti-arrhythmic potency of diltiazem in aorta-coronary bypass grafting. *Eur Heart J* 1992; **13:** 158.

Solomon AJ, Kouretas PC, Hopkins RA et al. Early discharge of patients with new-onset atrial fibrillation after cardiovascular surgery. *Am Heart J* 1998; **135:** 557–63.

Taylor J, Malik SA, Colliver JA. Usefulness of atrial fibrillation as a predictor of stroke after isolated coronary artery bypass grafting. *Am J Cardiol* 1987; **60:** 905–7.

Tisdale JE, Padhi ID, Goldberg AD et al. A randomized, double-blind comparison of intravenous diltiazem and digoxin for atrial fibrillation after coronary artery bypass surgery. *Am Heart J* 1998; **135:** 739–47.

Tittelbach V, Schwab M, Volff JN et al. Atrial fibrillation after coronary artery bypass surgery: association with changes in G protein levels in mononuclear leukocytes. *Naunyn Schmiedebergs Arch Pharmacol* 1999; **359:** 204–11.

Vecht RJ, Nicolaides EP, Ikweuke JK et al. Incidence and prevention of supra-ventricular tachyarrhythmias after coronary bypass surgery. *Int J Cardiol* 1986; **13:** 125–34.

Vogt PR, Brunner-LaRocca HP, Rist M et al. Preoperative predictors of recurrent atrial fibrillation late after successful mitral valve reconstruction. *Eur J Cardiothorac Surg* 1998; **13:** 619–24.

Wahr JA, Parks R, Boisvert D et al. Preoperative serum potassium levels and perioperative outcomes in cardiac surgery patients. Multicenter Study of Perioperative Ischemia Research Group. *JAMA* 1999; **281:** 2203–10.

Weber UK, Osswald S, Huber M et al. Selective versus non-selective antiarrhythmic approach for prevention of atrial fibrillation after coronary surgery: is there a need for pre-operative risk stratification? A prospective placebo-controlled study using low-dose sotalol. *Eur Heart J* 1998; **19:** 794–800.

6

Lone atrial fibrillation

Introduction

"Lone" atrial fibrillation (AF) is defined as AF without "overt" structural heart disease, as defined by physical examination, ECG, chest radiography, and in more recent series, the echocardiogram (Table 6.1). There are implications of labelling patients with this diagnosis, as this group is often considered as being "at low risk", although recent data have been inconclusive. Indeed, it is still uncertain whether some or all patients with lone AF should receive prophylactic anticoagulation in an attempt to prevent stroke and thromboembolisation.

This is a diagnosis of exclusion, only if

- No history of cardiovascular disease or hypertension.
- No abnormal cardiac signs on physical examination.
- A normal CXR and ECG (apart from AF, with no evidence of prior MI or LVH).
- Atria, valves and left ventricular size (and function) are normal on echocardiography.

Table 6.1
Idiopathic or "lone" AF.

Epidemiology

Patients with lone AF are generally male, have few symptoms, are refractory to maintaining sinus rhythm, and generally have a good prognosis, particularly if they are under the age of 60 years.

The prevalence of lone AF varies according to the population studied and the definition applied (Table 6.2). For example, the Framingham study showed that 31% of patients with AF had "lone" AF, but many had a history of hypertension (Brand et al, 1985). One study from the Mayo Clinic found that 2.7% of patients with AF were under the age of 60 and had no apparent heart disease, hypertension, precipitating illness (Kopecky et al, 1987). Our survey of patients with known AF in two general practices in the west of Birmingham only found six cases of AF without any associated predisposing factor (Lip et al, 1997).

Since nearly 50% of patients with paroxysmal AF can be classed as "lone" AF, this will have implications for the epidemiology of lone AF, since many patients with paroxysmal AF are actually symptom-free, or they may be in sinus rhythm at the time of screening. Furthermore, as patients get older, associated comorbidity will intervene — when the dividing line between lone AF and "non-lone" AF changes those who are not lone AF is still uncertain.

Study, y	Average Age, y	Patient-Years Observation	Thromboembolic Events, %/y
Framingham Study†	70	327	2.6
Mayo Clinic	44	1440	0.4
E. Anglia, UK	55	540	0.2
Reykjavik	...	112	0.0

* Adapted from Kopecky et al (1987), Close et al (1979) Brand et al (1985) and Onundarson et al (1987)
† Included patients with hypertension and lone atrial fibrillation

Table 6.2
Lone atrial fibrillation.*

Natural history

Importantly, the incidence of stroke in young patients (age <60 years) with lone AF in the study by Kopecky and colleagues (1987) was only 1.3%, with a 94% probability of survival at 15 years. There was no difference in survival or in survival free of stroke among the patients with the three types of lone AF (that is, isolated, recurrent, and chronic). Thus, lone AF in patients under the age of 60 at diagnosis is associated with a very low risk of stroke, suggesting that routine anticoagulation may not be warranted.

However, the relatively benign prognosis in lone AF may not apply to older patients. The prospective study from the Framingham group assessed patients who were primarily (90%) over the age of 60, some of whom were also hypertensive, and showed a 4-fold to 5-fold increase in stroke compared with an age-matched and sex-matched control population (Brand et al, 1985). Nevertheless, 56% of patients were older than 70 years, and 32% had a history of hypertension. The subsequent report from Kopecky and colleagues (1999) concluded that lone AF occurring after age 60 years was a risk marker for a substantial increase in cardiovascular events that warrants consideration for antithrombotic therapy. The event rates (% per person-year) in patients with lone AF were 0.9% for stroke, 1.1% for transient cerebral ischaemia, and 2.6% for myocardial infarction, for a total cardiovascular event rate of 5.0% per person-year; corresponding rates for the age-matched and sex-matched control group were 0.2%, 0%, and 1.1%, for a total of 1.3% per person-year. The incidence of total cardiovascular events was significantly greater in those with lone AF, although there was no difference in survival. However, in those under the age of 60 years in whom hypertension was excluded there was a very low risk of stroke and an overall survival similar to that of an age-matched and sex-matched control population over a mean follow-up of about 17 years.

A recent analysis of 23 years' follow-up of 7746 middle-aged men from the Paris Prospective Study suggested that even idiopathic AF was an independent risk factor for cardiovascular mortality and total deaths (Jouven et al, 1999). A recent Italian study has provided further information on lone AF and age (Scardi et al, 1999). The risk of stroke in that study was low in persons under age 70 and higher in the more elderly, although still not different from age-matched controls. The older patients with lone AF had a higher incidence of sudden death, raising the issue that these individuals do have underlying heart disease. There appears to be some difference between paroxysmal and chronic lone AF, with the latter being associated with increased risk of thromboembolism and higher mortality after 10 years' follow-up.

Why does lone AF develop?

The precise reasons why patients develop lone AF are still uncertain. There is the possibility of misclassification, with some patients having symptom-free vascular disease or hypertension leading to AF.

Some patients may have a familial tendency to develop AF. Brugada and colleagues (1997) studied a family of 26 members, ten of whom had AF that segregated as an autosomal dominant disease; there were two additional families in which the disease was linked to the same locus, 10q22-q24. Identification of the gene for familial AF will help to elucidate the molecular basis of the disease and provide some insights into acquired forms and the complications of AF. For example, Carter and colleagues (1999) recently reported that the alpha-fibrinogen Thr312Ala gene polymorphism, which occurs close to several sites important for factor XIIIa-dependent cross-linking, may give rise to an increased susceptibility for thromboembolism of intra-atrial clot, and is associated with an increase in post-stroke mortality in patients with AF.

Whether this genetic tendency to develop AF (or its complications) is manifest by abnormalities in the electrophysiological or anatomical substrate is still uncertain. These findings could have important implications for identifying subjects most at risk of developing thromboembolic complications. Indeed, anatomical and electrophysiological abnormalities leading to the development and initiation of AF have been described (see chapter 7) in animal models and by limited clinical data. In particular, abnormalities in left atrial histology have been reported in patients with lone AF: one study of 12 patients with lone AF showed that all atrial biopsy specimens were abnormal, with pathological evidence of healed myocarditis, active myocarditis, patchy fibrosis, or a non-inflammatory localised cardiomyopathy (Frustaci et al, 1997).

Some patients with lone AF may have an underlying "sick sinus syndrome". Such patients have underlying electrophysiological abnormalities of the atrial myocardium, and it is possible that AF is related to an escape or end-stage arrhythmia consequent upon sinus node dysfunction (Tanigawa et al, 1991). Atrial pacing may help stabilise the atria electrically, and reduce or prevent paroxysms of AF. Abnormalities of autonomic tone may also precipitate paroxysms of AF (see chapter 13). Indeed, some differences in clinical electrophysiological properties have been identified between patients with recurrent episodes of lone paroxysmal AF and controls, some of which may be related to autonomic changes (Capucci et al, 1995; Padeletti et al, 1995).

Some patients with lone AF develop arrhythmia at night, whilst asleep. This suggests a possible role for enhanced vagal tone in individuals who are already predisposed to AF, because of abnormalities in electrophysiological properties of the atrial myocardium. In animal models, Geddes and colleagues (1996) suggested that vagal tone may be important, in which direct vagal stimulation, reflex vagal activation with the alpha agonist, phenylephrine, or increased vagal activity induced by an acetylcholinesterase inhibitor will prolong episodes of AF or result in sustained AF, perhaps due to shortening of the atrial refractory period. In the setting of myocardial ischaemia, reduction of vagal tone is also arrhythmogenic, related to calcium influx and uptake of calcium by the sarcoplasmic reticulum (Wang et al, 1997). This overload of cellular calcium can alter atrial electrophysiology and result in delayed afterdepolarisations that trigger atrial arrhythmias. Taking clinical history carefully may help to decide on appropriate drug therapy.

References

Brand FN Abbott RD, Kannel WB, Wolf PA. Characteristics and prognosis of lone atrial fibrillation: 30 year follow-up in the Framingham study. *JAMA* 1985; **254:** 3449.

Brugada R, Tapscott T, Czernuszewicz GZ et al. Identification of a genetic locus for familial atrial fibrillation. *N Engl J Med* 1997; **336:** 905–11.

Capucci A, Biffi M, Boriani G et al. Dynamic electrophysiological behavior of human atria during paroxysmal atrial fibrillation. *Circulation* 1995; **92:** 1193.

Carter AM, Catto AJ, Grant PJ. Association of the alpha-fibrinogen Thr312Ala polymorphism with poststroke mortality in subjects with atrial fibrillation. *Circulation* 1999; **99:** 2423–6.

Close JB, Evans DW, Bailey SM. Persistent lone atrial fibrillation: its prognosis after clinical diagnosis. *J R Coll Gen Pract* 1979; **29:** 547–9.

Frustaci A, Chimenti C, Bellocci F et al. Histologic substrate of atrial biopsies in patients with lone atrial fibrillation. *Circulation* 1997; **96:** 1180.

Geddes LA, Hinds M, Babbs CF et al. Maintenance of atrial fibrillation in anesthetized and unanesthetized sheep using cholinergic drive. *Pacing Clin Electrophysiol* 1996; **19:** 165.

Jouven X, Desnos M, Guerot C, Ducimetiere P. Idiopathic atrial fibrillation as a risk factor for mortality. The Paris Prospective Study I. *Eur Heart J* 1999; **20:** 896–9.

Kopecky SL, Gersh BJ, McGoon MD et al. The natural history of lone atrial fibrillation. A population-based study over three decades. *N Engl J Med* 1987 **317:** 669–74.

Kopecky SL, Gersh BJ, McGoon MD et al. Lone atrial fibrillation in elderly persons: a marker for cardiovascular risk. *Arch Intern Med* 1999; **159:** 1118–22.

Lip GYH, Golding DJ, Nazir M et al. A survey of atrial fibrillation in general practice: the West Birmingham Atrial Fibrillation Project. *Br J Gen Pract* 1997; **47:** 285–9.

Onundarson PT, Thorgeirsson G, Jonmundsson E et al. Chronic atrial fibrillation epidemiologic features and 14-year-follow-up. *Eur Heart J* 1987; **8:** 521–7.

Padeletti L, Michelucci A, Giovannini T et al. Wavelength index at three atrial sites in patients with paroxysmal atrial fibrillation. *Pacing Clin Electrophysiol* 1995; **18:** 1266.

Scardi S, Mazzone C, Pandullo C et al. Lone atrial fibrillation: prognostic differences between paroxysmal and chronic forms after 10 years of follow-up. *Am Heart J* 1999; **137:** 686–91.

Tanigawa M, Fukatani M, Konoe A et al. Prolonged and fractionated right atrial electrograms during sinus rhythm in patients with paroxysmal atrial fibrillation and sick sinus syndrome. *J Am Coll Cardiol* 1991; **17:** 403.

Wang YG, Huser J, Blatter LA et al. Withdrawal of acetylcholine elicits Ca^{2+}-induced delayed afterdepolarizations in cat atrial myocytes. *Circulation* 1997; **96:** 1275.

III
Pathophysiology

7

Pathophysiology of atrial fibrillation: haemodynamics, thromboembolic risk, hypercoagulability

Introduction

The pathogenesis of atrial fibrillation (AF) requires an interaction between electrophysiological processes and anatomical substrate. Details of electrophysiological mechanisms leading to AF are detailed in chapter 8, but AF can be related to several coexisting re-entrant wavefronts continuously sweeping around the atria, repeatedly encountering excitable myocardium. It is likely that the continued maintenance of AF, once initiated, is related to the depolarisation waveforms and the size of the atria, allowing a critical mass of anatomical substrate for AF to be sustained. This is supported by the observation that atrial hypertrophy and dilatation predispose to AF, and reduction of this substrate by electrophysiological or surgical procedures, such as the "maze" procedure and catheter ablation, can "cure" AF.

The left atrium

Left atrial enlargement is common in AF, but chronic AF itself can lead to a progressive left atrial dilatation (Sanfillipo et al, 1990). The latter has been shown to be reversible with cardioversion and long-term maintenance of sinus rhythm (Manning et al, 1989). Many disorders predisposing to AF also have effects on the left atrium, predisposing to AF. For example, mitral valve disease can lead to increased left atrial pressure and dilatation, coronary disease can result in atrial ischaemia or infarction, and hypertension can result in reduced left ventricular compliance and increased stiffness, leading to increased left atrial pressures.

Nevertheless, left atrial enlargement can be important prognostically in AF. For example, a dilated left atrium decreases the probability that long-term maintenance of sinus rhythm post-cardioversion will be successful (Hoglund et al, 1985). In the Framingham Heart Study, left atrial enlargement was shown to precede and predispose to AF (Benjamin et al, 1995). After multivariate adjustment, for every 10 mm increase in left atrial size, the relative risk of stroke was 2.4 in men (95% CI 1.6–3.7) and 1.4 in women (0.9–2.1); the relative risk of death was 1.3 in men (1.0–1.5) and 1.4 in women (1.1–1.7). Nevertheless, the relation of left atrial enlargement to stroke and death appears to be partially mediated by left ventricular mass.

The first Stroke Prevention in Atrial Fibrillation study reported that a left atrial size corrected for body surface area was an independent echocardiographic predictor for stroke, in which the risk increased with increasing atrial size (SPAF, 1992b). Left atrial dilatation is also related to increased spontaneous echocontrast and in turn, the risk of intra-atrial thrombus and stroke risk. In the study by Heppel and colleagues (1997), left atrial thrombus was related to reduced left atrial appendage flow velocities, which were in turn associated with haemostatic abnormalities and spontaneous echocontrast. However, the most recent meta-analysis of echocardiographic data from 3 trials suggested that isolated left atrial dilatation per se was not an independent risk factor on multivariate analysis, and only left ventricular systolic dysfunction on 2-dimensional echocardiography was an independent risk factor (AF Investigators, 1998).

Anatomical substrate

It is seldom possible to identify the underlying anatomical processes that cause AF. However, histological examination of atrial tissue of patients with AF have shown patchy fibrotic changes, perhaps contributing to the differences in atrial refractoriness or acting as excitable foci. These fibrotic changes may be a reaction to an inflammation or degenerative process; the latter may account for the increased incidence of AF in the elderly. The sino-atrial node may also be involved by fibrosis or fatty infiltration. It is therefore unsurprising that AF has been referred to as the "Alzheimer's disease" of the atria.

The remodelling of the structure of atrial myocardium in a goat model of sustained AF was investigated by Ausma and colleagues (1997), who reported that a substantial proportion of the atrial myocytes (up to 92%) revealed marked changes in their cellular substructures, such as loss of myofibrils, accumulation of glycogen, changes in mitochondria shape and size, fragmentation of sarcoplasmic reticulum, and dispersion of nuclear chromatin. These changes were accompanied by an increase in size of the myocytes (up to 195%). There were virtually no signs of cellular degeneration, and the interstitial space remained unaltered. The duration of sustained AF did not significantly affect the degree of myolytic cell changes. Thus, sustained AF in goats may lead to predominantly structural changes in the atrial myocytes similar to those seen in ventricular myocytes from chronic hibernating myocardium. These structural changes may explain the depressed contractile function of atrial myocardium after cardioversion. Morillo and colleagues (1995) reported an experimental dog model in which sustained AF was readily inducible in most dogs (82%) after rapid atrial pacing. Biatrial myopathy and marked changes in atrial vulnerability were consistently found, especially in one area at the posterior left atrium, suggesting that this area may be important in the maintenance of AF.

Frustaci and colleagues' (1997) investigation into the histological substrate of atrial biopsies in patients with lone AF revealed different patterns: two patients had a severe hypertrophy with vacuolar degeneration of the atrial myocytes and ultrastructural evidence of fibrillolysis occupying more than 50% of the areas assessed morphometrically; eight had lymphomononuclear infiltrates with necrosis of the adjacent myocytes; and two had only non-specific patchy fibrosis. However, abnormal atrial histology was uniformly found in multiple biopsy specimens in all patients with (lone) AF in that study, perhaps compatible with a diagnosis of myocarditis in 66% of patients and a non-inflammatory localised cardiomyopathy.

Pathophysiology

The clinical manifestations of AF can broadly be related to the loss of atrial systolic function and the presence of an irregular, fast ventricular response. These lead to the main sequelae of AF, that is, the haemodynamic and thromboembolism effects.

Loss of atrial systole

The loss of atrial systolic function has two main results: firstly, impaired haemodynamic function of the heart, and secondly, intra-atrial stasis and thrombogenesis. The presence of AF is associated with a fall in overall stroke volume compared with sinus rhythm (Figure 7.1). This fall in stroke volume varies from about 10% in normal individuals (although there is a greater fall at fast ventricular rates) to over a third in the elderly. The contribution of atrial systolic function ("atrial kick") is particularly important with increasing age, due to progressive impairment of left ventricular contraction and/or diastolic dysfunction associated with left ventricular hypertrophy. Even several minutes of AF may be sufficient to induce atrial contractile dysfunction after cardioversion, suggesting that calcium loading during AF may be at least partially responsible for AF-induced electrical remodelling (Daoud et al, 1997; 1999).

Loss of atrial systolic function also results in increased stasis within the left atrium, leading to intra-atrial thrombus formation and an increased risk of stroke and thromboembolism. This is illustrated by the phenomenon of spontaneous echocontrast, which is commonly present within the left atrial cavity in patients with AF on transoesophageal echocardiography, especially if thrombus is present. Spontaneous echocontrast has also been documented during paroxysms of AF in patients with known paroxysmal AF (Obarski et al, 1990). Furthermore, stasis within the left atrium has been closely related to haemostatic abnormalities, with abnormalities of coagulation factors, endothelial function, and platelet

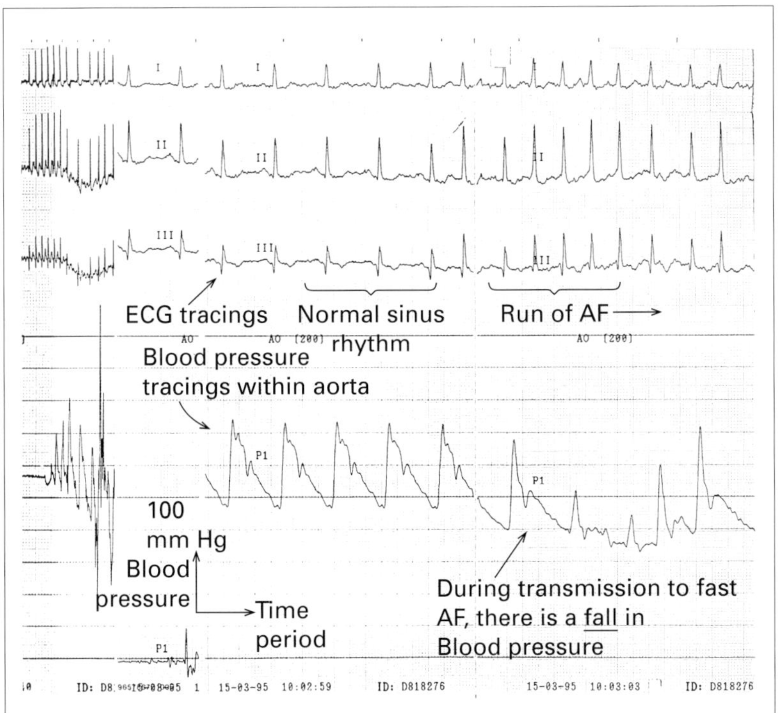

Figure 7.1
Tracing during cardiac catheterisation, showing fall in aortic blood pressure by transition from sinus rhythm to fast AF.

function suggestive of hypercoagulable factors, endothelial function, and platelet function suggestive of hypercoagulable state (Lip 1995; Lip 1997). Atrial natriuretic peptide levels are also increased in patients with AF, which may be contributable to haemoconcentration and an increased risk of thrombus formation (Peterson et al, 1988).

Irregular and uncontrolled ventricular response

The irregular and uncontrolled ventricular response in AF can result in an overall reduction in cardiac efficacy, with a consequent loss of cardiac output. A fast, uncontrolled heart rate in AF can lead to ultra-structural and microscopic changes within the myocardium, resulting in progressive left ventricular dilatation and reduction of left ventricular systolic function, now referred to as a "tachycardia-induced cardiomyopathy" (Spinale et al, 1991; Gallagher et al, 1997). The precise mechanisms for tachycardiomyopathy are uncertain, but the irregularity is judged to be a factor, since this problem is not seen in patients with fast, uncontrolled atrial flutter, where some coordinated electrical atrial activity remains. A rapid heart rate also reduces the diastolic filling interval, and the additional loss of the sequential atrio-ventricular contraction mechanism in AF leads to a dramatic reduction in stroke volume and other haemodynamic consequences.

These observations are supported by evidence of a significantly improved cardiac output and exercise capacity after cardioversion of AF to sinus rhythm (Van Gelder et al, 1993). Patients also feel easily tired and have lower quality-of-life scores, which are corrected by cardioversion to sinus rhythm. In addition, some patients commonly present with symptoms after their rhythm change from sinus rhythm to AF, as the irregularity of the heart rate seems to play an important part in the genesis of symptoms and the clinical manifestations.

Haemodynamic aspects

AF and heart failure

The adverse haemodynamic effects of AF are primarily manifest as symptoms of reduced exercise tolerance and exertional dyspnoea. It is therefore not surprising that AF is related to heart failure in 20–50% of case series. In some cases, AF precipitates heart failure, but there is evidence that heart failure may also lead to AF. Cardioversion from AF to sinus rhythm results in improved exercise capacity and left ventricular ejection fraction (see chapter 14). Furthermore, the presence of heart failure adds to the stroke and thromboembolic risks associated with AF (AF Investigators, 1994).

AF may lead to heart failure by loss of atrial transport, but in fast, uncontrolled heart rates, a "tachycardia-induced cardiomyopathy" may occur (Gallagher et al, 1997). The increased intra-cardiac pressures in congestive heart failure or post-myocardial infarction may lead to atrial stretch and dilatation, predisposing to AF. In patients after-myocardial infarction, the new development of AF is related to significant underlying cardiac dysfunction, and is a poor prognostic sign. If diastolic dysfunction is present, for example in left ventricular hypertrophy or hypertrophic cardiomyopathy, a change in rhythm from sinus rhythm to AF, with loss of atrial "kick" may also precipitate heart failure.

Thrombogenesis and AF

Clinical risk factors

The basic pathophysiological mechanism for thrombus formation and embolism appears to be abnormalities in blood flow within the fibrillating (and possibly dilated) left atrium, which predisposes to thrombus formation and arterial embolism, especially in the presence of underlying heart disease. The presence of the latter, including valvular heart disease, hypertensive heart disease, a dilated left atrium, and poor left ventricular function, is a significant risk factor for stroke and thromboembolism in patients with atrial fibrillation (SPAF 1992a; SPAF 1992b; Cabin et al, 1990).

For example, the thromboembolic risk of AF is 18 times greater if rheumatic heart disease is present (Cairns and Connolly, 1991). In analyses of clinical and echocardiographic data from the Stroke Prevention in Atrial Fibrillation (SPAF) study, the presence of recent (within 3 months) congestive heart failure and left ventricular dysfunction also contributes to an increased risk of stroke in AF (SPAF 1992a; SPAF 1992b). The presence of left ventricular hypertrophy secondary to hypertension is another important risk factor for stroke, and AF may add to this risk.

The importance of congestive heart failure in thromboembolic risk has long been recognised, since thromboembolism is a common cause of death in patients with congestive heart failure. Death occurs in nearly a third of patients, but this figure is partly reduced by prophylactic anticoagulation (Griffith et al, 1952). Despite this, anticoagulant prophylaxis has not been widely used in patients with heart failure or echocardiographic left ventricular dysfunction.

A previous history of stroke, transient ischaemic attack, or other thromboembolic episodes substantially adds to the risk of stroke in AF (relative risk 2.5, AF Investigators, 1994). Hypertension and diabetes are risk factors for stroke, and the presence of these disorders also increases (by nearly 2-fold) the risk of stroke and thromboembolism in AF.

Anatomical aspects — the left atrium

Morphological changes in the left atrial endocardium, predisposing to thromboembolism, have been investigated in 21 cases with AF, in which "rough endocardium" due to a granular and wrinkled appearance of the endocardium associated with oedematous and fibrous thickening was seen (Masawa et al, 1993). Mural thrombi and oedema with neutrophil infiltration in the subendocardium could be seen on microscopy, and small areas of endothelial denudation and thrombotic aggregations were commonly observed by scanning electron microscopy (SEM).

An increased left atrial size in patients with AF contributes to an increased risk of intra-atrial thrombi formation and thromboembolism. Although previous evidence had suggested that left atrial enlargement was the cause rather than a consequence of AF, recent studies have suggested the converse — that left atrial enlargement may be consequent upon the duration of AF (Takahashi et al, 1982; Sanfilippo et al, 1990; Sosa-Suarez et al, 1989; Petersen et al, 1987). This is relevant since the risk of thromboembolism increases with the duration of AF (Cabin et al, 1990; Caplan et al, 1986).

A left atrial size of 4.0 cm or more has also been previously identified as the single strongest predictor of increased risk for thromboembolisation (Cabin et al, 1990), but atrial dilatation rarely occurs in isolation without the presence of associated clinical risk factors such as hypertension. Thus in the most recent analysis from the AF Investigators, isolated left atrial dilatation was not predictive of stroke and thromboembolism on multivariate analysis (AF Investigators, 1998). Nevertheless, patients with lone AF (that is, those who have no underlying cause for their arrhythmia) have a low risk of stroke and usually have an atrial size of less than 4.0 cm (Davidson et al, 1989). Left atrial enlargement has also been associated with the presence of "spontaneous echocontrast" on transoesophageal echocardiography. This refers to the presence of a smoke-like appearance of blood within the enlarged atrial cavity, suggesting stasis of intra-atrial blood flow, which causes erythrocyte and platelet aggregation, and thrombus formation (Daniel et al, 1988). The rheological mechanism for spontaneous echocontrast is thought to involve plasma fibrinogen and aggregates of platelets and erythrocytes (Sigel et al, 1981). By contrast, the absence of spontaneous echocontrast has been associated with a low thromboembolic risk. Early cardioversion has been done in such patients without oral anticoagulant therapy, with no excess in embolic events (Manning et al, 1993) (see chapter 14).

Mechanical aspects

The loss of atrial systolic function results in a reduction in stroke volume, leading to a corresponding reduction in cardiac output and increased atrial stasis. The latter results in increased propensity to thrombus formation. Thrombus usually forms within the left atrial appendage, and this has been associated with stasis within this structure, as illustrated by abnormal doppler profiles (Heppell et al, 1997). The prevalence of left atrial appendage thrombus has been reported as high as 15% using transoesophageal echocardiography (TOE), in patients admitted with acute AF (Stoddard et al, 1995).

In patients with paroxysmal AF, there appears to be a cluster of thromboembolic events during transition from AF to sinus rhythm, perhaps reflecting embolisation of pre-formed clot. Indeed, after cardioversion from AF to sinus rhythm, there is risk of thromboembolism of about 7% if anticoagulation is not used, with the highest risk within the first week after cardioversion. This increased risk may again reflect mechanical reasons leading to embolisation of pre-formed thrombus), but it is more likely that it is related to post-cardioversion atrial dysfunction ("stunning") and the delay in return of atrial systolic function, which can be up to 3 weeks after cardioversion (Manning et al, 1994). The latter varies according to the duration of prior AF. Atrial "stunning" post-cardioversion is related to the reorganisation of electrical activity, resulting in increased intra-atrial stasis and echocontrast.

Mitral valve function can influence the pathophysiology of AF, especially in relation to thrombogenesis. For example, moderate to severe mitral regurgitation appears to protect against clinical thromboembolism in chronic AF and intracardiac thrombus, presumably by reduction of stasis in the left atrium and atrial appendage by a "stirring" effect (Beppu et al, 1985; Tsai et al, 1992; Black et al, 1991; Chen et al, 1990). Nevertheless, irrespective of the presence of mitral regurgitation, a patient with a grossly enlarged left atrium and poor left ventricular function will still have an increased risk of thrombogenesis. By contrast, mitral regurgitation does not appear to be protective against thrombus formation in patients with new onset AF. AF occurs in the late stages in patients with aortic stenosis, especially if heart failure is present, and is generally poorly tolerated.

Whilst most of the factors leading to thrombus formation are known, those leading to actual embolism are uncertain. In the Copenhagen study, stroke and thromboembolism was more common soon after the transition from paroxysmal AF to chronic AF (Petersen and Godtfredsen, 1986; Godtfredsen, MD thesis, 1975). Anticoagulation before cardioversion would allow endothelisation of pre-existing thrombi or dissolution by the body's pre-existing fibrinolytic systems; the precise time needed for this is uncertain, but is judged to require 3 weeks.

Duration of AF

The duration and onset of AF may also be of importance. The onset of AF may be temporally related to the occurrence of stroke. In the Framingham study, for example, AF was present at the time of stroke onset in 24% of patients, and about a third of the strokes associated with AF occurred within 6 months of onset of the arrhythmia (Wolf et al, 1983). In addition, stroke recurrence in the first 6 months after the initial event was more common in patients with chronic AF (47% compared with 20% in non-AF group). However, this finding was not confirmed in the Oxfordshire study.

AF and hypercoagulability

For over 150 years it has been well recognised that abnormalities in the blood vessel wall, blood flow, and blood constituents may result in an increased propensity towards thrombus formation (Virchow's triad). Clinical and echocardiographic criteria may help identify the first two of Virchow's basic postulates for thrombogenesis — namely, abnormalities of blood flow and vessels, for example, valvular heart disease and cardiac impairment. As discussed above, both valve disease and cardiac impairment increase the risk of stroke in AF.

Kumagai and colleagues (1990) described a cross-sectional study of 73 patients with chronic AF in whom increased fibrin D-dimer levels (an index of fibrin turnover and thrombogenesis) were found compared with controls in sinus rhythm. This finding seemed to be irrespective of the presence of underlying structural heart disease. A similar cross-sectional study of patients with AF by Yamauchi and colleagues (1986) showed increased levels of beta-thromboglobulin and platelet factor 4, which were markers of platelet activation. A Swedish study by Gustafsson and colleagues (1990) compared 20 stroke patients who had non-valvular AF, 20 patients who had non-valvular AF without stroke, 20 stroke patients in sinus rhythm, and 40 healthy controls, and found that both groups of patients with AF had abnormal elevations in plasma haemostatic markers such as fibrinogen, fibrin D-dimer, beta-thromboglobulin, von Willebrand factor and platelet factor IV which were confirmed by Lip and colleagues (1995, 1996a) (Figures 7.2a and 7.2b) and Li Saw Hee et al (2000b).

Other studies in patients with AF have also suggested abnormalities in other markers of increased thrombogenesis, such as plasma fibrinopeptide A — where levels were reduced by heparin (Uno et al, 1988) — thromboxane β2 and platelet factor 4 (Panchenko et al, 1991), and prothrombin fragment F1 + 2 and thrombin-antithrombin III (Asakura et al, 1992).

Importantly, there appears to be no significant relations to aetiology of AF, left atrial size, valvular heart disease, or ventricular function as determined by echocardiography. In the study by Lip et al (1995) was also a significant (positive) correlation of plasma fibrin D-dimer levels with plasma von Willebrand factor (a marker of endothelial dysfunction) in keeping with the role of the endothelium in thrombogenesis. In a study of 20 patients with chronic lone AF after treadmill exercise, plasma fibrinogen and beta-thromboglobulin levels were increased in association with enhanced platelet activation, but with lower levels of intrinsic anticoagulant and antifibrinolytic activity (Furui et al, 1987).

Recent concerns that measurement of peripheral blood levels of these markers may

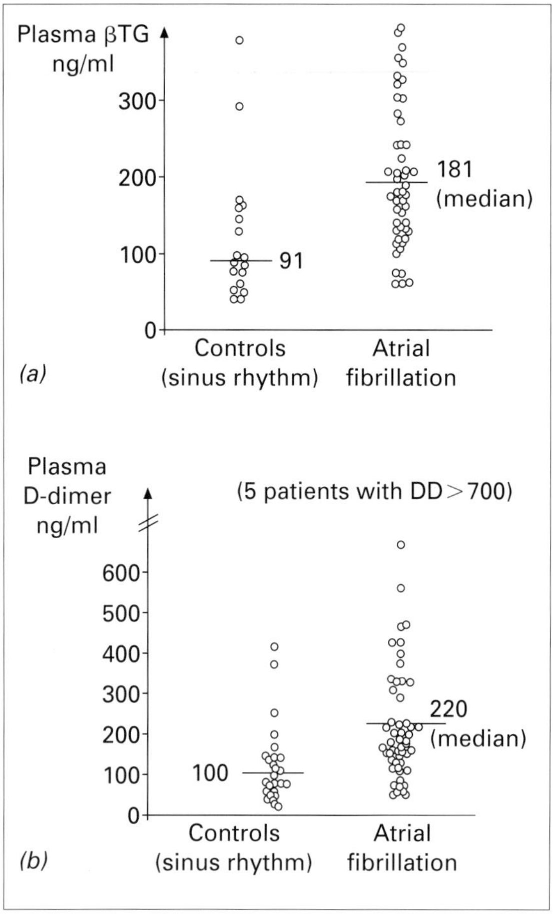

Figure 7.2

(a) Plasma βTG in chronic AF. (b) Plasma fibrin D-dimer in chronic AF. Reproduced with permission of Lip et al (1996).

not reflect intracardiac levels of thrombogenesis (Peverill et al, 1996; Yamamoto et al, 1995) have not been confirmed by our group (Li Saw Hee et al, 1999) (Figure 7.3). In the latter study there were no significant differences in markers of thrombogenesis, platelet activation, endothelial dysfunction, and fibrinogen between femoral vein and artery, and the left and right atria in patients with AF and mitral stenosis undergoing percutaneous balloon mitral valvuloplasty, indicating that peripheral levels did reflect intracardiac levels of these markers. There also does not appear to be any significant circadian or diurnal variation in levels of these markers, indicating a constant hypercoagulable state (Li Saw Hee et al, 2000a); this would be in keeping with the lack of any significant diurnal variation in presentation of stroke or thromboembolism in patients with AF.

The studies by Kumagai and colleagues (1990) and Lip and colleagues (1995) suggest that with identical underlying structural heart disease, AF was perhaps a discriminating factor for abnormal intravascular haemostasis. In patients with paroxysmal AF intermediate levels of plasma fibrinogen and fibrin D-dimer have been found, compared with similar patients with chronic AF and controls in sinus rhythm (Lip et al, 1996b). A study by Sohara and colleagues (1997) also reported abnormal haemostasis in paroxysmal AF, which was related to the duration of paroxysms and whether the subjects were in AF at the time of blood sampling. The association of spontaneous echocontrast on transoesophageal echocardiography with haemostatic abnormalities in patients with AF is further "visual" evidence for stasis being related to a hypercoagulable state (Black et al, 1993; Fatkin et al, 1994). Indeed, the mechanism of spontaneous echocontrast formation is thought to be due to erythrocyte aggregation in low shear rate conditions, with a possible interaction of platelets and plasma fibrinogen (Sigel et al, 1981; Merino et al, 1992).

If AF confers a hypercoagulable state, these markers should be altered by the introduction of antithrombotic therapy or by cardioversion to sinus rhythm. In the cross-sectional study by Lip and colleagues (1995), median fibrin D-dimer levels were highest in patients who were not on any antithrombotic therapy;

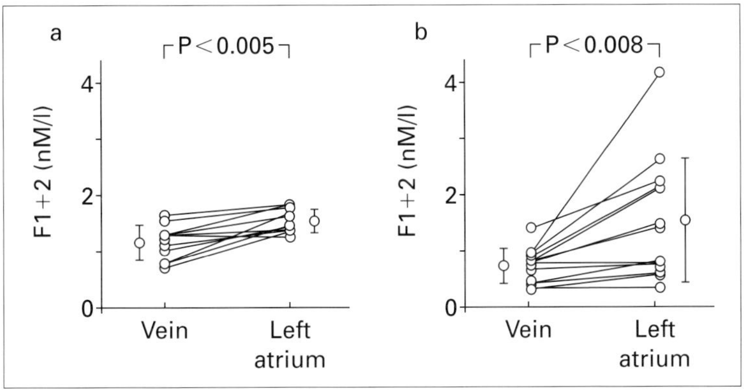

Figure 7.3
Prothrombin fragment 1 + 2 (F1 + 2) levels in peripheral venous and left atrial blood samples in patients with mitral stenosis and mild (a) or marked (b) left atrial spontaneous echo-contrast. Reproduced with permission from Peverill et al (1996).

whilst those were established on warfarin had the lowest fibrin D-dimer levels. Patients established on aspirin alone had intermediate levels of fibrin D-dimer, but this was not a significant difference from those without any antithrombotic therapy. Asakura and colleagues (1992) reported lower prothrombin fragment F1 + 2 and thrombin-antithrombin III levels in patients on warfarin, compared with those on aspirin or those without any antithrombotic therapy. In the BAATAF study, anticoagulation therapy reduced prothrombin fragment F1 + 2 by 71%, while aspirin had little effect on prothrombin activation (Kistler et al, 1993). In patients with AF who were randomised to aspirin (300 mg daily) alone or ultra-low dose warfarin (using a fixed-dose 1 mg daily regimen), no significant alterations in plasma fibrin D-dimer or beta-thromboglobulin levels were shown after 6 weeks' follow-up (Lip et al, 1996a). Similarly, fixed low dose warfarin, and aspirin-warfarin combination therapy does not reduce haemostatic markers (Li Saw Hee et al, 2000b). These changes were therefore consistent with the prophylactic benefits of warfarin therapy and the lower efficacy of other aspirin regimes in reducing stroke in patients with AF.

Patients with chronic AF who were not on anticoagulants and who were cardioverted to sinus rhythm show a sequential fall in fibrin D-dimer levels (but not plasma fibrinogen levels), which were reduced to normal levels 2 weeks after cardioversion (Lip et al, 1995). Although that study was a small, non-randomised study, the results do suggest that intracardiac blood flow abnormalities in AF were probably responsible for the increased haemostatic state.

If the mechanisms of thromboembolism are not simply mechanical but related to an underlying prothrombotic state, measurement of suitable markers of thrombogenesis may be useful in identifying "high risk" patients and determining the duration and intensity of anticoagulant therapy required. In view of the potential value of clotting factor abnormalities in assessing the hypercoagulable state in patients with AF, prospective studies are required to assess the predictive nature of these markers for stroke and thromboembolic risk. We need to know, for example, whether or not an abnormal marker of a hypercoagulable state, such as a high fibrin D-dimer level, will predict stroke or death in patients with AF. Lack of such prognostic data in patients with chronic AF raises the question whether these abnormalities of haemostasis in patients with AF are a "cause or effect" phenomenon. Indeed, a prothrombotic state is unlikely to be the sole mechanism, as it is also recognised that there may be an increased risk of thromboembolism around the time of onset of AF.

The abnormalities of haemostatic markers in patients with AF that are unrelated to aetiology and underlying structural heart disease (and alter with antithrombotic therapy and cardioversion) point towards a hypercoagulable state in this common arrhythmia. These abnormalities in haemostasis may perhaps complement clinical and echocardiographic risk stratification for thromboembolism. The value of these markers in assisting the monitoring of anticoagulation intensity or efficacy also needs to be established. However, the value of haemostatic markers in assessing long-term prognosis in many cardiovascular disorders (including AF) still requires further, larger studies.

References

Asakura H, Hifumi S, Jokaji H et al. Prothrombotic fragment F1 + 2 and thrombin-antithrombin III complex are useful markers of the hypercoagulable state in atrial fibrillation. *Blood Coag Fibrinolys* 1992; **3:** 469–73.

Atrial Fibrillation Investigators. Echocardiographic predictors of stroke in patients with atrial fibrillation: a prospective study of 1066 patients from three clinical trials. *Arch Intern Med* 1998; **158:** 1316–20.

Atrial Fibrillation Investigators. Risk factors for stroke and efficacy of antithrombotic treatment in atrial fibrillation: analysis of pooled data from randomized controlled trials. *Arch Intern Med* 1994; **154:** 1449–57.

Ausma J, Wijffels M, Thone F et al. Structural changes of atrial myocardium due to sustained atrial fibrillation in the goat. *Circulation* 1997; **96:** 3157–63.

Benjamin EJ, D'Agostino RB, Belanger AJ et al. Left atrial size and the risk of stroke and death. The Framingham Heart Study. *Circulation* 1995; **92:** 835–41.

Beppu S, Ninura Y, Sakakibara H et al. Smoke-like echo in the left atrial cavity in mitral valve disease: its features and significance. *J Am Coll Cardiol* 1985; **6:** 744–9.

Black IW, Chesterman CN, Hopkins AP et al. Hematologic correlates of left atrial spontaneous echo contrast and thromboembolism in nonvalvular atrial fibrillation. *J Am Coll Cardiol* 1993; **21:** 451–7.

Black IW, Hopkins AP, Lee LC et al. Left atrial spontaneous echo contrast: a clinical and echocardiographic analysis. *J Am Coll Cardiol* 1991; **18:** 398–404.

Cabin HS, Clubb S, Hall C et al. Risk for systemic embolization of atrial fibrillation without mitral stenosis. *Am J Cardiol* 1990; **65:** 1112–16.

Cairns JA, Connolly SJ. Nonrheumatic atrial fibrillation. Risk of stroke and role of antithrombotic therapy. *Circulation* 1991; **84:** 469–81.

Caplan LR, D'Cruz I, Hier DB et al. Atrial size, atrial fibrillation and stroke. *Ann Neurol* 1986; **19:** 158–61.

Chen YT, Kan MN, Chen JS et al. Contributing factors to formation of left atrial spontaneous echo contrast in mitral valvular disease. *J Ultrasound Med* 1990; **9:** 151–5.

Daniel WG, Nellessen U, Schroder E et al. Left atrial spontaneous echo contrast in mitral valve disease: an indicator for an increased thromboembolic risk. *J Am Coll Cardiol* 1988; **11:** 1204–11.

Daoud EG, Knight BP, Weiss R et al. Effect of verapamil and procainamide on atrial fibrillation-induced electrical remodeling in humans. *Circulation* 1997; **96:** 1542–50.

Daoud EG, Marcovitz P, Knight BP et al. Short-term effect of atrial fibrillation on atrial contractile function in humans. *Circulation* 1999; **99:** 3024–7.

Davidson E, Rotenberg Z, Wienberger I et al. Diagnosis and characteristics of lone atrial fibrillation. *Chest* 1989; **95:** 1048–50.

Fatkin D, Herbert E, Feneley MP. Hematologic correlates of spontaneous echo contrast in patients with atrial fibrillation and implications for thromboembolic risk. *Am J Cardiol* 1994; **73:** 672–6.

Frustaci A, Chimenti C, Bellocci F et al. Histological substrate of atrial biopsies in patients with lone atrial fibrillation. *Circulation* 1997; **96:** 1180–4.

Furui H, Taniguchi N, Yamauchi K et al. Effects of treadmill exercise on platelet function, blood coagulability and fibrinolytic activity in patients with atrial fibrillation. *Jpn Heart J* 1987; **28:** 177–84.

Gallagher MM, Obel OA, Camm JA. Tachycardia-induced atrial myopathy: an important mechanism in the pathophysiology of atrial fibrillation? *J Cardiovasc Electrophysiol* 1997; **8:** 1065–74.

Godtfredsen J. Atrial fibrillation. Etiology, course and prognosis. MD thesis. Copenhagen: Munksgaard, 1975.

Griffith GC, Stragnell R, Levinson DC et al. Study of beneficial effects of anticoagulant therapy in congestive heart failure. *Ann Intern Med* 1952; **37:** 867–87.

Gustafsson C, Blomback M, Britton M et al. Coagulation factors and the increased risk of stroke in nonvalvular atrial fibrillation. *Stroke* 1990; **21:** 47–51.

Heppell RM, Berkin KE, McLenachan JM, Davies JA. Haemostatic and haemodynamic abnormalities associated with left atrial thrombosis in non-rheumatic atrial fibrillation. *Heart* 1997; **77:** 407–11.

Hoglund C, Rosenhame G. Echocardiographic left atrial dimension as a predictor of maintaining sinus rhythm after conversion of atrial fibrillation. *Acta Med Scand* 1985; **217:** 411.

Kistler JP, Singer DE, Millenson MM et al. Effect of low-intensity warfarin anticoagulation on level of activity of the hemostatic system in patients with atrial fibrillation. BAATAF Investigators. *Stroke* 1993; **24:** 1360–5.

Kumagai K, Fukunami M, Kitabatake A et al. Increased cardiovascular clotting in patients with chronic atrial fibrillation. *J Am Coll Cardiol* 1990; **16:** 377–80.

Li Saw Hee FL, Blann AD, Lip GYH. A cross-sectional and diurnal study of thrombogenesis among subjects with chronic atrial fibrillation. *J Am Coll Cardiol* 2000a; **35:** 1926–31.

Li Saw Hee FL, Blann AD, Lip GYH. Effects of fixed low dose warfarin, aspirin-warfarin combination therapy, and dose-adjusted warfarin on thrombogenesis in chronic atrial fibrillation. *Stroke* 2000b; **31:** 828–33.

Li Saw Hee FL, Blann AD, Goldsmith I, Lip GYH. Indices of hypercoagulability measured in peripheral blood reflect levels in intracardiac blood in patients with atrial fibrillation secondary to mitral stenosis. *Am J Cardiol* 1999; **83:** 1206–9.

Lip GYH, Lip PL, Zarifis J et al. Fibrin D-dimer and beta-thromboglobulin as markers of thrombogenesis and platelet activation in atrial fibrillation: effects of introducing ultra-low dose warfarin and aspirin. *Circulation* 1996a; **94:** 425–31.

Lip GYH, Lowe GDO, Rumley A, Dunn FG. Plasma fibrinogen and fibrin D-dimer levels in paroxysmal atrial fibrillation: Evidence for intermediate levels of intravascular thrombogenesis. *Am Heart J* 1996b; **131:** 724–30.

Lip GYH, Lowe GDO, Rumley A, Dunn FG. Increased markers of thrombogenesis in chronic atrial fibrillation: effects of warfarin therapy. *Br Heart J* 1995; **73:** 527–33.

Lip GYH, Rumley A, Dunn FG, Lowe GDO. Plasma fibrinogen and fibrin D-dimer levels in a trial fibrillation: effect of cardioversion to sinus rhythm. *Int J Cardiol* 1995; **51:** 245–53.

Lip GYH. Does atrial fibrillation confer a hypercoagulable state? *Lancet* 1995; **346:** 1313–4.

Lip GYH. Hypercoagulability and haemodynamic abnormalities in atrial fibrillation. *Heart* 1997; **77:** 395–6.

Manning WJ, Silverman DI, Gordon SPF et al. Cardioversion from atrial fibrillation without prolonged anticoagulation with use of transesophageal echocardiography to exclude the presence of atrial thrombi. *N Engl J Med* 1993; **328:** 750–5.

Manning WJ, Leeman DE, Gotch PJ et al. Pulsed Doppler evaluation of atrial mechanical function after electrical cardioversion of atrial fibrillation. *J Am Coll Cardiol* 1989; **13:** 617.

Manning WJ, Silverman DI, Katz SE et al. Impaired left atrial mechanical function after cardioversion: relationship to the duration of atrial fibrillation. *J Am Coll Cardiol* 1994; **23:** 1535.

Masawa N, Yoshida Y, Yamada T et al. Diagnosis of cardiac thrombosis in patients with atrial fibrillation in the absence of macroscopically visible thrombi. *Virchows Arch A Pathol Anat Histopathol* 1993; **422:** 67–71.

Merino A, Hauptman P, Badimon L et al. Echocardiographic 'smoke' is produced by an interaction of erythrocytes and plasma proteins modulated by shear forces. *J Am Coll Cardiol* 1992; **20:** 1661–8.

Morillo CA, Klein GJ, Jones DL, Guiraudon CM. Chronic rapid atrial pacing. Structural, functional, and electrophysiological characteristics of a new model of sustained atrial fibrillation. *Circulation* 1995; **91:** 1588–95.

Obarski TP, Salcedo EE, Castle LW, Stewart WJ. Spontaneous echo contrast in the left atrium during paroxysmal atrial fibrillation. *Am Heart J* 1990; **120:** 988–90.

Panchenko VM, Smoliar MI, Zhivoderov VM et al.

Thromboxane, prostacyclin and platelet factor 4 in patients with atrial fibrillation. *Klin Med Mosk* 1991; **69:** 80–2.

Petersen P, Kastrup J, Brinch K et al. Relation between left atrial dimension and duration of atrial fibrillation. *Am J Cardiol* 1987; **60:** 382–4.

Petersen P, Kastrup J, Wilhelmsen R, Schutten HJ. Atrial natriuretic peptide in atrial fibrillation before and after electrical cardioversion therapy. *Eur Heart J* 1988; **9:** 639–41.

Petersen P, Godtfredsen J. Embolic complications in paroxysmal atrial fibrillation. *Stroke* 1986; **17:** 622–5.

Peverill RE, Harper RW, Gelman J. Determinants of increased regional left atrial coagulant activity in patients with mitral stenosis. *Circulation* 1996; **94:** 331–9.

Sanfilippo AJ, Abascal VM, Sheehan M et al. Atrial enlargement as a consequence of atrial fibrillation. A prospective echocardiographic study. *Circulation* 1990; **82:** 792–7.

Sigel B, Coelho JCU, Spigos DG et al. Ultrasonography of blood during stasis and coagulation. *Invest Radiol* 1981; **16:** 71–6.

Sohara H, Amitani S, Kurose M, Miyhara K. Atrial fibrillation activates platelets and coagulation in a time-dependent manner: a study in patients with paroxysmal atrial fibrillation. *J Am Coll Cardiol* 1997; **29:** 106–12.

Sosa-Suarez G, Lampert S, Graboys TB et al. Changes in left atrial size due to chronic atrial fibrillation. *J Am Coll Cardiol* 1989; **13:** 206A.

Spinale FG, Tomita M, Zellner JL et al. Collagen remodelling and changes in LV function during development and recovery from supraventricular tachycardia. *Am J Physiol* 1991; **261:** H308–18.

Stoddard ME, Dawkins PR, Prince CR, Ammash NM. Left atrial appendage thrombus is not uncommon in patients with acute atrial fibrillation and a recent embolic event: a transesophageal echocardiographic study. *J Am Coll Cardiol* 1995; **25:** 452–9.

Stroke Prevention in Atrial Fibrillation Investigators. Predictors of thromboembolism in atrial fibrillation: I. Clinical features of patients at risk. *Ann Intern Med* 1992a; **116:** 1–5.

Stroke Prevention in Atrial Fibrillation Investigators. Predictors of thromboembolism in atrial fibrillation: II. Echocardiographic features of patients at risk. *Ann Intern Med* 1992b; **116:** 6–12.

Takahashi N, Umataka K, Seki A, Fujii J. Left atrial enlargement in patients with paroxysmal atrial fibrillation. *Jpn Heart J* 1982; **23:** 677–83.

Tsai LM, Chen JH, Fang CJ et al. Clinical implications of left atrial spontaneous echo contrast in nonrheumatic atrial fibrillation. *Am J Cardiol* 1992; **70:** 327–31.

Uno M, Tsuji H, Sawada S et al. Fibrinopeptide A (FPA) levels in atrial fibrillation and the effects of heparin administration. *Jpn Circ J* 1988; **52:** 9–12.

Van Gelder IC, Crijns HJ, Blanksma PK et al. Time course of hemodynamic changes and improvement of exercise tolerance after cardioversion of chronic atrial fibrillation unassociated with cardiac valve disease. *Am J Cardiol* 1993; **72:** 560–6.

Wolf PA, Kannel WB, McGee DL et al. Duration of atrial fibrillation and imminence of stroke: the Framingham study. *Stroke* 1983; **14:** 664–7.

Yamamoto K, Ikeda U, Seino Y et al. Coagulation activity is increased in the left atrium of patients with mitral stenosis. *J Am Coll Cardiol* 1995; **25:** 107–12.

Yamauchi K, Furui H, Taniguchi N, Sotobata I. Plasma beta-thromboglobulin and platelet factor 4 concentrations in patients with atrial fibrillation. *Jpn Heart J* 1986; **27:** 481–7.

8

Electrophysiology

The ECG in AF

The ECG in atrial fibrillation (AF) typically shows the following:

- P waves that usually characterise synchronised atrial depolarization in normal sinus rhythm are absent, and are replaced by fibrillatory (f) waves
- f waves are present at a rate that is generally between 350 and 600 beats/min, varying in amplitude morphology, and intervals
- The R-R intervals are irregularly irregular
- narrow QRS complexes unless AV conduction is abnormal due to functional (rate-related) aberration, pre-existing bundle branch or fascicular block, pre-excitation with ventricular activation via an accessory pathway.

Atrial fibrillatory activity is usually seen in precordial lead V1 and in the inferior standard leads, II, III, and aVF. The amplitude of the f waves varies, and may be especially prominent (or "coarse") in lead V1. The fibrillation may be fine (amplitude <0.5 mm on ECG), coarse (amplitude >0.5 mm), or, on occasion, inapparent. The f waves may be inapparent on the standard and precordial leads, especially in chronic AF. Occasionally, some artifacts, such as tremors as in Parkinson's disease, may simulate f waves.

Rapid AF with a rapid ventricular response may be easily mistaken for other supraventricular arrhythmias, for example, atrial flutter or supraventricular tachycardias. Subtle variation in the R-R interval is the important clue: this may be made more obvious by carotid sinus massage or by increasing the speed of the ECG trace. AF with a bundle branch block pattern on the QRS may also prove a diagnostic problem, and may be difficult to distinguish from ventricular tachycardia: again, the important difference is the irregularity of the R-R interval. AF with widening of the QRS complex is present with a pre-existing conduction defect (left or right bundle branch block), a functional (generally rate-related) block in a portion of the infranodal conduction system that results in asynchronous or aberrant activation, or with pre-excitation through an atrioventricular (AV) bypass tract that is capable of antegrade conduction.

Nevertheless, AF should be distinguished from other rhythms in which the R-R intervals are irregularly irregular, for example, multifocal atrial tachycardia, wandering atrial pacemaker, multifocal atrial premature beats, and atrial tachycardia or atrial flutter with varying AV block. However, the R-R interval may be regular with AV dissociation or block — for example with digoxin toxicity, a setting in which a ventricular pacemaker assumes control of the ventricles.

In a young patient with fast AF, an under-

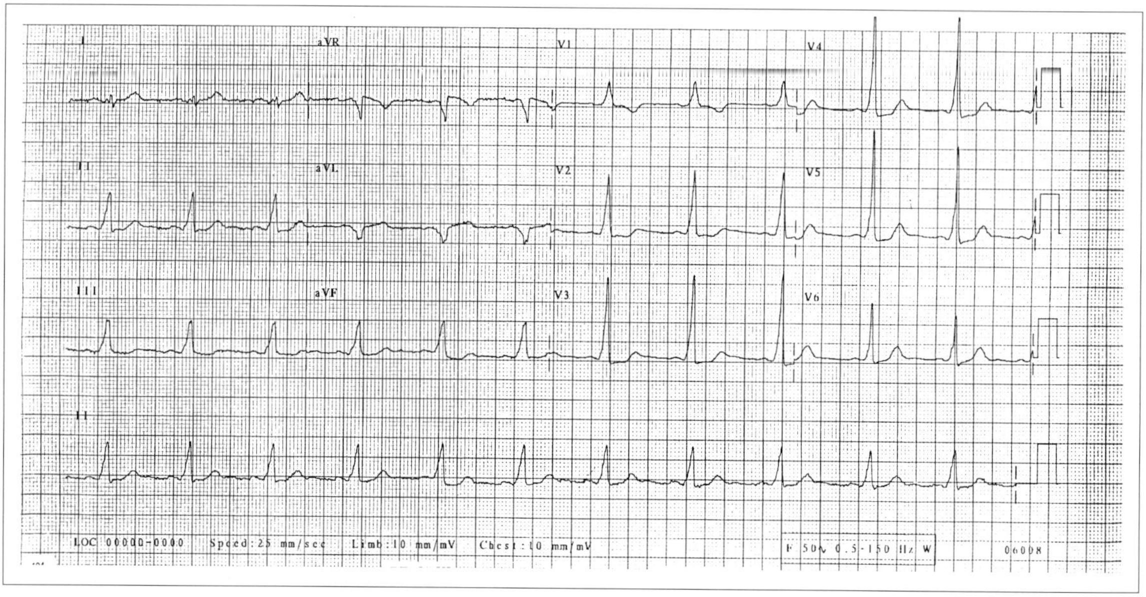

Figure 8.1
ECG showing Wolff-Parkinson-White syndrome.

lying pre-excitation syndrome such as Wolff-Parkinson-White syndrome should be considered (Figure 8.1). This is important since "traditional" drugs that block atrioventricular node conduction, such as digoxin or verapamil, will accelerate the ventricular response by increasing conduction through the accessory pathway.

Electrophysiology of AF

Several potential electrophysiological mechanisms may cause AF. Several factors predispose to, and allow long-term maintenance of the arrhythmia: these can include atrial enlargement (secondary to mitral valve disease, hypertension, etc), fibrosis of atrial tissue (resulting in slowing of intra-atrial conduction), and altered autonomic tone, especially increased sympathetic activity. AF may also be initiated by atrial premature beats, atrial flutter, or supraventricular tachycardias, suggesting a re-entrant mechanism for the arrhythmia (Allessie et al, 1996). In the electrophysiology laboratory, electrically-induced atrial beats and rapid atrial pacing can induce AF.

Two theories have been suggested as the underlying mechanism for AF

- enhanced automaticity, involving one or more foci firing rapidly
- re-entry involving one or more circuits

In addition, heterogeneity of atrial refractoriness and slow conduction times (allowing time for the myocardium to regain excitability between each wavefront) lead to AF being sustained in the long-term (Figures 8.2 and 8.3).

The most widely accepted mechanism is the multiple wavelet re-entry hypothesis of Moe (1962), in which a critical number of coexisting wavefronts continuously sweep through the atria in a random, irregular, shifting fash-

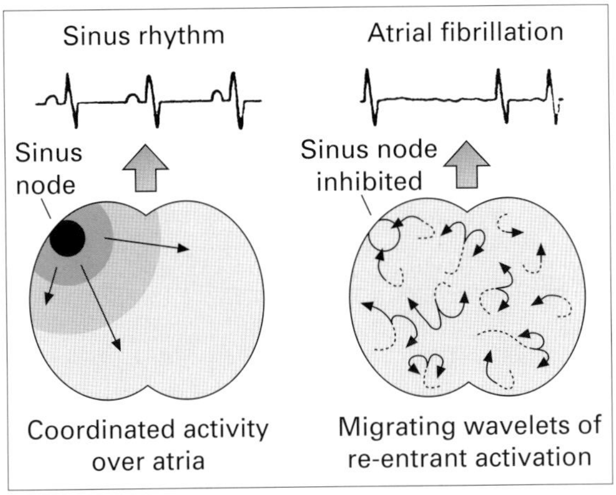

Figure 8.2
AF compared with sinus rhythm. AF is characterised by multiple electrical wavelets in the atria. Disorders that increase atrial size, decrease tissue wavelength or affect both may increase propensity for AF. Reproduced with permission from Narayan et al (1997).

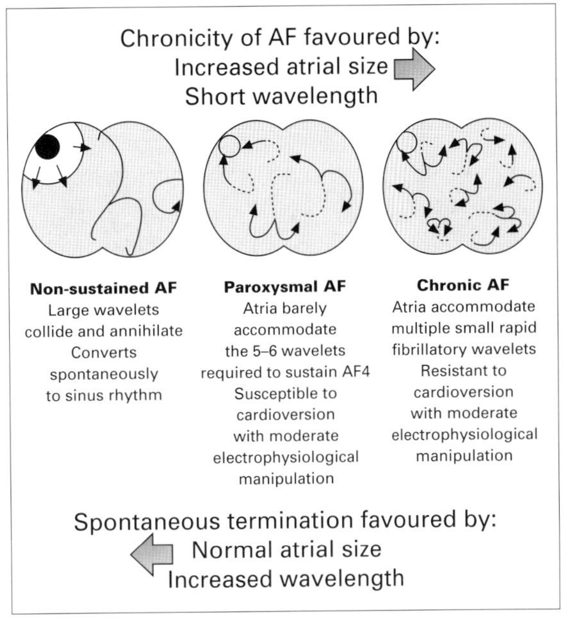

Figure 8.3
Subtypes of AF. Non-sustained AF reverts spontaneously to sinus rhythm. Paroxysmal AF may resolve with modest electrophysiological intervention. Chronic AF resists cardioversion. Reproduced with permission from Narayan et al (1997).

ion, repeatedly encountering excitable myocardium. This hypothesis requires a minimum number (4–6) of independent wavefronts and enough atrial tissue to permit their simultaneous propagation. However, Allessie's model (Allessie et al, 1996) suggests that AF is due to multiple wavelets continuously sweeping around the atria in patterns. There are usually multiple wavefronts of activation that may collide with each other, extinguishing themselves or creating new wavelets and wavefronts, thereby perpetuating the arrhythmia. With normal AV nodal conduction, there is a resultant irregularly irregular ventricular response of 90 to 140–170 beats/min.

In selected patients, AF is produced by rapid tachycardias from either focal sources or stable re-entrant circuits that drive the remaining atrial tissue until degeneration to AF occurs. The study by Jais and colleagues (1997) reported nine patients with drug-resistant paroxysmal AF in whom a single, rapidly firing focus was identified by electrophysiological mapping, with a centrifugal and consistent pattern of atrial activation and striking and abrupt changes in atrial cycle lengths. In these relatively young patients, ablation of these foci, near the ostia of great vessels, may result in the cure of AF. The same group (Haissaguerre et al, 1998) subsequently reported that the pulmonary veins were an important source of ectopic beats, initiating frequent paroxysms of AF, and that these foci also responded well to treatment with radiofrequency ablation.

The electrophysiology of the AV node plays an important part in the clinical manifestations of AF. The rate of AV nodal conduction is dependent upon multiple factors, including the following

- AV nodal blocking agents such as digoxin, calcium channel blockers, or beta blockers
- the channels responsible for activation and inactivation
- the electrophysiological characteristics of cell-cell communication, nodal geometry, dead-end pathways
- the influence of the autonomic nervous system

The atrial cycle length in AF is short (<160 msec). Multiple impulses bombard the AV node during its refractory period and are not conducted. Nevertheless, some impulses, although not fully conducted, partially penetrate the AV node and reset the refractory period for subsequent impulses ("concealed conduction"), which in turn creates a refractory wave that affects succeeding impulses.

The ventricular response in AF is typically irregularly irregular, with a ventricular rate that may be slow, moderate, or rapid depending on the capacity of the AV node to conduct impulses from the fibrillating atria to the ventricle. Anatomically distinct AV nodal inputs, called the slow and fast pathways, are involved in the ventricular response to AF. Modulation of AV conduction can be done by ablation of the "slow" AV node pathway, representing a therapeutic option in patients with drug refractory AF or flutter (Della Bella et al, 1995). When AF occurs in patients with pre-excitation, extremely rapid ventricular rates may occur since the refractory period of the accessory connection may be the chief determinant of AV conduction; indeed, the AV node is bypassed by "fast" tracts that activate and reactivate much faster than the AV node, resulting in rapid conduction (Kriner et al, 1996) and rarely, ventricular fibrillation (Klein et al, 1979).

The ventricular response to AF is characteristically irregularly irregular, although it may appear regular in the presence of complete AV block, as may occur with digoxin toxicity. The usual ventricular rate in AF is between 90 and 170 beats/min in the absence of AV node disease, drugs that affect conduction, or enhanced vagal inputs. A ventricular rate below 60 beats/min in the absence of AV nodal blocking agents suggests AV nodal disease that may be associated with the sick sinus syndrome. A ventricular rate above 170 beats/min suggests thyrotoxicosis, catecholamine excess, parasympathetic withdrawal, or the existence of an accessory bypass tract in the pre-excitation syndrome.

AF begets AF

AF is self-perpetuating via a process termed "electrical remodelling". As shown in animal models and clinical experiments, AF results in a number of electrophysiological changes by which "AF begets AF" (Wijffels et al, 1995; Wijffels et al, 1997; Goette et al, 1996). Wijfells and colleagues (1995) used a goat model in which initial pacing-induced AF terminated spontaneously, but, after repetitive induction, progressively longer episodes occurred, leading finally to a sustained AF and an increase in atrial rate (Figure 8.4). This increasing propensity for long-lasting AF is related to progressive shortening of effective refractive periods with an increasing duration of AF episodes. A greater effect occurs at longer cycle lengths, to allow the reinitiation of AF with single extrastimuli; this is a phenomenon known as "electrophysiological remodelling". These changes are reversible over time with restoration of sinus rhythm. In response to periods of AF, the atrial refractory period shortens. Repeat episodes of AF result in a longer duration of each episode until the arrhythmia becomes persistent and sinus node

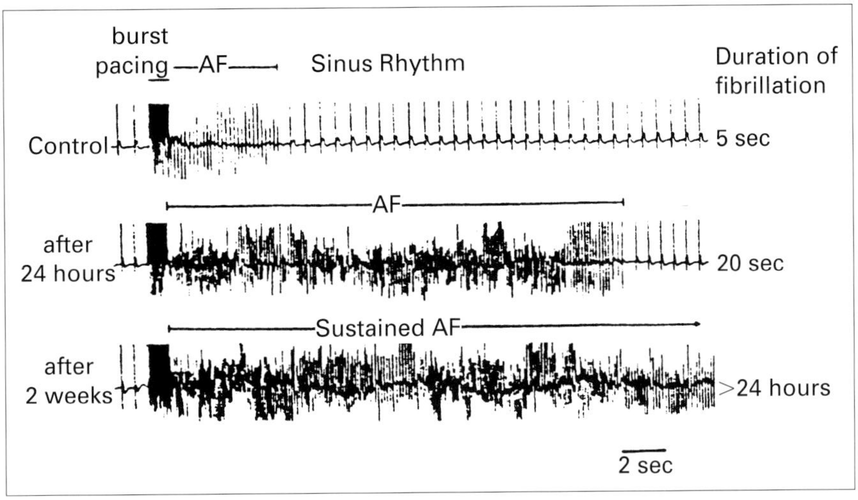

Figure 8.4
Prolongation of the duration of episodes of electrically induced AF after maintaining AF for respectively 24 hours and 2 weeks. The three tracings show a single atrial electrogram recorded from the same goat during induction of AF by a 1-sec burst of stimuli (50 Hz, 4 × threshold). In the upper tracing the goat has been in sinus rhythm all the time and atrial fibrillation self-terminated within 5 sec. The second tracing was recorded after the goat had been connected to the fibrillation pacemaker for 24 hours showing a clear prolongation of the duration of AF to 20 sec. The third tracing was recorded after 2 weeks of electrically maintained atrial fibrillation. After induction of AF this episode became sustained and did not terminate. Reproduced with permission from Wijffels et al (1995).

function becomes depressed (Elvan et al, 1996). Indeed, the changes in atrial refractory period observed after an episode of AF predispose to the spontaneous recurrence of AF in the days after cardioversion. An animal study by Goette and colleagues (1996) showed that electrical remodelling begins quickly, within the first 30 min after the onset of AF, and continues for several minutes; quick resolution of these electrophysiological changes also occurs, being virtually complete after 30 min of sinus rhythm. These changes appear to be mediated by cytosolic calcium overload, since verapamil seems to prevent electric remodelling and hasten complete recovery without influencing in the inducibility of AF, whilst hypercalcemia appears to accentuate the phenomenon (Tieleman et al, 1997).

These experimental data are in keeping with clinical observations that suggest that the presence of paroxysms of AF persisting for longer periods results in prolongation of subsequent episodes of AF and a reduction in the ability to restore and maintain sinus rhythm. Paroxysmal AF commonly precedes the development of chronic AF. The role of cytosolic calcium is illustrated by the report from Daoud and colleagues (1997) in which verapamil but not procainamide prevented remodelling when given before the electrophysiological induction of AF. Van Gelder and colleagues (1999) recently reported AF-induced alterations in mRNA contents of proteins and ion channels involved in calcium handling, which seem to occur in relation to the previous duration of AF. Lai and colleagues (1999) recently investigated the gene expression of calcium-handling genes including L-type calcium channel, sarcoplasmic reticular calcium adenosine triphosphatase (Ca^{2+}-ATPase), ryanodine receptor, calsequestrin, and phospholamban in atrial tissue from patients with AF who were undergoing open heart surgery. The researchers showed that L-type calcium channel and the sarcoplasmic reticular (Ca^{2+})-ATPase gene were down-regulated in AF as a consequence of, and as a contributory factor for, AF. Overall, these alterations in gene expression of proteins involved in calcium handling in patients with AF may have a role in electrical remodelling in AF.

Electromechanical feedback

Some of the structural abnormalities associated with AF may be related to or predispose to the electrophysiological abnormalities seen in this arrhythmia. For example, dilatation and an increase in intra-atrial pressure can alter atrial electrophysiological properties, a phenomenon known as "electromechanical feedback". The amplitude of the f waves on the ECG also appears to correlate with increasing atrial size in some studies (Henry et al, 1976; Aronow et al, 1987), but not all studies (Morganroth et al, 1979), although there may be a correlation with the duration of AF. Recently, Ravelli and colleagues (1997) reported that left atrial enlargement and increased left atrial pressure in the isolated Lanfendorff-perfused rabbit heart decreased the atrial refractory period and action potential duration, thereby predisposing to AF; conversely, lowering left atrial pressure resulted in reversion of the arrhythmia.

The microarchitecture and anisotropic properties of the atrium may influence patterns of impulse propagation. For example, the signal averaged electrocardiogram (SAECG) detects abnormal potentials related to conduction delays in the myocardium that can lead to re-entry. Indeed, a prolonged signal-averaged P wave duration and the presence of low voltage atrial late potential may potentially identify patients at risk of developing AF (Jukunami et al, 1991), including after ablation of an accessory bypass tract (Maia et al, 1995) or after CABG surgery (Stafford et al, 1997). Stafford and colleagues (1997) studied 201 patients after CABG and showed that the signal-averaged P wave duration (>141 ms) was a far better predictor of AF than the P wave duration or terminal vector obtained from lead II or V1 on the standard ECG or left atrial dimension on echocardiography.

Gaspo and colleagues (1997) recently suggested functional mechanisms underlying tachycardia-induced sustained AF in a chronic dog model. In that model, rapid atrial activation caused time-dependent decreases in refractory period, conduction velocity, and wavelength, which, along with increased regional heterogeneity, provided a substrate for AF. Thus the conduction abnormalities and increased regional heterogeneity previously noted in patients with AF may be a consequence, as well as a cause, of the tachyarrhythmia.

Lone AF

The electrophysiological basis of lone AF still remains uncertain. Differences in clinical electrophysiological properties have been identified in patients with recurrent lone paroxysmal AF. An enhanced vagal tone, resulting in shortening of the atrial refractory period, may be relevant, since many of these patients develop AF at night whilst asleep. Abnormalities in left atrial histology have also been observed in patients with lone AF (Frustaci et al, 1997), including healed myocarditis, active myocarditis, patchy fibrosis, or a non-inflammatory localised cardiomyopathy.

Poret and colleagues (1996) reported five cases of apparently lone AF in the same family from three generations, and raised the question of a genetic predisposition to lone AF. The AF had occurred at an early age and rapidly became permanent in all cases. In 1997, Brugada and colleagues described a family of 26 members in which ten had familial AF, segregating as an autosomal dominant disease, with the responsible gene localised to chromosome 10. One study failed to find any significant association between lone AF and ACE gene polymorphism (Yamashita et al, 1997).

References

Allessie MA, Konings K, Kirchhoff CJHJ, Wijffels M. Electrophysiologic mechanisms of perpetuation of atrial fibrillation. *Am J Cardiol* 1996; **77:** 10A–23A.

Aronow WS, Schwartz KS, Koenigsberg M. Prevalence of enlarged left atrial dimension by echocardiography and its correlation with atrial fibrillation and an abnormal P terminal force in lead V1 of the electrocardiogram in 588 elderly persons. *Am J Cardiol* 1987; **59:** 1003.

Brugada R, Tapscott T, Czernuszewicz GZ et al. Identification of a genetic locus for familial atrial fibrillation. *N Engl J Med* 1997; **336:** 905–11.

Daoud EG, Knight BP, Weiss R et al. Effect of verapamil and procainamide on atrial fibrillation-induced electrical remodeling in humans. *Circulation* 1997; **96:** 1542–50.

Della Bella P, Carbucicchio C, Tondo C, Riva S. Modulation of atrioventricular conduction by ablation of the "slow" atrioventricular node pathway in patients with drug refractory atrial fibrillation or flutter. *J Am Coll Cardiol* 1995; **25:** 39.

Elvan A, Wylie K, Zipes DP. Pacing-induced chronic atrial fibrillation impairs sinus node function in dogs: electrophysiological remodeling. *Circulation* 1996; **94:** 2953–60.

Frustaci A, Chimenti C, Bellocci F et al. Histologic substrate of atrial biopsies in patients with lone atrial fibrillation. *Circulation* 1997; **96:** 1180.

Gaspo R, Bosch RF, Talajic M, Nattel S. Functional mechanisms underlying tachycardia-induced sustained atrial fibrillation in a chronic dog model. *Circulation* 1997; **96:** 4027–35.

Goette A, Honeycutt C, Langberg JJ. Electrical remodeling in atrial fibrillation. *Circulation* 1996; **94:** 2968–74.

Haissaguerre M, Jais P, Shah DC et al. Spontaneous initiation of atrial fibrillation by ectopic beats originating in the pulmonary veins. *N Engl J Med* 1998; **339:** 659–66.

Henry WL, Morganroth J, Pearlman AS et al. Relation between echocardiographically determined left atrial size and atrial fibrillation. *Circulation* 1976; **53:** 273–9.

Jais P, Haissaguerre M, Shah DC et al. A focal source of atrial fibrillation treated by discrete radiofrequency ablation. *Circulation* 1997; **95:** 572–6.

Jukunami M, Yamada T, Ohmori M et al. Detection of patients at risk for atrial fibrillation during sinus rhythm by P wave triggered signal-averaged electrocardiogram. *Circulation* 1991; **83:** 162–9.

Klein GJ, Bashore TM, Sellers TD et al. Ventricular fibrillation in the Wolff-Parkinson-White syndrome. *N Engl J Med* 1979; **301:** 1080.

Kriner G, Heinz G, Siostrzonek P, Gossinger HD. Effect of slow pathway ablation on ventricular rate during atrial fibrillation: dependence on electrophysiologic properties of the fast pathway. *Circulation* 1996; **93:** 277.

Lai LP, Su MJ, Lin JL et al. Down-regulation of L-type calcium channel and sarcoplasmic reticular Ca^{2+}-ATPase mRNA in human atrial fibrillation without significant change in the mRNA of ryanodine receptor, calsequestrin and phospholamban: an insight into the mechanism of atrial electrical remodeling. *J Am Coll Cardiol* 1999; **33:** 1231–7.

Maia IG, Cruz-Filho FES, Fagundes MLA et al. Signal averaged P wave in patients with Wolff-Parkinson-White syndrome after successful radiofrequency catheter ablation. *J Am Coll Cardiol* 1995; **26:** 1310–14.

Moe GK. On the multiple wavelet hypothesis of atrial fibrillation. *Arch Int Pharmacodyn Ther* 1962; **140:** 183.

Morganroth J, Horowitz LN, Josephson ME, Kastor JA. Relationship of atrial fibrillatory wave amplitude to left atrial size and etiology of heart disease. *Am Heart J* 1979; **97:** 184–6.

Narayan SM, Cain ME, Smith JM. Atrial fibrillation. *Lancet* 1997; **350:** 943–50.

Poret P, Mabo P, Deplace C et al. Is isolated atrial fibrillation genetically determined? Apropos of a familial history. *Arch Mal Coeu Vaiss* 1996; **89:** 1197–203.

Ravelli F, Allessie M. Effects of atrial dilatation on refractory period and vulnerability to atrial fibrillation in the isolated Langendorff-perfused rabbit heart. *Circulation* 1997; **96:** 1686–95.

Stafford PJ, Kolvekar S, Cooper J et al. Signal averaged P wave compared with standard electrocardiography for prediction of atrial fibrillation after coronary bypass grafting. *Heart* 1997; **77:** 417–22.

Tieleman RG, De Langen CDJ, Van Gelder IC et al. Verapamil reduces tachycardia-induced electrical remodeling of the atria. *Circulation* 1997; **95:** 1945–53.

Wijffels MC, Kirchhof CJHJ, Dorland R et al. Electrical remodeling due to atrial fibrillation in chronically instrumented conscious goats. Roles of neurohumoral changes, ischemia, atrial stretch, and high rate of electrical activation. *Circulation* 1997; **96:** 3710–20.

Wijffels MCEF, Kirchhof CJHJ, Dorland R et al. Atrial fibrillation begets atrial fibrillation. A study in awake chronically instrumented goats. *Circulation* 1995; **92:** 1954.

Van Gelder IC, Brundel BJ, Hening RH et al. Alterations in gene expression of proteins involved in the calcium handling patients with atrial fibrillation. *J Cardiovasc Electrophysiol* 1999; **10:** 552–60.

Yamashita T, Hayami N, Ajiki K et al. Is ACE gene polymorphism associated with lone atrial fibrillation? *Jpn Heart J* 1997; **38:** 637–41.

IV
Clinical Features

9

Clinical features, presenting symptoms, and complications of atrial fibrillation

Clinical classification

No general agreement on the terminology for classifying atrial fibrillation (AF) is available. There are many definitions of the different types of AF, which are of varying usefulness and consistency. One proposed clinical definition of AF divides patients into acute-onset and chronic AF; the latter are further divided into paroxysmal and sustained AF. Sustained AF is further divided into persistent and permanent AF (Figure 9.1). This "3P" classification (that is, paroxysmal, persistent, and permanent) allows adequate division along the lines of clinical objectives of management and can assist treatment strategies, but many patients change from one category to another. The differentiation between these clinical categories is dependent upon the history given by the patient, ECG documentation of the current episode, and the duration of the last episode of AF. Although this classification is helpful, there is much inter-patient and intra-patient variability in the temporal pattern of AF episodes, and therapy must be individualised.

The term "acute AF" is used to describe either an episode of AF related to a transient and reversible cause or the first onset of AF. The term "chronic AF" implies either recurrent or prolonged episodes. Chronic AF can then be subclassified as either paroxysmal (self-terminating) or sustained. Persistent AF is sustained AF that can be successfully cardioverted, whereas permanent AF is sustained AF that is either resistant to or not appropriate for cardioversion (Sopher and Camm, 1996; Lip, 1999).

Amongst the more chronic forms of AF, clinical classification can assist management strategies. For example, in paroxysmal AF, episodes are generally self-terminating, and thus the main objective of management is the prevention of paroxysms and long-term maintenance of sinus rhythm. In persistent AF, the possibility of cardioversion from AF to sinus rhythm remains, and the objective of management is appropriate anticoagulation to reduce

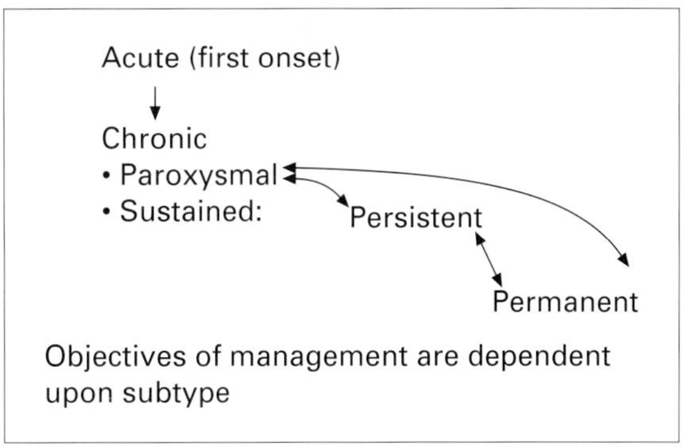

Figure 9.1
AF classification.

the risk of thromboembolism, and antiarrhythmic therapy to maintain long-term sinus rhythm. In permanent AF, cardioversion is not feasible, and the objective of management is heart-rate control and appropriate antithrombotic therapy. The term "permanent" also implies that AF has been present for a long time and that cardioversion is unlikely to be successful, or that one or several attempts of cardioversion have failed to restore sinus rhythm. If cardioversion is the management objective for patients with persistent AF, appropriate use of antiarrhythmic therapy to maintain sinus rhythm, and anticoagulation to reduce the risk of thromboembolism, should be considered.

In the paroxysmal form, an episode lasting more than 48 h may be called persistent AF. This timeframe is the duration beyond which formal anticoagulation should be taken before cardioversion. A period of 7 days has been proposed as a cut-off point to differentiate paroxysmal (less than 7 days) from chronic AF (more than 7 days) (Levy et al, 1999). The paroxysmal form of AF is also heterogeneous, in that AF may be defined by its frequency, duration, mode of termination, and the presence and severity of symptoms. Patients with paroxysmal AF may also be classed as vagally-induced or adrenergic-induced (Coumel, 1994). For example, paroxysms of AF may result from increased vagal tone (vagally-induced AF) recurring usually at night or after meals, especially in male patients without organic heart disease. By contrast, some patients have adrenergic AF, with paroxysms of AF induced by exercise, emotion, and stress. Generally, no clear distinction can be made between the two components based on a single history. The mode of initiation of AF may also differ in the same patient over time.

Clinical features and presenting symptoms

AF is probably the most common cardiac arrhythmia responsible for hospital admissions in the USA, representing 34% of all hospital admissions for cardiac arrhythmias (Bialy et al, 1992). The prevalence of AF amongst acute hospital admissions ranges from 3–6% (Zarifis et al, 1997; Lip et al, 1994), and these tend to be related to an acute illness, exacerbation of chronic symptoms, or the development of a complication of AF (Figure 9.2). However, hospital-based surveys may give an incomplete picture; indeed, only one third of patients in one general-practice survey had ever been admitted to hospital (Lip et al, 1997), suggesting that many patients with AF could be managed in the community, with few problems needing hospital admission.

AF may be symptomatic or symptom-free. Both symptomatic and symptom-free episodes of AF can occur in the same patient. In a com-

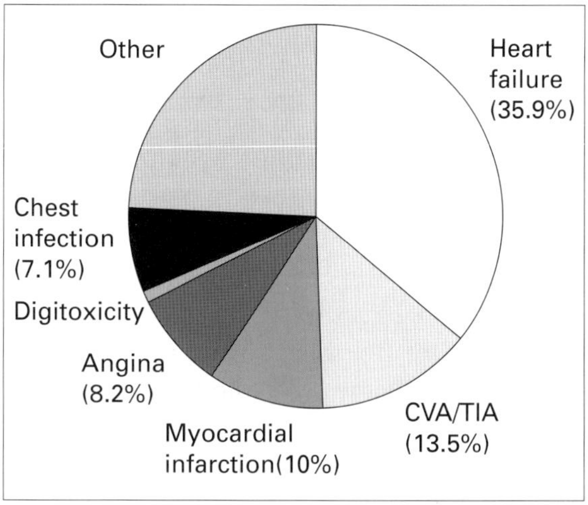

Figure 9.2
Presenting clinical features of admissions with AF to a Scottish district general hospital. Reproduced with permission from Lip et al (1994).

Symptoms	Total Population (n = 756)	Paroxysmal AF (n = 167)	Chronic AF (n = 389)	Recent Onset AF (n = 200)
Palpitations (%)	409 (54.1)	132 (79.0)	174 (44.7)	103 (51.5)
Chest pain (%)	76 (10.1)	22 (13.2)	32 (8.2)	22 (11.0)
Dyspnea (%)	336 (44.4)	38 (22.8)	182 (46.8)	116 (58.00)
Syncope, dizzy spells (%)	79 (10.4)	29 (17.4)	31 (8.0)	19 (9.5)
Fatigue (%)	108 (14.3)	21 (12.6)	51 (13.1)	36 (18.0)
Other (%)	7 (0.9)	0	7 (1.8)	0
None (%)	86 (11.4)	9 (5.4)	63 (16.2)	14 (7.0)

Reproduced with permission from Levy et al (1999).

Table 9.1
Complaints and symptoms.

parison of patients with paroxysmal supraventricular tachycardia (PSVT) and patients with paroxysmal AF, most episodes of PSVT tend to be symptomatic, whilst only 1 in 12 of paroxysms of AF are symptomatic (Page et al, 1994). Symptom-free AF is usually discovered incidentally during cardiac auscultation, 12-lead ECG recording, of 24 h Holter recording undertaken for unrelated reasons. Very often the patient may have presented because of associated medical problems such as heart failure. The duration of AF may be unknown in such patients, and whether AF was the cause of effect of heart failure may be uncertain.

Most symptomatic patients with recent-based AF present with symptoms related to the arrhythmia. Patients admitted with AF can have a wide variety of cardio-respiratory presenting symptoms and clinical features, including syncope and stroke (Lip et al, 1994, Levy et al, 1999) (Tables 9.1 and 9.2). Symptoms associated with AF can vary depending on several factors, including the ventricular rate, cardiac function, concomitant medical problems, and individual patient perception.

Occasionally, certain patterns to patients' symptoms may give a clue to the underlying pathophysiology. For example, Coumel and colleagues (1994) have described a vagal and adrenergic form of AF based upon differences in clinical presentation. In brief, the vagal form is predominant in men, with age of onset at 40 to 50 years, and a higher prevalence of lone AF. Vagal AF is usually preceded by bradycardia, and there is a tendency for its occurrence at night, during rest, after eating, or with absorption of alcohol. Importantly, beta-blockers and digoxin may increase the frequency of the vagal form of AF. By contrast, the adrenergic form of AF form is less common than the vagal type, and tends to occur only during daytime, being preceded by exercise, adrenergic stimuli (such as exercise), and emotional stress. Beta-blockers are usually the treatment of choice in adrenergic AF.

Broadly, the clinical features and presenting symptoms associated with AF can be divided into those related to haemodynamic effects and thromboembolism.

	Total (n = 591)						
	Total	*SR (n = 181)*	*AF (n = 410)*	*P value SR/AF*	*Paroxysmal*	*Chronic*	*Recent Onset*
LA diameter, mm	43.8 ± 8.6	39.7 ± 7.6	45.5 ± 8.5	$p < 0.001$	40.0 ± 7.9	46.5 ± 8.8	41.5 ± 7.1
LVM-index, g/m^2	133.7 ± 52.6	130.7 ± 58.6	134.9 ± 50.1	NS	138.2 ± 70.0	136.9 ± 46.4	122.3 ± 45.5
EF, %	58.7 ± 12.9	61.4 ± 12.5	57.3 ± 12.9	$p < 0.01$	63.3 ± 11.1	56.9 ± 12.4	58.4 ± 13.7
FS, %	32.1 ± 8.2	33.9 ± 7.7	31.5 ± 8.2	$p < 0.001$	34.7 ± 8.7	31.6 ± 8.3	31.1 ± 7.8
Calcification of MV annulus, No. (%) of patients	156 (26.4)	. . .	. . .		22 (18.0)	86 (26.1)	48 (28.2)

SR indicates sinus rhythm; LA, left atrium; LVM, left ventricular mass index calculated using the Devereux and Reichek formula; FS, fractional shortening; and mV, mitral valve.
Reproduced with permission from Levy et al (1999).

Table 9.2
Echocardiographic findings.

Haemodynamic effects

Mild symptoms associated with AF include palpitation, a sense of the heart racing, fatigue, lightheadedness, increased urination, or mild shortness of breath. Pre-syncope, dizziness, fatigue, exercise intolerance, and dyspnoea are not uncommon. These symptoms are usually related to loss of atrial transport, but prolonged uncontrolled irregular ventricular rates can lead to ventricular dilatation and reduced left ventricular function — the so-called "tachycardia-induced cardiomyopathy".

More severe symptoms related to the haemodynamic effects of AF include congestive heart failure, angina, hypotension, presyncope, or (infrequently) syncope. Angina may develop consequent upon fast heart rates in uncontrolled AF, whilst cardiac ischaemia may cause angina and occasionally precipitate AF. Since both heart failure and AF are commonly associated with heart disease, and both conditions are common and co-exist, it is often difficult to distinguish whether the development of AF lead to heart failure, or whether high intracardiac (or intra-atrial) pressures in heart failure led to the development of AF.

Syncope is a rare but serious complication of AF, and is common in patients with sinus node disease or structural heart disease such as hypertrophic cardiomyopathy. In one study, patients with AF who present with syncope often showed periods of ventricular standstill with 24 h Holter monitoring, and such patients would benefit from pacemaker therapy (Rebello and Brownlie, 1987).

Thromboembolic sequelae

AF may nevertheless present for the first time with symptoms relating to a stroke or thromboembolism. The latter may include systemic thromboembolisation to the leg (leading to acute limb ischaemia) or to organs such as the kidneys (causing infarction). This topic is addressed in detail in Chapter 16. Very rarely, right sided thrombi may lead to pulmonary thromboemboli.

AF and acute myocardial infarction (AMI)

Occasionally, AF can be present in a patient admitted with AMI. In such patients, the presence of AF is an adverse feature, with a higher mortality compared with those who do not develop AF; this is due to the association of AF with large infarctions and significant left ventricular impairment (Sakata et al, 1997; Pedersen et al, 1999; Behar et al, 1992; Crenshaw et al, 1997; Rathore et al, 2000).

In the TRAndolapril Cardiac Evaluation (TRACE) study, a total of 1395 (21%) patients had AF or atrial flutter during hospital admission: they were significantly older, with a significantly greater proportion of women, more extensive left ventricular systolic dysfunction, less frequent use of thrombolytic therapy, and more anterior Q wave myocardial infarction. The unadjusted in-hospital mortality rate was significantly higher in patients with AF or atrial flutter (18%) than in patients without AF or atrial flutter (9%, $p < 0.001$). After adjustment for baseline characteristics, the presence of AF or atrial flutter was still associated with increased in-hospital mortality (odds ratio 1.5 [95% CI 1.2–1.8]). In patients surviving beyond their hospital stay, the unadjusted 5-year mortality rate was also significantly higher in patients with AF or atrial flutter (56%) than in patients without AF or atrial flutter (34% $p < 0.001$). After adjustment for important prognostic baseline characteristics, the presence of AF or atrial flutter was still associated with an increased mortality (relative risk 1.3 [95% CI 1.2–1.4]).

Sustained AF or atrial flutter during hospital stay was associated with the highest risk of dying after AMI (relative risk 1.4 [95% CI 1.2–1.7]). Thus, AF or atrial flutter often occurs after AMI and is an independent predictor of an increased short and long-term mortality (Pedersen et al, 1999).

In the study by Sakata (1997), patients with AF and AMI were divided into three groups: AF group 1 (n = 45) who developed AF within 24 h of the onset of AMI; AF group 2 (n = 41) who developed AF more than 24 h after the onset of AMI; and AF group 3 (n = 14), who developed AF before the onset of AMI. The infarct-related lesion was most common (67%) in the proximal right coronary artery in AF group 1. In the acute phase, the frequencies of heart failure, cardiogenic shock, and in-hospital mortality were higher for all three AF groups than for patients in sinus rhythm ($p < 0.01$). Importantly, the long-term survival rate was significantly lower in AF group 1 and AF group 2 than in the sinus group, with AF being an independent predictor of cardiac death in AF group 1 (odds ratio 2.5 [95% CI 1.2–5.0]); $p = 0.0012$) and AF group 2 (3.7 [1.8–7.5]); $p = 0.0005$), but not in AF group 1. Thus the onset time of AF in AMI appears to be a useful measurement to assess the cardiac status and prognosis of patients with AMI.

AF in the setting of AMI may also independently predict stroke. In the GUSTO-I (Global Utilization of Streptokinase and TPA for Occluded Coronary Arteries) trial, the clinical predictors and the angiographic and clinical outcomes associated with AF in the setting of AMI reported that patients with AF more often had three-vessel coronary artery disease and initial thrombolysis in myocardial infarction (TIMI) grade <3 flow than those without the arrhythmia (Crenshaw et al, 1997). In-hospital stroke was significantly increased in patients with AF (3.1% *vs* 1.3%), with mainly ischemic stroke (1.8% *vs* 0.5%). Other significant multivariable predictors of later AF included advanced age, higher peak creatine kinase levels, worse Killip class, and increased heart rate. The unadjusted mortality rate was significantly higher at 30 days (14.3% *vs* 6.2%) and at 1 year (21.5% *vs* 8.6%) in patients with AF. More aggressive treatment strategies in this subgroup may be warranted and deserve further study.

Similar observations were made in the SPRINT study (Behar et al, 1992) with respect to paroxysmal AF: the incidence of paroxysmal AF among 5803 consecutive hospital admitted patients with myocardial infarction was 9.9%, especially in patients who were older, female, or had congestive heart failure. Hospital mortality was significantly higher (25.5%) in patients with paroxysmal AF than in those without (16.2%), although the effect of paroxysmal AF disappeared when other factors influencing the short term prognosis (ie, heart failure) were taken into account by multivariate logistic regression analysis. The 1-year and 5-year mortality rates were 18.6% and 43.3% in patients with paroxysmal AF, compared with 8.2% and 25.4%, respectively, in patients free of paroxysmal AF. Thus, the net risk of dying among patients with paroxysmal AF complicating the acute myocardial infarction is estimated at 1.28 (90% CI 1.12–1.46) relative to those patients free of the complication.

Complications of AF

Mortality

The presence of non-rheumatic AF is associated with a 5-fold increase in mortality, especially from stroke and thromboembolism, heart failure, and other cardiovascular events. AF is also associated with concomitant heart disease, and hence much of the morbidity and mortality associated with AF can be related to the cardiovascular system. The most recent analysis from the Framingham study reported that AF was independently associated with an odds ratio for death of 1.5 for men and 1.9 for women, which did not vary by age (Benjamin et al, 1998). Most of the excess of mortality attributed to AF occurred soon after diagnosis of AF, and there was a significant interaction between AF and sex with respect to mortality.

Mortality is also greater amongst patients with AF who present with a stroke. Reports from the Copenhagen Stroke Study (Jorgensen et al, 1997) and the Framingham study (Lin et al, 1996) have also suggested that patients with AF who develop a stroke have higher mortality, greater disability, and more severe strokes, with a longer duration of in-hospital stay and lower rate of discharge to their own homes (also Chapter 16). In one Glasgow study, patients admitted with acute severe stroke who also had AF (25%) had a significantly higher hospital mortality than patients in sinus rhythm (67% *vs* 44%) (Lowe et al, 1983). The Oxfordshire community stroke project also found that patients with acute stroke and AF (17%) had a threefold higher 30-day mortality than patients in sinus rhythm (Sandercock et al, 1992).

Heart failure

AF is present in about a third (range 10–50%) of patients with chronic heart failure, and it may be a cause or a consequence of the heart failure (Figure 9.3). In a survey of AF amongst AF acute medical admissions to a district general hospital in Glasgow, heart failure was present in 36% (Lip et al, 1995). Predisposing causes for AF in patients with heart failure should be considered, including mitral valve disease, thyrotoxicosis, and sinus node disease. Importantly, sinus node disease may be associated with bradycardias, which might be exacerbated by antiarrhythmic treatment. The presence of heart failure is of particular relevance since it increases the risk of stroke and thromboembolism in AF (SPAF Investigators, 1992). The most recent meta-analysis from the AF Investigators suggested that only moderate to severe left ventricular systolic dysfunction on two-dimensional transthoracic echocardiography independently predicted stroke (AF Investigators, 1998). As previously discussed, AF in the context of severe left ventricular dysfunction after myocardial infarction also leads to a bad prognosis.

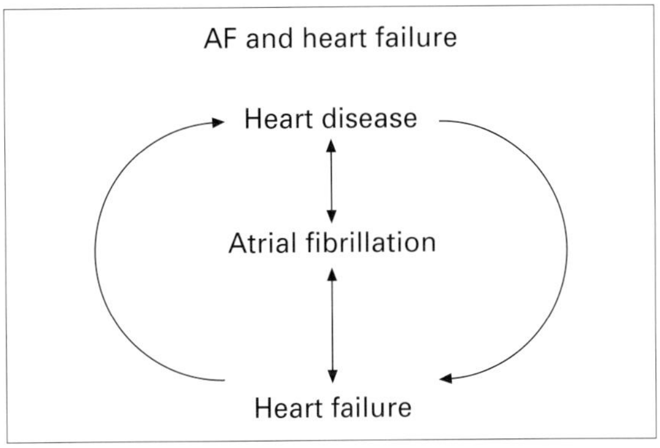

Figure 9.3
AF and heart disease.

In a recent report from the Study of Left Ventricular Dysfunction (SOLVD) group, the presence of AF was significantly associated on multivariate analysis with an increase in all-cause mortality (relative risk 1.34 [95% CI 1.12–1.62], p = 0.002), an increase risk of progressive pump failure death (1.42 [1.09–1.85], p = 0.01) and risk of death or hospital readmission (1.26 [1.03–1.42], p = 0.02); (Dries et al, 1998) (Table 9.3). Thus, the presence of AF in patients with symptom-free and symptomatic left ventricular

%	AF	SR	p
All cause mortality	34	23	<0.001
Death from pump failure	16.7	9.4	<0.001
Death or hospitalization for HF	45	33	<0.001
Arrhythmic death	2.5	2.2	0.36
Multivariate analysis	AF significantly associated with		
• All cause mortality	RR 1.34 [1.12–1.62, p = 0.002]		
• Progressive pump failure death	1.42 [1.09–1.85, p = 0.01]		
• Death or rehospitalisation	1.26 [1.03–1.42, p = 0.02]		

Table 9.3
Af and LV dysfunction ± symptoms. Reproduced for SOLVD Investigators (1998).

Study and country of origin	*Stroke rate AF vs no AF (%/year) Relative risk (RR)*	*Mortality AF vs AF (%/year); Relative risk (RR)*	*Comment*
British Regional Heart,	0.3; RR 2.3	–	General practice sample
Busselton, Australia	–	RR 1.92	Prospective study in elderly population; 2–17 year follow-up
Edinburgh, Scotland, UK	–	67.0 vs 27.3; RR 2.3	Prospective study of elderly population; 5 year follow-up
Framingham, USA	4.1; RR 5.6	(All cause) men 59.2 vs 34.3; RR 1.7 women: 44.9 vs 25.3; RR 1.8	Population sample, 24 year follow-up
Manitoba Follow-up Study, Canada	RR 2.07	RR 1.31	Prospective study amongst male air crew recruits; 44 year follow-up
Reykjavik, Iceland	4.4; RR 7.1	32.0 vs 20.0; RR 1.9	Population sample, 14 year follow-up
Shibata, Japan	RR 5.56	–	Prospective population study of stroke, 6.5 year follow-up
Whitehall, UK	1.8; RR 6.9	RR 2.6	Male civil servants screened; 18 year follow-up

Table 9.4
Stroke rates and mortality in AF: examples of studies in the literature.

systolic dysfunction is associated with an increased risk for all-cause mortality, largely explained by an increased risk for pump-failure death, consistent with the possibility that AF is associated with progression of left ventricular systolic dysfunction.

Nevertheless, the recent report by Mahoney and colleagues (1999) on 234 consecutive

	Patients with atrial fibrillation at any time			Patients with atrial fibrillation before stroke		
	No	%	95% Confidence interval	No	%	95% Confidence interval
Types of stroke:						
Cerebral infarction (n = 545)	97	18	15 to 21	61	63	52 to 72
Primary intracerebral haemorrhage (n = 66)	7	11	4 to 11	5	71	29 to 96
Subarachnoid haemorrhage (n = 33)	0	0	0 to 11	0	0	
Transient ischaemic attack (n = 184)	26	14	9 to 19	Not known	Not known	

Reproduced with permission from Sandercock et al (1992).

Table 9.5
Prevalence of atrial fibrillation in different types of stroke and subtypes of cerebral infarction: Oxfordshire Community Stroke Project.

patients (27% with AF) referred for heart transplantation found that the 1-year event-free survival was 48%, with no difference in event-free survival between patients with and without AF. Predictors of decreased event-free survival included: advanced New York Heart Association class; higher pulmonary capillary wedge pressure; lower cardiac index; lower maximum exercise oxygen consumption; use of inotropic therapy; and greater pulmonary artery systolic pressure. Thus, AF in patients with advanced heart failure is not associated with decreased event-free survival, suggesting that AF may simply reflect other adverse haemodynamic effects related to heart failure.

Stroke and thromboembolism

Non-rheumatic AF has generally been associated with a 5-fold increase in the risk of ischaemic stroke compared with that of sinus rhythm, and with a 5–7% yearly risk that increases with age (Chesebro et al, 1990). In the Framingham study, for example, the annual rate of stroke for patients in AF was about 4% (Wolf et al, 1987), which was similar to those in two other studies — the Copenhagen AFASAK study and the Stroke Prevention in Atrial Fibrillation Study — in which the annual incidence of stroke among patients on placebo was 4.9% (Petersen et al, 1989; SPAF 1991).

In several large epidemiological studies (Table 9.4), the stroke rate varied between 0.3% and 4.6% per year. In the Oxfordshire Community Stroke Project, prior AF was noted in about 15% of patients with thrombotic stroke, although up to 11% of patients had stroke due to intracerebral haemorrhage had AF (Sandercock et al, 1992) (Table 9.5). Hence caution is needed in immediately anticoagulating all patients presenting with cerebrovascular event who also have AF, because it is inaccurate to presume that all patients with AF have thromboembolic stroke. This also poses the question of whether AF predisposes to stroke (as is likely in most cases) or whether in some cases, the acute illness leads to AF. Systemic thromboembolism in AF is not uncommon, although it is given less prominence compared with strokes.

As discussed above, the presence of AF in a patient with a stroke is associated with a higher mortality and morbidity, with greater disability, longer hospital stays, lower Barthel scores, and a lower discharge rate to the patient's own home (Lin et al, 1996; Jorgensen et al, 1997; Lowe et al, 1983). AF in association with acute stroke is also associated with a 1.5–3.0-fold higher mortality than that for stroke patients who are in sinus rhythm.

There is a clear relation between stroke rate and age in patients with AF. In the pooled analysis of the AF trials, for example, the annual stroke rate in patients with AF but without coexistent cardiac disease was 1.6% in those aged 60–69 years old, 2.1% in those aged 70–79 years, and 3.0% in those over age 80 (AF Investigators, 1994). In elderly patients (mean age 79.3 years), the presence of non-valvular AF is also an important factor in fatal massive cerebral infarction (Yamanouchi et al, 1989). Computed tomography studies have also shown that silent ischaemic cerebral infarction is present in 26% of patients with non-rheumatic AF (Petersen et al, 1987).

References

Atrial Fibrillation Investigators. Echocardiographic predictors of stroke in patients with atrial fibrillation: a prospective study of 1066 patients from three clinical trials. *Arch Intern Med* 1998; **158:** 1316–20.

Atrial Fibrillation Investigators. Risk factors for stroke and efficacy of antithrombotic therapy in atrial fibrillation. *Arch Intern Med* 1994; **154:** 1449–57.

Behar S, Zahavi Z, Goldbourt U, Reicher-Reiss H. Long-term prognosis of patients with paroxysmal atrial fibrillation complicating acute myocardial infarction. SPRINT Study Group. *Eur Heart J* 1992; **13:** 45–50.

Benjamin EJ, Wolf PA, D'Agostino RB et al. Impact of atrial fibrillation on the risk of death. *Circulation* 1998; **98:** 946–52.

Bialy D, Lehmann MH, Schumacher DN et al. Hospitalisation for arrhythmias in the United States: importance of atrial fibrillation. *J Am Coll Cardiol* 1992; **19:** 41A.

Chesebro JH, Fuster V, Halperin HL. Atrial fibrillation — risk marker for stroke. *N Engl J Med* 1990; **323:** 1556–8.

Coumel P. Paroxysmal atrial fibrillation: a disorder of autonomic tone? *Eur Heart J* 1994 **15(suppl A):** 9–16.

Crenshaw BS, Ward SR, Granger CB et al. Atrial fibrillation in the setting of acute myocardial infarction: the GUSTO-I experience. Global Utilization of Streptokinase and TPA for Occluded Coronary Arteries. *J Am Coll Cardiol* 1997; **30(2):** 406–13.

Dries DL, Exner DV, Gersh BJ et al. Atrial fibrillation is associated with an increased risk for mortality and heart failure progression in patients with asymptomatic and symptomatic left ventricular dysfunction: a retrospective analysis of the SOLVD trials. *J Am Coll Cardiol* 1998; **32:** 695–703.

Jorgensen HS, Nakajama H, Reith J et al. Stroke recurrence: predictors, severity, and prognosis. The Copenhagen Stroke Study. *Neurology* 1997; **48:** 891–5.

Levy S, Maarek M, Coumel P et al. Characterization of different subsets of atrial fibrillation in general practice in France. The ALFA study. *Circulation* 1999; **99:** 3028–35.

Lin HJ, Wolf PA, Kelly-Hayes M et al. Stroke severity in atrial fibrillation. The Framingham Study. *Stroke* 1996; **27:** 1760–4.

Lip GYH. How would I manage a 60-year-old woman presenting with atrial fibrillation? *Proc R Coll Physicians Edinb* 1999; **29:** 301–6.

Lip GYH, Golding DJ, Nazir M et al. A survey of atrial fibrillation in general practice: The West Birmingham Atrial Fibrillation Project. *Br J Gen Pract* 1997; **47:** 285–9.

Lip GYH, Tean KN, Dunn FG. Treatment of atrial fibrillation in a district general hospital. *Br Heart J* 1994; **71:** 92–5.

Lowe GDO, Jaap AJ, Forbes CD. Relation of atrial fibrillation and high haematocrit to mortality in acute stroke. *Lancet* 1983; **1:** 784–6.

Mahoney P, Kimmel S, DeNofrio D et al. Prognostic significance of atrial fibrillation in patients at a tertiary medical center referred for heart transplantation because of severe heart failure. *Am J Cardiol* 1999; **83:** 1544–7.

Page RL, Wilkinson WE, Clair WK et al. Asymptomatic arrhythmias in patients with symptomatic paroxysmal atrial fibrillation and paroxysmal supraventricular tachycardia. *Circulation* 1994; **89:** 224–7.

Pedersen OD, Bagger H, Kober L, Torp-Pedersen C. The occurrence and prognostic significance of atrial fibrillation/-flutter following acute myocardial infarction. *Eur Heart J* 1999; **20:** 748–54.

Petersen P, Boysen G, Godtfredsen J et al. Placebo controlled, randomised trial of warfarin and aspirin for prevention of thromboembolic complications in chronic atrial fibrillation: the Copenhagen AFASAK study. *Lancet* 1989; **1:** 175–9.

Petersen P, Madsen EB, Brun B et al. Silent cerebral infarction in chronic atrial fibrillation. *Stroke* 1987; **18:** 1098–100.

Rathore SS, Berger AK, Weinfurt KP et al. Acute myocardial infarction complicated by atrial fibrillation in the elderly. *Circulation* 2000; **101:** 969–74.

Rebello R, Brownlee WC. Intermittent ventricular standstill during chronic atrial fibrillation in patients with dizziness or syncope. *PACE* 1987; **10:** 1271–6.

Sakata K, Kurihara H, Iwamori K et al. Clinical and prognostic significance of atrial fibrillation in acute myocardial infarction. *Am J Cardiol* 1997; **80:** 1522–7.

Sandercock P, Bamford J, Dennis M et al. Atrial fibrillation and stroke: prevalence in different types of stroke and influence on early and long term prognosis (Oxfordshire Community Stroke Project). *BMJ* 1992; **305:** 1460–5.

Sopher SM, Camm AJ. Atrial fibrillation: maintenance of sinus rhythm versus rate control. *Am J Cardiol* 1996; **77:** 24A–37A.

Stroke Prevention in Atrial Fibrillation Investigators. Stroke Prevention in Atrial Fibrillation Study. Final results. *Circulation* 1991; **84:** 527–39.

Stroke Prevention in Atrial Fibrillation Investigators. Predictors of thromboembolism in atrial fibrillation: I. Clinical features of patients at risk. *Ann Intern Med* 1992; **116:** 1–5.

Wolf PA, Abott RD, Kannell WB. Atrial fibrillation: a major contributor to stroke in the elderly. The Framingham Study. *Arch Intern Med* 1987; **147:** 1561–4.

Yamanouchi H, Tomonaga M, Shimada H et al. Novalvular atrial fibrillation as a cause of fatal massive cerebral infarction in the elderly. *Stroke* 1989; **20:** 1653–6.

Zarifis J, Beevers DG, Lip GYH. Acute admissions with atrial fibrillation in a British multiracial hospital population. *Br J Clin Pract* 1997; **51:** 91–6.

V
Investigation of Atrial Fibrillation

10

Basic investigations and initial assessment

Basic investigations and initial assessment

Basic investigations and initial assessment of the new patient with atrial fibrillation (AF) will address the following: whether it is actually AF; if so, why has the patient developed it; what management strategy should be followed; and how should we approach the patient. Inconsistencies are common, even amongst consultant physicians, over the management of AF, with wide variation in treatment options and more cardiologists than non-cardiologists considering cardioversion and antithrombotic therapy (Lip et al, 1996).

Thus, the approach to a patient with AF requires a careful clinical history (including past medical history) with emphasis on certain clinical features, for example, whether the symptoms are sustained or intermittent, and whether any complications (such as heart failure, stroke, or thromboembolism) are present. The date of the first episode, precipitants, relief of the occurrence, the type of AF (for example recent onset, paroxysmal, persistent, or permanent), the frequency or duration of symptomatic AF episodes, the duration of the current or last episode, and previous drug treatments are useful information. In addition, it is important to assess the patient for potentially reversible causes of AF such as thyroid disease. Associated problems, such as congestive heart failure, stroke or thromboembolism, pulmonary problems, hypertension, or hyperthyroidism should be managed. An assessment of the urgency of heart rate slowing is needed, for example, in a patient presenting with fast AF.

Initial basic investigations and assessment in a patient presenting de novo with AF should include blood tests, chest radiography and ECG (Table 10.1). As with any arrhythmia, AF should first be documented before treatment is begun. Transthoracic (and in some cases, transoesophageal) echocardiography is generally desirable to assess cardiac size and valvular function, to refine risk stratification for thromboprophylaxis, and, in patients about to undergo cardioversion, to detect the possible presence of left atrial thrombi.

Blood tests and chest radiography

At the initial consultation, basic blood tests including full blood count, biochemistry (renal function, electrolytes), and thyroid-function tests should be done. A full blood count is useful, especially when anticoagulants are considered. Serum urea and electrolytes are relevant for consideration of drug therapy (for example, electrolyte abnormalities may interfere with antiarrhythmic drug use, and reduced dose of digoxin may be needed in renal

Blood tests
- Full blood count — especially when anticoagulants considered
- Urea and electrolytes — baseline, and for consideration of drug therapy (e.g. reduced dose of digoxin in renal impairment)
- Thyroid function tests

ECG and Ambulatory ECG recording
- 12-lead ECG
- Consider 24-hour Holter monitor — if patients presents with syncope, and paroxysmal atrial fibrillation or sick sinus syndrome suspected
- Consider Cardiomemo — if symptoms only intermittent and infrequent

Chest X-ray

Echocardiography
- Standard transthoracic echocardiography and Doppler
- Consider transoesophageal echocardiography — if prosthetic mitral valve in situ, endocarditis or atrial thrombi suspected.

Table 10.1
Atrial fibrillation — "standard investigations".

impairment). The risk of AF is increased in subclinical hyperthyroidism, and thus the serum thyroid stimulating hormone (TSH) level should be measured in all patients with AF, even if there are no symptoms to suggest thyrotoxicosis. This is particularly important in the elderly, in whom the signs and symptoms of thyroid disease may be masked. Patients with low TSH values (<0.5 mU/L with the newer sensitive assays) and normal thyroid hormone levels probably have subclinical hyperthyroidism (Forfar and Toft, 1982; Forfar 1997).

Chest radiography may occasionally be useful in patients with AF. For example, in the young patient with AF, it may give a clue to the presence of underlying congenital heart disease, such as atrial septal defect. In older patients, chest radiography can give some information on heart size and the presence of heart failure or intrathoracic pathology. Chest radiography may also give clues about the underlying cause of AF, such as a lung tumour, pneumonia, or pleural effusion. For example, a large globular heart on chest radiography may suggest a pericardial effusion, whilst pericardial calcification raises the suspicion of constrictive pericarditis.

Documentation of the arrhythmia

The arrhythmia should be documented, initially with a 12-lead standard ECG if possible. In AF, the ECG characteristically shows rapid oscillations of "f" waves that vary in size, shape, and timing, and the absence of consistent P wave before each QRS complex. There is usually an irregularly irregular ventricular rate, although fairly regular "R-R" intervals are still possible in the presence of idioventricular or idiojunctional rhythms associated with the conduction system disease or drug therapy, and in patients with ventricular pacemakers. Nevertheless, the ECG may provide a clue to the aetiology or electrophysiological features that may have caused AF, for example, the presence of ischaemic heart disease (prior myocardial infarction), left ventricular hypertrophy, or pre-excitation (delta wave in Wolff-Parkinson-White syndrome if in sinus rhythm).

A 24 h Holter monitor may be required to document paroxysmal AF or the sick sinus syndrome (Figure 10.1). However, this investigation is unlikely to be useful in patients who have only intermittent and infrequent symptoms, for example palpitations. In such patients, a cardiomemo (or transtelephonic event monitor) may be preferred. This is a device that allows the transmission of an ECG trace via telephone, whereby the patient may record an ECG during an episode of palpitations.

Echocardiography

Most cardiologists would request on echocardiogram for their patients with AF. In most patients with AF, echocardiography would help diagnose the presence of structural heart disease and document cardiac function. The information from echocardiography may also be helpful in determining the cause of AF.

Echocardiography is useful for the detection of left ventricular hypertrophy, assessment of focal wall motion abnormalities (secondary to myocardial infarction), and detection of infrequent causes of AF, such as pericardial disease (pericardial effusion, etc), cardiac tumours (myxoma), and pulmonary thromboemboli (dilated and poorly functioning right ventricle). Echocardiography can also detect occult mitral valve disease, which may initially present with AF, often in the setting of a stroke or acute thromboembolism. Indeed, doppler echocardiography is particularly useful for the careful assessment of valvular heart disease.

Echocardiography can potentially refine risk stratification for stroke and thromboembolism in AF (Lip, 1999). The most recent meta-analyses from the AF Investigators (1998) reported that only left ventricular function was an independent risk factor for stroke and thromboembolism on multivariate analysis. Contrary to previous reports, isolated left atrial enlargement was not an independent risk factor, as discussed further below. Nevertheless the value of adding echocardiography to clinical risk factors for stroke risk stratification has been subject to much discussion. The Newcastle survey reported that echocardiography would be useful in the minority of (mainly younger) patients with AF who did not have any clinical risk factors for stroke and thromboembolism (Sudlow et al, 1998). Echocardiography may also help to stratify the likelihood of successful cardioversion to sinus rhythm, and the risk of recurrent AF after cardioversion (for example, poor left ventricular function or mitral stenosis would be an unfavourable sign).

Recently, transoesophageal echocardiography (TOE) has provided a useful means of identifying left atrial appendage thrombi, especially if a mitral prosthetic valve is in situ. Additionally, the role of TOE in guiding cardioversion management, by detecting atrial appendage thrombi, and shortening and simplifying anticoagulation regimes, is being evaluated (Klein et al, 1997; Manning et al, 1993; Manning et al, 1995a/b).

Left atrial size and atrial thrombi

Transthoracic echocardiography is particularly helpful in assessing left atrial size in AF. Left atrial dilatation is common in AF, especially in patients with mitral valve disease or hypertension. Although a dilated left atrium can lead to

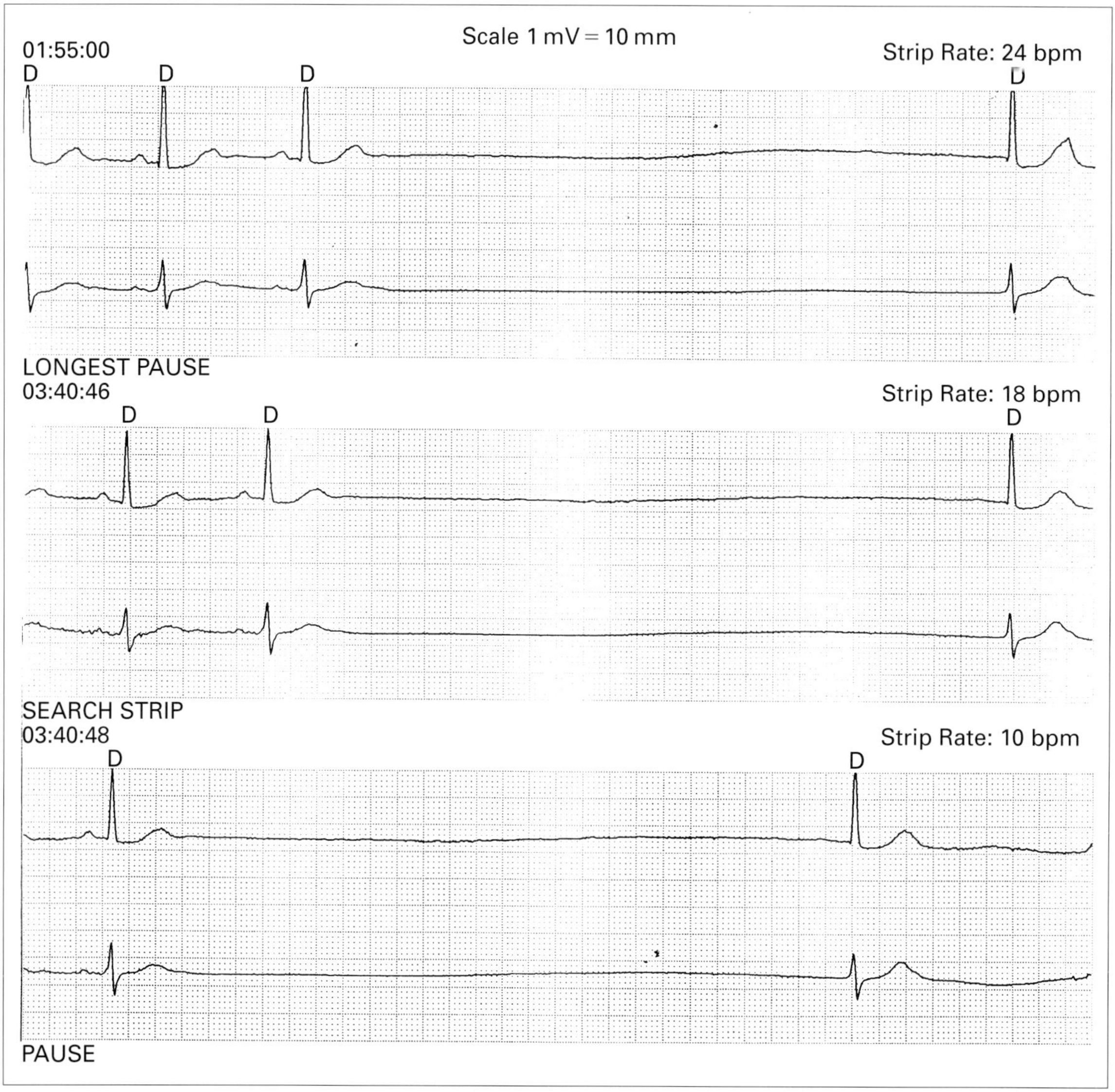

Figure 10.1
24° Holter trace showing sick sinus syndrome.

AF, sustained AF itself can itself lead to a further increase in left atrial size, which is reversible with cardioversion and maintenance of sinus rhythm (Sanfillippo, 1990; Manning, 1989). Transthoracic echocardiography is less useful for imaging left atrial thrombi and assessing left atrial appendage anatomy and function, and a TOE is preferred (Silverman and Manning, 1998).

The presence of left atrial enlargement probably reduces the chances of successful cardioversion and long-term maintenance of sinus rhythm, although not all series are consistent on this point (Dittrich 1989; Hoglund et al, 1985). It is more likely that the duration of prior AF is the more important consideration when assessing the likelihood of successful cardioversion (Lip, 1996). Left atrial dilatation was reported to increase the risk of stroke in the SPAF-1 study (SPAF Investigators, 1992), and this finding is in keeping with increased left atrial spontaneous echocontrast on transoesophageal echocardiography (indicating greater stasis) in more dilated atria (Fatkin et al, 1994; Tsai 1992). Nevertheless, the most recent meta-analysis from the AF Investigators of 1066 patients from three clinical trials suggested that isolated left atrial dilatation was not an independent predictor of stroke risk on multivariate analysis (AF Investigators, 1998).

The sensitivity and specificity of TOE for left atrial thrombi in patients in whom the left atrium was directly examined at surgery are 93–100% and 99–100%, respectively (Silverman and Manning, 1998) (Table 10.2). The prevalence of left atrial thrombi is increased in patients with mitral stenosis, left ventricular systolic dysfunction, dilatation of the left atrium or left atrial appendage, reduced left atrial appendage doppler velocities, dense spontaneous echocontrast, or a recent thromboembolic event (Fatkin et al, 1994; Verhorst et al, 1993; Fatkin et al, 1997; Black et al, 1991). However, TOE evidence of left atrial thrombi is seen in up to 27% of patients presenting with AF of more than 3 days' duration (Manning et al, 1995b, Rubin et al, 1996). Even in patients with acute-onset AF (≤48 h), the prevalence of left atrial appendage thrombi can be as high as 15%, with important implications for antithrombotic therapy usage (Stoddard et al, 1995).

Spontaneous echocontrast

Spontaneous echocontrast (or "smoke") refers to the presence of dynamic, smoke-like echoes seen during TOE in over 50% of all patients with AF and in over 80% if left atrial appendage thrombi are present (Manning et al, 1995b). The presence of "smoke" is associated with an increased risk of stroke and thromboembolism, but neither aspirin nor warfarin affects the presence of echocontrast. Spontaneous echocontrast is believed to represent stasis and is formed by erythrocyte aggregation in low shear rate conditions, mediated by plasma proteins (especially fibrinogen) promoting red cell rouleaux formation (Fatkin, 1997). The intermittent development of spontaneous echocontrast has been noted to correspond to paroxysms of AF, indicating intermittent atrial stasis during these paroxysms (Obarski et al, 1990).

Mitral valve function

Mitral valve disease is common in AF, and transthoracic echocardiography is useful in the assessment of valvular function. Moderate to severe mitral regurgitation appears to protect against clinical thromboembolism in chronic AF, presumably by reducing stasis within the left atrium and atrial appendage (Manning et al, 1995a), but it does not appear to be protective against thrombus formation in new onset AF (Manning et al, 1995b). AF may also be the initial presentation of occult mitral stenosis.

Left ventricular morphology and function

Echocardiographic assessment of cardiac structure and function helps to guide the choice of therapy for ventricular rate control and antithrombotic therapy in chronic AF. For example, a beta-blocker or calcium channel blocker (diltiazem or verapamil) is recommended for rate control in patients with preserved left ventricular systolic function, whilst

Study	Probe	n	Sensitivity %	Specificity %	Accuracy
Mugge 1990	M	12	100		100
Olson 1992	M	20	100	100	100
Hwang 1993	M/B	213	93	100	99
Manning 1995	M/B/Mu	231	100	99	99
Fatkin 1996	B	60	100	93	93

M = mono; B = biplane; Mu = multiplane
i.e. Excellent sensitivity and predictive accuracy of TOE for identification and exclusion of LA thrombus

Table 10.2
TOE for left atrial thrombi. Adapted from Silverman and Manning (1998).

those with depressed systolic function may need digoxin or amiodarone. Moderate to severe left ventricular systolic dysfunction via 2-dimensional echocardiography independently predicts stroke risk in patients with AF (AF Investigators, 1998).

Other investigations

If the patient complains of angina, it should be established whether the angina occurs only during attacks of AF in view of an uncontrolled ventricular rate, or whether angina occurs independently of the arrhythmia. Exercise testing may occasionally be needed in order to clarify the severity of underlying cardiac ischaemia. However, caution with interpretation of the exercise ECG must be made if digoxin therapy is taken, as this can result in false-positive ST segment changes, making the diagnosis less reliable. AF may also limit the patient's exercise capacity. Exercise testing may also have a role in assessing the adequacy of drug treatment in heart-rate control.

If an accessory pathway is suspected (eg, AF secondary to the Wolff-Parkinson-White syndrome) electrophysiology testing is useful. Occasionally, more complex electrophysiology assessment may be needed, especially in patients with pre-excitation syndromes or focal paroxysmal AF. This may also lead to a "cure" of the disorder by transcatheter ablation of the accessor pathway. Situations in which referral to an electrophysiologist for further assessment and management may be indicated are summarised in Table 10.3.

Initial assessment

If a patient presents with acute de novo AF, it is important to assess their haemodynamic status. Indications for urgent cardioversion include the presence of haemodynamic compromise, as shown by significant hypotension. The presence of a pre-excitation syndrome may also lead to an extremely rapid ventricular rate, which could result in cardiac ischemia and cardiovascular collapse.

If the patient has only mild to moderate symptoms, treatment directed at slowing the ventricular rate will usually result in improvement or resolution of symptoms. Pharmaco-

- Poorly controlled ventricular rate despite antiarrhythmic drugs
- Congestive heart failure due to tachyarrhythmia? tachycardiomyopathy
- When medical therapy entails a higher risk than interventional options
- Poorly managed Paroxysmal AF? atrial defibrillator
- Accessory pathway suspected, e.g. WPW
- Electrophysiological studies needed e.g. focal AF, familial AF

Table 10.3
Atrial arrhythmias — When is a specialist opinion required?

logical agents that slow or block conduction through the atrioventricular node are useful, such as beta-blockers, calcium channel blockers (primarily verapamil and diltiazem), and digoxin. Appropriate antithrombotic therapy, such as intravenous heparin, should be initiated. The next step after control of the ventricular rate in patients with mild to moderate symptoms involves a decision about whether cardioversion to sinus rhythm is needed. The role for cardioversion depends upon the duration of the arrhythmia as well as the presence of a reversible aetiological factor.

AF is rarely the manifestation of an symptom-free acute cardiac ischemic event or myocardial infarction. There is therefore no reason to admit the patient to a coronary care unit to "rule out myocardial infarction", unless there are other clinical reasons to consider this diagnosis such as chest pain or an ECG that shows an acute infarct or ongoing cardiac ischaemia. Nevertheless, hospital admission is usually necessary for the treatment of other comorbidity or associated medical problems, such as a chest infection or pulmonary thromboembolism, and for treatment of those at risk of developing complications resulting from therapy.

References

Atrial Fibrillation Investigators. Echocardiographic predictors of stroke in patients with atrial fibrillation: A prospective study of 1066 patients from three clinical trials. *Arch Intern Med* 1998; **158:** 1316–20.

Black IW, Hopkins AP, Lee LC et al. Left atrial spontaneous echo contrast: a clinical and echocardiographic analysis. *J Am Coll Cardiol* 1991; **18:** 398.

Dittrich HC, Ericksson JS, Schneiderman T et al. Echocardiographic and clinical predictors for outcome of elective cardioversion of atrial fibrillation. *Am J Cardiol* 1989; **63:** 193.

Fatkin D, Kelly RP, Feneley MP. Relations between left atrial appendage blood flow velocity, spontaneous echocardiographic contrast and thromboembolic risk in vivo. *J Am Coll Cardiol* 1994; **23:** 961.

Fatkin D, Loupas T, Low J et al. Inhibition of red cell aggregation prevents spontaneous echocardiographic contrast formation in human blood. *Circulation* 1997; **96:** 889.

Forfar JC, Atrial fibrillation and the pituitary-thyroid axis—a re-evaluation. *Heart* 1997; 77(**1**): 3–4.

Forfar JC, Toft AD. Thyrotoxic atrial fibrillation: an underdiagnosed condition? *BMJ* 1982; **285:** 909–10.

Hoglund C, Rosenhame G. Echocardiographic left atrial dimension as a predictor of maintaining sinus rhythm after conversion of atrial fibrillation. *Acta Med Scand* 1985; **217:** 411.

Klein AL, Grimm RA, Black IW et al. Cardioversion guided by transoesophageal echocardiography: the ACUTE Pilot Study. A randomized, controlled trial. Assessment of Cardioversion Using Transesophageal Echocardiography. *Ann Intern Med* 1997; **126:** 200–9.

Lip GYH, Zarifis J, Watson RD, Beevers DG. Physician variation in the management of patients with atrial fibrillation. *Heart* 1996; **7:** 200–5.

Lip GYH. Thromboprophylaxis for atrial fibrillation. *Lancet* 1999; **353:** 4–6.

Manning WJ, Leeman DE, Gotch PJ et al. Pulsed Doppler evaluation of atrial mechanical function after electrical cardioversion of atrial fibrillation. *J Am Coll Cardiol* 1989; **13:** 617.

Manning WJ, Silverman DI, Gordon SPF et al. Cardioversion from atrial fibrillation without prolonged anticoagulation with use of transesophageal echocardiography to exclude the presence of atrial thrombi. *N Engl J Med* 1993; **328:** 750.

Manning WJ, Silverman DI, Keighley CS et al. Prevalence of residual left atrial thrombi in patients presenting with acute thromboembolism and newly recognized atrial fibrillation. *Arch Intern Med* 1995a; **155:** 2193.

Manning WJ, Silverman DI, Keighley CS et al. Transesophageal echocardiographically facilitated early cardioversion from atrial fibrillation using short-term anticoagulation: final results of a prospective 4.5 year study. *J Am Coll Cardiol* 1995b; **25:** 1354.

Obarski TP, Salcedo EE, Castle LW, Stewart WJ. Spontaneous echo contrast in the left atrium during paroxysmal atrial fibrillation. *Am Heart J* 1990; **120:** 988.

Rubin DN, Katz SE, Riley MF et al. Evaluation of left atrial appendage anatomy and function in recent-onset atrial fibrillation by transesophageal echocardiography. *Am J Cardiol* 1996; **78:** 774.

Sanfillippo AJ, Abascal VM, Sheehan M et al. Atrial enlargement as a consequence of atrial fibrillation. A prospective echocardiographic study. *Circulation* 1990; **82:** 792–7.

Silverman DI, Manning WJ. Role of echocardiography in patients undergoing elective cardioversion of atrial fibrillation. *Circulation* 1998; **98:** 479–86.

Stoddard ME, Dawkins PR, Prince CR, Ammash NM. Left atrial appendage thrombus is not uncommon in patients with acute atrial fibrillation and a recent embolic event: a transesophageal echocardiographic study. *J Am Coll Cardiol* 1995; **25:** 452–9.

Stroke Prevention in Atrial Fibrillation Investigators. Predictors of thromboembolism in atrial fibrillation II. Echocardiographic features of patients at risk. *Am Intern Med* 1992; **116:** 6–12.

Sudlow M, Thomson R, Thwaites B et al. Prevalence of atrial fibrillation and eligibility for anticoagulants in the community. *Lancet* 1998; **325:** 1167–71.

Tsai LM, Chen JH, Fang CJ et al. Clinical implications of left atrial spontaneous echo contrast in nonrheumatic atrial fibrillation. *Am J Cardiol* 1992; **70:** 327–31.

Verhorst PM, Kamp I, Visser CA et al. Left atrial appendage flow velocity assessment using transesophageal echocardiography in nonrheumatic atrial fibrillation and systemic embolism. *Am J Cardiol* 1993; **71:** 192.

VI
Management

11

Non-pharmacological strategies for atrial fibrillation

Introduction

If pharmacological measures fail to prevent recurrence of atrial fibrillation (AF) and control the ventricular rate, non-pharmacological strategies should be considered. These include pacemakers, electrophysiological techniques (atrioventricular node modification or ablation), and surgery. In patients with paroxysmal AF, the atrial defibrillator is a new device for treating paroxysms of AF and to maintain sinus rhythm.

Pacemaker therapy

Pacemaker therapy in AF is indicated for symptomatic low heart rates where anti-bradycardia pacing is considered. Chronic AF with symptomatic bradycardia that is related to atrioventricular block or the use of antiarrhythmic drugs may also require pacing; rate-responsive ventricular pacing (VVIR pacing mode) is usual. Patients with chronic AF and symptomatic chronotropic incompetence during exercise, resulting in limitation of exercise capacity, may require implantation of a rate adaptive VVIR pacemaker even in the absence of significant bradycardia at rest. Acquired atrioventricular block from atrioventricular nodal ablation, or from an attempt at atrioventricular nodal modification for control of ventricular rate in patients with chronic or paroxysmal AF, requires permanent pacing, usually with VVIR pacing mode, which may improve heart rate control (Figure 11.1)

In patients with the sick sinus syndrome, there is significant decrease in the incidence of AF with atrial pacing, perhaps by stabilising the atrium electrically. Atrial pacing may also prevent the development of AF that occurs during bradycardia, by reducing the atrial premature beats that may initiate AF. The average annual incidence of chronic AF is 1.5% in atrially-paced patients with sick sinus syndrome, compared with 12% in ventricular paced groups. The prospective study by

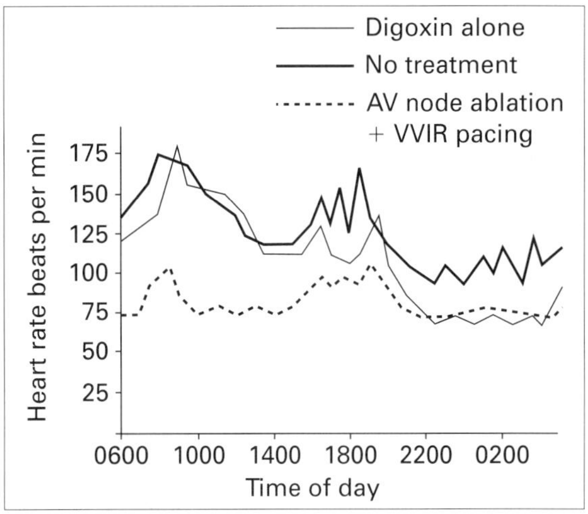

Figure 11.1
Permanent AF: heart rate over 24h on different treatments.

Andersen and colleagues (1994) of 225 patients with sick sinus syndrome showed that atrial pacing decreased the frequency of AF and the likelihood of thromboembolism (5% *vs* 17%) at a 3-year follow-up, perhaps by maintaining atrioventricular synchrony. Atrial pacing continued to give a significantly lower risk for AF, thromboembolism, heart failure, and mortality compared with ventricular pacing after 8 years of follow-up, with a low incidence of progression to atrioventricular block (Andersen et al, 1997) (Figures 11.2–11.4). Indeed, only four of 110 patients in the atrial pacing group developed grade 2 to 3 AV block that required upgrading of the pacemaker (0.6% per year), and two of these four patients had right bundle-branch block at pacemaker implantation. Furthermore, AV conduction, estimated as PQ interval and atrial stimulus-Q interval at atrial pacing rates of 100 and 120 beats/min and the Wenckebach block point, remained stable during long-term follow-up, suggesting that single-chamber atrial pacing is safe and can be recommended to patients with sick sinus syndrome but without bundle-branch block (Andersen et al, 1998).

The same investigators also reported that arterial thromboembolism in patients with sick sinus syndrome is very common, and is associated primarily with brady-tachy syndrome at randomisation and with ventricular pacing. Importantly, the risk of thromboembolism was small in atrial paced patients in whom AF had never been shown (Andersen et al, 1999).

In patients who have evidence of atrioventricular nodal disease, a dual-chamber pacemaker is often preferred. Nevertheless, the use of dual-chamber pacemakers may result in tracking of atrial rates to the upper rate limit of the pacemaker, which can be overcome by the use of a pacemaker with mode-switching capability. Such a pacemaker changes from DDDR (or DDD) to a non-tracking but atrial sensing mode (DDIR, DDI, VDIR or VDI) in the presence of an atrial tachyarrhythmia. The use of mode-switching pacemakers in patients with paroxysmal atrial tachyarrhythmia

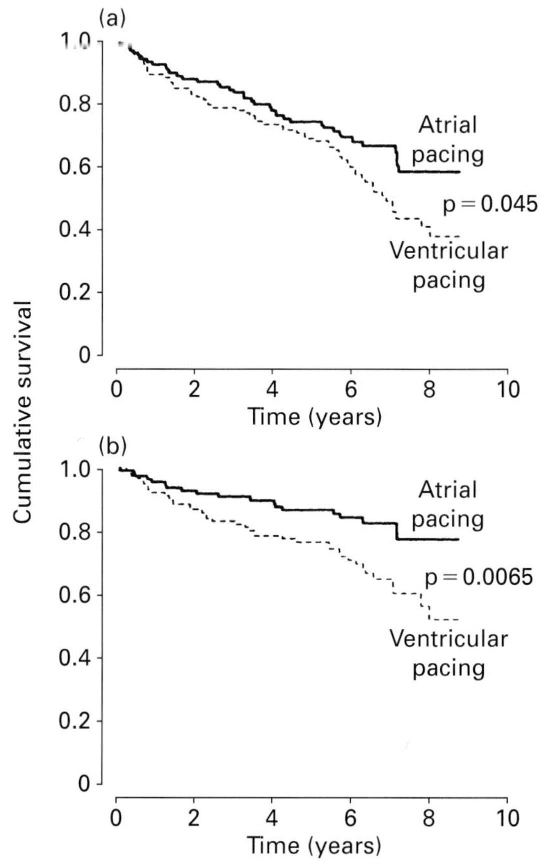

Number of patients at risk during follow-up

Atrial pacing	110	102	97	92	86	82	59	38	13
Ventricular pacing	115	103	96	91	85	80	56	29	12

Figure 11.2
Kaplan-Meier survival plots of overall survival (a) and survival from cardiovascular death (b). Reproduced with permission from Andersen et al (1997).

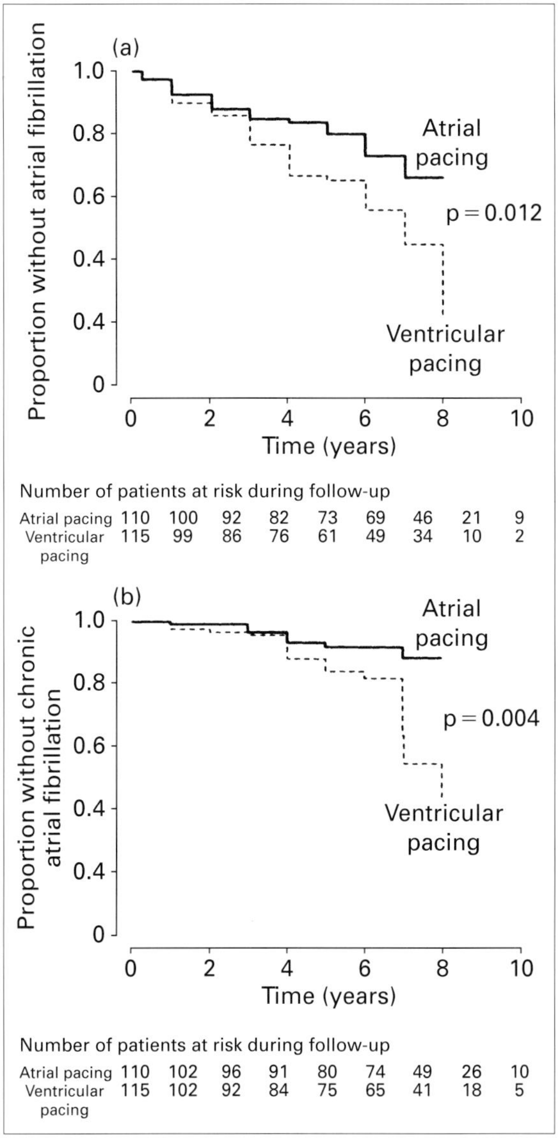

Figure 11.3
Kaplan-Meier plots of freedom from atrial fibrillation (a) and chronic AF (b) during follow-up. Reproduced with permission from Andersen et al (1997).

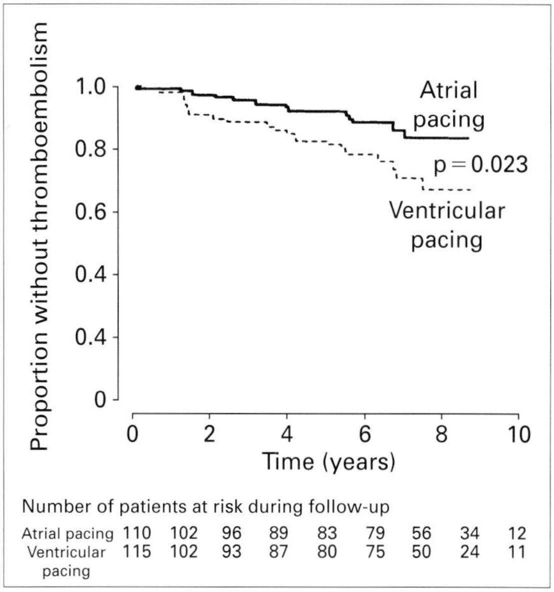

Figure 11.4
Kaplan-Meier plots of thromboembolic events (stroke and peripheral arterial embolus). Reproduced with permission from Andersen et al (1997).

improves symptoms and prolongs exercise times when compared with conventional DDDR or VVIR modes of pacing (Kamalvand, 1997).

Dual versus single site pacing may also allow suppression of AF by a reduction in atrial conduction delay (Saksena et al, 1996; Yu et al, 1997). In the study by Saksena and colleagues (1996) of patients with paroxysmal AF refractory to drug therapy alone, the frequency of AF during dual-site right atrial pacing was compared prospectively with that during single-site atrial pacing. Both forms of pacing were effective, but dual-site pacing was the more effective therapy for reducing the recurrence rate and lengthening the AF-free period.

Pacing for the prevention of AF with atrial pacing may prevent the arrhythmogenic effect of bradycardias (especially in vagally-mediated AF) and of marked heart-rate variation causing dispersion of refractoriness. Multi-site atrial pacing may also be useful in AF prevention, by increasing the coupling interval of the initiating premature beat in the abnormal substrate, either by pre-exciting the re-entry zone or by pacing at one or more sites opposite to the activation of the premature beat. Multisite atrial pacing has kept 75% of patients free of arrhythmias at a 2-year follow-up (Daubert et al, 1994).

Atrial implantable defibrillator (atrioverter)

This new therapy is currently under evaluation but initial experience is extremely encouraging. Using technology similar to that used for suppression of ventricular tachyarrhythmias, the standalone atrial defibrillator delivers low energy shocks (less than 6 joules) designed to re-establish sinus rhythm with a minimum risk of ventricular arrhythmias. The Metrix system 3020 (InControl, Redmond, USA) uses three electrodes — one in the right atrium, one in the coronary sinus (for atrial defibrillation), and one in the ventricule (for R-waves synchronisation and post-shock ventricular pacing, if necessary). The use of an atrial defibrillator is based on the concept that "AF begets AF" and that prompt reversion of AF should reduce recurrences and the risk of persistent AF.

The effectiveness of the atrioverter is illustrated by a recent prospective multicentre study of an implantable defibrillator connected to right atrial and coronary sinus defibrillation, allowing prompt restoration of sinus rhythm by a low-energy shock (Wellens et al, 1998). In 51 patients with recurrent AF who were followed-up for a mean of 259 days, 96% of 227 spontaneous episodes of AF in 41 patients were successfully converted to sinus rhythm by the atrioverter. In 27% of episodes, several shocks were required because of early recurrence of AF. Importantly, the shocks did not induce ventricular arrhythmias.

The major problems with the atrioverter are pain and the potential risk of inducing ventricular tachycardia or fibrillation. For example, one joule produces pain in a fifth of patients, and two joules produce pain in 40%. The incidence of induced ventricular fibrillation after shocks of 0.1–5.0 joules ranges from 2.0–6.5% in dogs, but this usually occurs when a shock is delivered at or just before the onset of a normal QRS complex (Keelan et al, 1997). The risk of this complication is increased if a right or left bundle branch block is present, especially if the preceding RR interval is 380 msec or less. An experimental study by Iskos and colleagues (1996) showed that use of a class III antiarrhythmic drug significantly reduced the atrial fibrillation threshold and defibrillation energy requirements. Nevertheless, use of atrioverter may provide significant symptom relief and improved quality of life in patients with paroxysmal AF who may have had severe symptoms of arrhythmia or have had many side-effects with drug therapy.

Atrioventricular node modification and atrioventricular nodal ablation

In drug-resistant, poorly tolerated AF, atrioventricular (AV) junction catheter ablation is an option. Technically, the procedure is easy and relatively safe. Atrioventricular node modification or ablation should be reserved for patients with AF in whom complete heart block and pacemaker therapy are an acceptable treatment risk. For patients with chronic

AF, a VVIR pacemaker is inserted. For those having severely symptomatic episodes of paroxysmal AF, DDDR mode-switching devices are more appropriate. This treatment is highly effective in controlling symptoms, improving general well-being, and increasing exercise capacity (Touboul, 1999). Left ventricular ejection fraction may increase after ablation, especially in patients with markedly depressed myocardial function. There is a small risk of sudden cardiac death, perhaps due to AV-block-related ventricular tachyarrhythmias, occurring early after ablation, but why some late sudden deaths occur is uncertain (Darpo et al, 1997; Twidale et al, 1998).

In the study by Darpo and colleagues (1997), 220 patients with paroxysmal AF (n = 105) or chronic AF (n = 115) were followed up for an average of 31 months after radiofrequency ablation of the AV junction and pacemaker implantation. In this study, 31 patients died, with six sudden unexplained deaths, 14 cardiovascular deaths, and 11 deaths from noncardiovascular causes; 11 patients, all with structural heart disease, died suddenly out of hospital and six of these had no obvious cause of death. The series by Geelen and colleagues (1997) showed that malignant ventricular arrhythmias and sudden death were possible complications of radiofrequency ablation of the atrioventricular function. These complications could have a bradycardia dependent nature. It seems that the occurrence of malignant arrhythmias can be prevented by temporarily pacing the heart at relatively fast rates immediately after ablation. Twidale and colleagues (1998) found that baseline ejection fraction of 30% less, presence of significant mitral regurgitation (>2+) before ablation, and failure to show improved cardiac performance by 1 month after ablation were independent predictors of death after AV node ablation in patients with heart failure and AF.

In the study by Brignole and colleagues (1997), ablation and VVIR pacemaker treatment was effective and better than drug therapy in controlling symptoms, although cardiac performance was not modified by the treatment. This was a multicentre, randomised, 6-month assessment of the clinical effects of AV junction ablation and DDDR mode-switching pacemaker ("ablate and pace") versus pharmacological treatment in 43 patients with intolerable, recurrent and resistant paroxysmal AF. At the end of 6 months, the 21 patients of the "ablate and pace" group who completed the study showed, by comparison with the 18 patients in the drug group, lower scores in the Living with Heart Failure Questionnaire (−51%), palpitations (−71%), effort dysponea (−36%), exercise intolerance score (−46%), and easy fatigue (−51%). At the end of the study, palpitations were no longer present in 81% of the "ablate and pace" group and in 11% of the drug group. AF was documented in 25% in the "ablate and pace" group and in 8% of the drug group. Chronic AF developed in 24% and 0% of the two groups, respectively.

The Ablate and Pace Trial (Kay et al, 1998) also prospectively assessed the effects of catheter ablation of the AV conduction system and permanent pacemaker implantation on health-related quality of life, survival, exercise capacity, and ventricular function in 156 patients with symptomatic AF. Survival over the first year of follow-up was significantly lower for patients with an impaired baseline left ventricular ejection fraction (LVEF <0.45), although these patients had the greatest improvement in LVEF (from 0.31 +/− 0.20 at baseline to 0.41 at 3 months and 0.41 at 12). The New York Heart Association functional class improved from 2.1 at baseline to 1.8 at 3 months and 1.9 at 12 months' follow-up

($p = 0.0001$), concurrent with significant improvements in quality of life scores and arrhythmia-related symptoms. There were no significant changes in treadmill exercise duration or VO_{2max}. Similar findings were reported by Manolis and colleagues (1998).

The recent study by Marshall and colleagues (1999) confirmed these observations, with improved quality of life, exercise tolerance, and symptoms at follow-up over 18 weeks in patients with paroxysmal AF, who had ablation and dual-chamber mode-switching (DDDR/MS) pacemakers fitted (slow algorithm [n = 19] or fast algorithm [n = 18]), compared with medical therapy (n = 19). There was a high rate of progression to persistent AF in the pacemaker group at 6 weeks (12 of 37 *vs* 0 of 19, $p < 0.01$). Thus, ablation and dual chamber mode-switching pacing produced more symptomatic benefit than medical therapy or ablation and VVIR pacing, but may result in early development of persistent AF. These observations were confirmed in a meta-analysis of 21 studies with 1181 patients (Wood et al, 2000), with 1 year total and sudden death mortality rates after "ablate and pace" of 6.3% and 2.0% respectively.

Radiofrequency ablation has been extended to develop a catheter-based technique that roughly reproduces the surgical "maze" procedure. Here, radiofrequency ablation is used to create linear non-conductive barriers to prevent intra-atrial re-entry, commonly referred to as a "catheter maze" procedure (Swartz et al, 1994; Haissaguerre et al, 1994). Ablation only in the right atrium is a safe technique with limited success, whereas linear lesions in the left atrium significantly increases the incidence of stable restoration of sinus rhythm, the inability to induce sustained AF, and the final success rate. Haissaguerre and colleagues (1996) reported 45 patients with frequent symptomatic drug-refractory episodes of paroxysmal AF in which progressively complex linear lesions were created by sequential applications of radiofrequency current to the right atrium and then to the left atrium if required. The researchers concluded that successful radiofrequency catheter ablation of drug-refractory daily paroxysmal AF was feasible using linear atrial lesions complemented by focal ablation targeted at arrhythmogenic foci. Whilst encouraging, the procedure is very long and the radiation exposure is substantial.

Some young patients with no detectable heart disease and AF due to a rapidly firing atrial foci located near the orifice or within the left pulmonary veins have been treated and cured by ablation of the atrial focus (Jais et al, 1997; Haissaguerre et al, 1998) (Figure 11.5). Jais and colleagues (1997) reported nine patients with paroxysmal focal AF resistant to drug therapy, who were free of structural heart disease. AF was commonly associated with runs of irregular atrial tachycardia or monomorphic extrasystoles, and electrophysiological study showed that all the atrial arrhythmias were due to the same focus firing irregularly and showing a consistent and centrifugal pattern of activation. Three foci were located in the right atrium, two near the sinus node, one in the ostium of the coronary sinus, and others in the left atrium at the ostium of the right and the left superior pulmonary veins. All atrial arrhythmias were successfully treated by radiofrequency ablation.

Surgery for AF

Surgery is not considered as a routine non-pharmacological treatment of AF and its application is limited to a select group of AF patients who are resistant to conventional treatment. The goals of surgery for AF include the abolition of AF, restoration of sinus rhythm, the re-establishment or maintenance

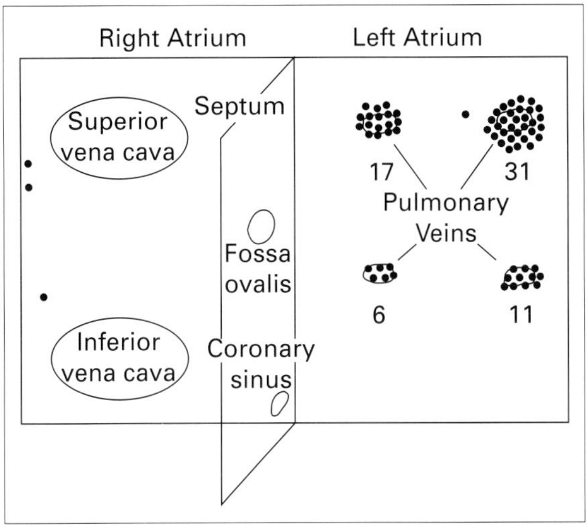

Figure 11.5
Diagram of the sites of 69 foci triggering atrial fibrillation in 45 patients. Note the clustering in the pulmonary veins, particularly in both superior pulmonary veins. Numbers indicate the distribution of foci in the pulmonary veins. Reproduced with permission from Haissaguerre et al (1998).

of atrioventricular synchrony (including restoration of atrial transport), and the reduction or elimination of the risk of stroke and thromboembolism by reducing intra-atrial blood stasis (Cox et al, 1991).

Since chronic AF usually occurs in the setting of mitral and aortic valve disease, and since these patients undergo valve replacement that improves cardiac function but does not prevent AF, some patients may benefit from additional surgery for the cure of AF done in combination with valve surgery (Crijns et al, 1996). The study by Crijns and colleagues (1996) showed that patients with a history of chronic AF before surgery (risk ratio 5.4, [95% CI 2.5–11.3]) had a poor arrhythmia outcome, with a lower success rate in patients with mitral valve disease than in those with aortic valve disease. Congestive heart failure and cardiovascular mortality were most common in patients with an unsuccessful cardioversion strategy, suggesting that patients scheduled for mitral valve surgery with a history of chronic AF should be considered as candidates for additional surgery for AF concomitant to valve surgery. However, Kim and colleagues (1998) suggest that whilst the maze operation could be safely added to standard open-heart surgery for the correction of underlying structural heart disease, the rate of conversion to sinus rhythm resulting solely from the operation might be lower than the rates previously reported for the procedure, and the duration of prior AF might adversely affect the subsequent restoration of left atrial mechanical function. Since not all patients who are converted to sinus rhythm after the procedure show atrial mechanical function, the role of the maze operation in the prevention of systemic embolism, with subsequent improvement in survival, is still uncertain.

Two surgical procedures, including the modified Cox maze procedure and the left atrial isolation or corridor procedure, have generally been used (Figures 11.6 and 11.7). In the maze operation, several small incisions are made in the atria, excising both atrial appendices and isolating the pulmonary veins, to obtain compartments that are small enough and unable to sustain AF. This results in interruption of the potential re-entrant pathways required for AF. Since AF is characterised by multiple re-entrant circuits in both atria, AF cannot be sustained after the maze procedure because the impulse is not able to re-enter upon itself. The procedure cures AF, restores atrioventricular synchrony, and preserves atrial transport function in 98% of patients, with 2% mortality and only 9% requiring antiarrhythmic medications (Cox et al, 1993), and is effective in patients undergoing mitral

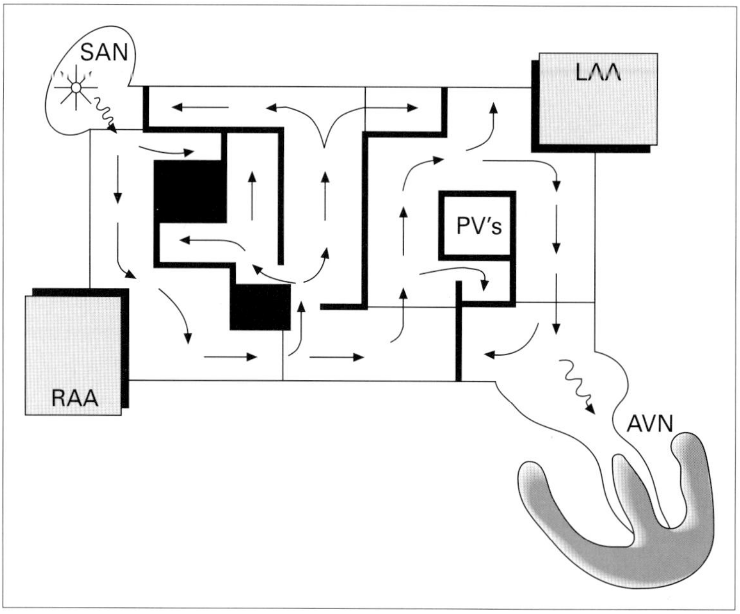

Figure 11.6
Maze procedure for AF. Because AF is characterised by the presence of multiple macroreentrant circuits that are fleeting in nature and can occur anywhere in the atria, a surgical procedure based on the principle of a maze was developed. Both atrial appendages are excised and the pulmonary veins are isolated. Appropriately placed atrial incisions not only interrupt the conduction routes of the most common reentrant circuits, but they also direct the sinus impulse from the SA node to the AV node along a specified route. The entire atrial myocardium (except for the atrial appendage and pulmonary veins) is electrically activated by providing for multiple blind alleys off the main conduction route between the SA node and the AV node, thereby preserving atrial transport function postoperatively. AVN = atrioventricular node; LAA = left atrial appendage; PV = pulmonary veins; RAA = right atrial appendage; SAN = sinoatrial node. Adapted from Cox et al (1991).

valve surgery (Isobe et al, 1998). Postoperative atrial pacemakers are needed in 40% of cases, mostly for preoperative sick sinus syndrome, but occasionally for iatrogenic sinus node injury. Indeed, the manifestations of sinus node dysfunction following the Cox-maze III procedure are time-dependent. Their frequency and intensity is progressively decreased and may disappear within 12 months of surgery, with the potential recovery of cardiac autonomic activity (Pasic et al, 1998).

Other adverse effects of surgery for AF include massive fluid retention (in approximately 5%), possibly related to loss of atrial natriuretic peptide, which may be prevented by the use of spironolactone after surgery. The resultant atrial dysfunction after surgery may also limit the haemodynamic benefit, although the modified maze procedure in patients undergoing surgery for mitral valve disease or an atrial septal defect was reported by Sandova (1996) to be effective in restoring sinus rhythm (85% of patients) and atrial contractility (71%).

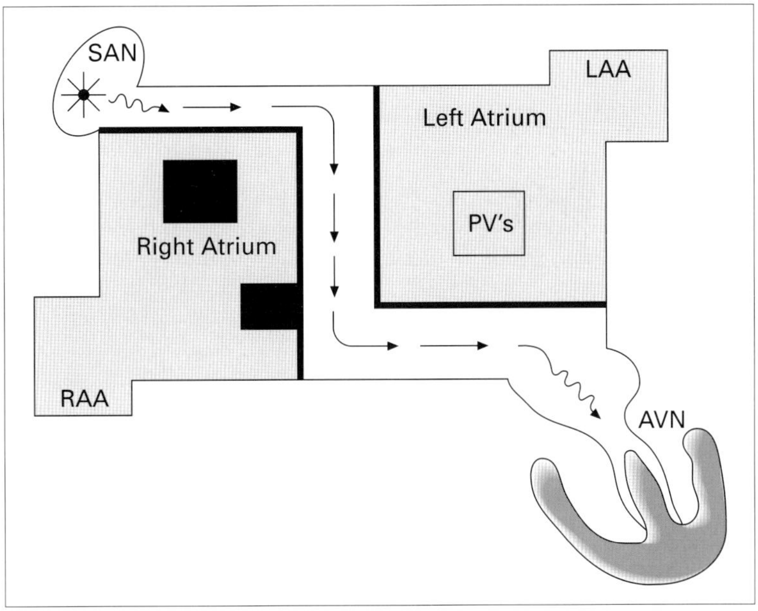

Figure 11.7
Schematic representation of the results of the corridor procedure for the surgical treatment of atrial fibrillation. Technically speaking, a sinus rhythm may follow this procedure in that the sinus node impulse drives the ventricles. However, because of loss of both right atrial and left atrial synchrony with the respective ventricles, the haemodynamic abnormalities associated with atrial fibrillation are not improved. In addition, the vulnerability to the development of left atrial thrombi is not alleviated. AVN = atrioventricular node; LAA = left atrial appendage; PV = pulmonary veins; RAA = right atrial appendage; SAN = sinoatrial node. Adapted from Cox et al (1991).

The corridor operation isolates the sinus node area, a strip of atrial tissue, and the atrioventricular node from the remaining atrium, thereby allowing sinus rhythm to be sustained. Sinus node function and physiological control of heart rate is restored, but atrial contraction or atrioventricular synchrony is not. Hence the risk of thromboembolism remains together with the requirement for anticoagulation. Most patients maintain sinus rhythm and achieve rate control at follow-up, but some patients may require a pacemaker due to postoperative sinus node dysfunction (Leitch et al, 1991). However, the corridor procedure does not eliminate the need for long-term anticoagulation nor does it re-establish atrial transport or atrioventricular synchrony, especially if a biatrial isolation procedure is used. It thus leaves the free wall tissue of the right and left atria fibrillating, while the ventricles are being activated by the sinoatrial node through the corridor (Defauw et al, 1992).

References

Andersen HR, Nielsen JC, Thomsen PE et al. Arterial thromboembolism in patients with sick sinus syndrome: prediction from pacing mode, atrial fibrillation, and echocardiographic findings. *Heart* 1999; **81:** 412–18.

Andersen HR, Nielsen JC, Thomsen PE et al. Atrioventricular conduction during long-term follow-up of patients with sick sinus syndrome. *Circulation* 1998; **98:** 1315–21.

Andersen HR, Nielsen JC, Thomsen PE et al. Long-term follow-up of patients from a randomised trial of atrial versus ventricular pacing for sick sinus syndrome. *Lancet* 1997; **350:** 1210.

Andersen HR, Thuesen L, Bagger JP et al. Prospective randomized trial of atrial versus ventricular pacing in sick sinus syndrome. *Lancet* 1994; **344:** 1523.

Brignole M, Gianfranchi L, Menozzi C et al. Assessment of atrioventricular junction ablation and DDDR mode-switching pacemaker versus pharmacological treatment in patients with severely symptomatic paroxysmal atrial fibrillation: a randomized controlled study. *Circulation* 1997; **96:** 2617–24.

Cox JL, Boineau JP, Schuessler RB et al. A review of surgery for atrial fibrillation. *J Cardiovasc Electrophysiol* 1991; **2:** 541.

Cox JL, Boineau JP, Schuessler RB et al. Five year experience with the maze procedure for atrial fibrillation. *Ann Thorac Surg* 1993; **56:** 814.

Crijns HJ, Van Gelder IC, Van der Woude HJ et al. Efficacy of serial electrical cardioversion therapy in patients with chronic atrial fibrillation after valve replacement and implications for surgery to cure atrial fibrillation. *Am J Cardiol* 1996; **78:** 1140–4.

Darpo B, Walfridsson H, Aunes M et al. Incidence of sudden death after radiofrequency ablation of the atrioventricular junction for atrial fibrillation. *Am J Cardiol* 1997; **80:** 1174–7.

Daubert C, Mabo P, Berder V et al. Atrial tachyarrhythmias associated with high degree interatrial conduction block: prevention by permanent atrial resynchronization. *Eur J Clin Pacing Electrophysiol* 1994; **4:** 435.

Defauw JJ, Guiraudon GM, van Hemel NM et al. Surgical therapy of paroxysmal atrial fibrillation with the "corridor" operation. *Ann Thorac Surg* 1992; **53:** 564.

Geelen P, Brugada J, Andries E, Brugada P. Ventricular fibrillation and sudden death after radiofrequency catheter ablation of the atrioventricular junction. *Pacing Clin Electrophysiol* 1997; **20:** 343–8.

Haissaguerre M, Jais P, Shah DC et al. Right and left atrial radiofrequency catheter therapy of paroxysmal atrial fibrillation. *J Cardiovasc Electrophysiol* 1996; **7:** 1132–44.

Haissaguerre M, Jaïs P, Shah DC et al. Spontaneous initiation of atrial fibrillation by ectopic beats originating in the pulmonary veins. *Mass Med Soc* 1998; **339:** 659–66.

Haissaguerre M, Gencel L, Fischer B et al. Successful catheter ablation of atrial fibrillation. *J Cardiovasc Electrophysiol* 1994; **5:** 1045.

Isobe F, Kawashima Y. The outcome and indications of the Cox maze III procedure for chronic atrial fibrillation with mitral valve disease. *Thorac Cardiovasc Surg* 1998; **116:** 220–7.

Iskos D, Lurie KG, Adler SW et al. Effect of parenteral d-sotalol on transvenous atrial defibrillation threshold in a canine model of atrial fibrillation. *Am Heart J* 1996; **132:** 116.

Jais P, Haissaguerre M, Shah DC et al. A focal source of atrial fibrillation treated by discrete radiofrequency ablation. *Circulation* 1997; **95:** 572–6.

Kamalvand K, Tan K, Kotaskis A et al. Is mode switching beneficial? A randomized study in patients with paroxysmal atrial tachyarrhythmias. *J Am Coll Cardiol* 1997; **30:** 496.

Kay GN, Ellenbogen KA, Giudici M et al. The Ablate and Pace Trial: a prospective study of catheter ablation of the AV conduction system and permanent pacemaker implantation for treatment of atrial fibrillation. APT Investigators. *J Interv Card Electrophysiol* 1998; **2:** 121–35.

Keelan ET, Krum D, Hare J et al. Safety of atrial defibrillation shocks synchronized to narrow and wide QRS complexes during atrial pacing protocols simulating atrial fibrillation in dogs. *Circulation* 1997; **96:** 2022.

Kim YJ, Sohn DW, Park DG et al. Restoration of atrial mechanical function after maze operation in patients with structural heart disease. *Am Heart J* 1998; **136:** 1070–4.

Leitch JW, Klein G, Yee R, Guiraudon G. Sinus node-atrioventricular node isolation: long term results with "corridor" operation for atrial fibrillation. *J Am Coll Cardiol* 1991; **17:** 970.

Manolis AG, Katsivas AG, Lazaris EE et al. Ventricular performance and quality of life in patients who underwent radiofrequency AV junction ablation and permanent pacemaker implantation due to medically refractory atrial tachyarrhythmias. *Interv Card Electrophysiol* 1998; **2:** 71–6.

Marshall HJ, Harris ZI, Griffith MJ et al. Prospective randomized study of ablation and pacing versus medical therapy for paroxysmal atrial fibrillation: effects of pacing made and mode-switch algorithm. *Circulation* 1999; **99:** 1587–92.

Pasic M, Musci M, Siniawski H et al. Transient sinus node dysfunction after the Cox-maze III procedure in patients with organic heart disease and chronic fixed atrial fibrillation. *J Am Coll Cardiol* 1998; **32:** 1040–7.

Saksena S, Prakash A, Hill M et al. Prevention of recurrent atrial fibrillation with chronic dual-site right atrial pacing. *J Am Coll Cardiol* 1996; **28:** 687.

Sandova IN, Velasco VM, Orjuela H et al. Concomitant mitral valve or atrial septal defect surgery and the modified Cox-maze procedure. *Am J Cardiol* 1996; **77:** 591.

Swartz JF, Pellersels G, Silvers J et al. A catheter-based curative approach to atrial fibrillation in humans (abstract). *Circulation* 1994; **90:** I.

Touboul P. Atrioventricular nodal ablation and pacemaker implantation in patients with atrial fibrillation. *Am J Cardiol* 1999; **83(5B):** 241D–245D.

Twidale N, Manda V, Nave K, Seal A. Predictors of outcome after radiofrequency catheter ablation of the atrioventricular node for atrial fibrillation and congestive heart failure. *Am Heart J* 1998; **136:** 647–57.

Wellens HJ, Lau CP, Luderitz B et al. Atrioverter: an implantable device for the treatment of atrial fibrillation. *Circulation* 1998; **98:** 1651–6.

Wood MA, Brown-Mahoney C, Kay N, Ellenbogen KA. Clinical outcomes after ablation and pacing therapy for atrial fibrillation. A meta-analysis. *Circulation* 2000; **101:** 1138–44.

Yu WC, Chen SA, Tai CT et al. Effects of different atrial pacing modes on atrial electrophysiology. Implicating the mechanism of biatrial pacing in the prevention of atrial fibrillation. *Circulation* 1997; **96:** 2992.

12

Management strategies for atrial fibrillation

Introduction

The management of patients with atrial fibrillation (AF) requires consideration of several points. Firstly, is the diagnosis of AF certain? The arrhythmia must be documented and it is important to distinguish between sustained and paroxysmal AF, as there are important management differences between the two conditions. Secondly, how did the arrhythmia develop, and why now? AF is associated with common heart problems, and thus a search for the underlying aetiological or predisposing factors should be made. Thirdly, the presence of complications, such as heart failure, stroke, and thromboembolism should be assessed and treated (Figure 12.1)

Management of AF depends on the subtype of AF that one is dealing with. Distinguishing between paroxysmal, persistent, and permanent AF helps decisions about management strategies (Table 12.1).

Acute AF

Acute AF usually describes an acute episode of AF related to an acute curable cause or an acute attack of AF. Patients presenting de novo with acute onset AF may do so with several cardiorespiratory symptoms such as chest pain, palpitations, dyspnoea, or syncope. Such patients usually feel very anxious, concerned that their heart may be "running away", and they may think that they are on the verge of dying. Patients may present acutely, but some patients may have had symptom-free AF present for a long time — thus a careful clinical history and assessment is important. Very fast AF may look like a fast narrow complex tachycardia such as supraventricular tachycardia; one clue may be subtle irregularity in the R-R interval on the ECG. However, intravenous adenosine may aid the diagnosis by transiently increasing the atrioventricular blockade and increasing the R-R interval, making the absence of P waves and the fine "f" (fibrillation) waves more easily discernible between the QRS complexes on the ECG.

For acute presentations of AF, consider whether or not there were any "acute" precipitating factors such as infection. In such patients, quick assessment of haemodynamic status, underlying cause(s) and associated complications is needed. Admissions with acute AF are usually admitted to a coronary care unit to rule out acute myocardial infarction, even in the absence of chest pain. In fact, such situations are rare, and unless the patient is haemodynamically compromised or gives a clear history of cardiac ischaemia, or if the patient requires treatment of an associated medical problem, monitoring in the coronary care unit may be unnecessary (Shlofmitz et al,

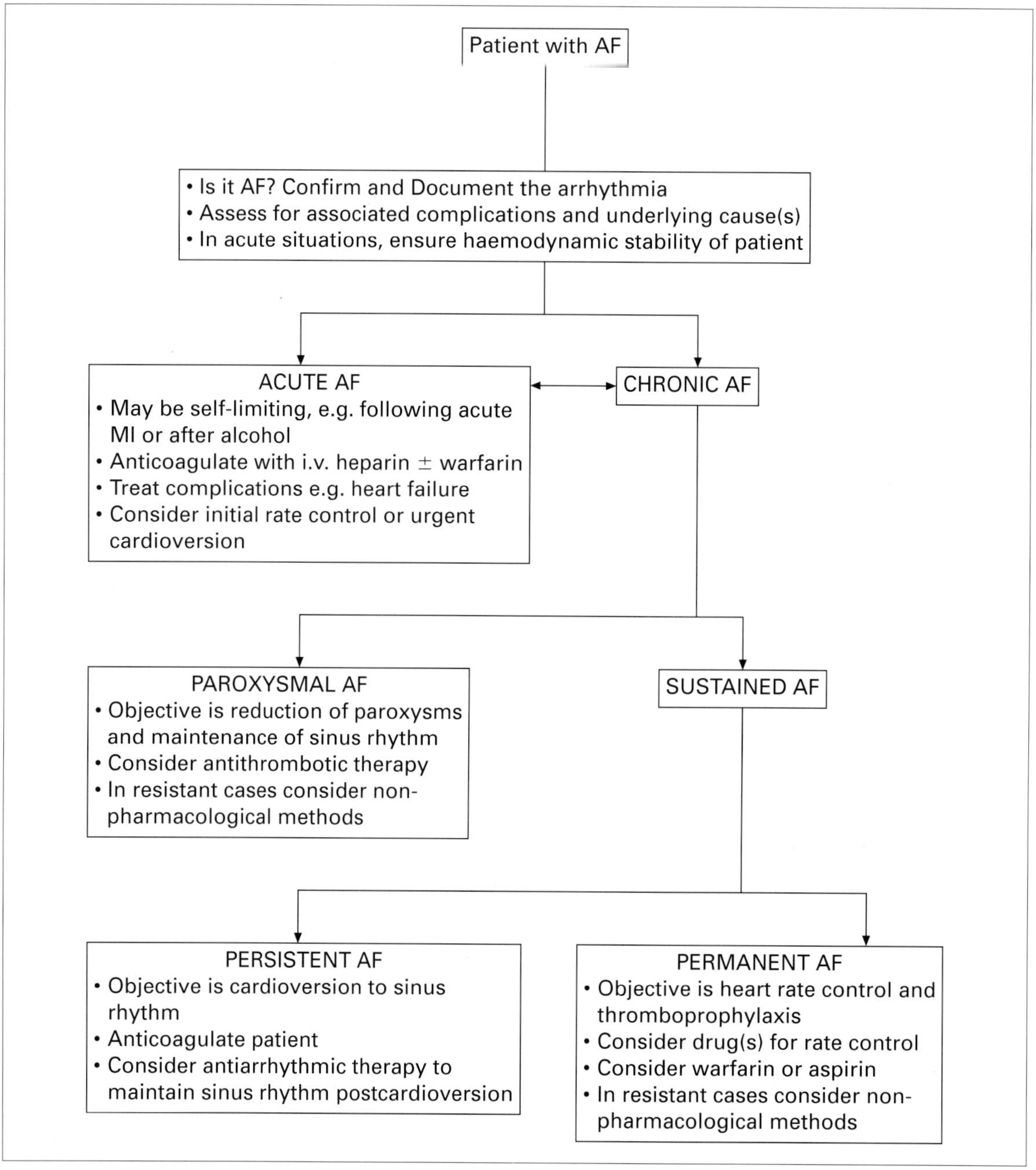

Figure 12.1
Management strategies for AF. Adapted from Lip (1999).

Pattern	Goal of Rx
Permanent AF	VR control
Persistent AF	Cardioversion to SR
Paroxysmal AF	↓ arrhythmia frequency (arrhythmia prevention) ↓ arrhythmia duration (arrhythmia termination) ↓ symptom frequency (control of VR, irregularity and neurohumoral responses)

Table 12.1
Goals of management in chronic AF. VR = ventricular rate.

1986; Friedman et al, 1987). Patients with significant underlying heart disease who have haemodynamic consequences from the AF, or who are at risk for a complication resulting from therapy of the arrhythmia (especially the elderly), may be more safely treated for AF in hospital. The main considerations in acute AF relate to haemodynamic stability, reducing the risk of thromboembolism, and an assessment of the urgency of heart-rate slowing.

The initial management strategy depends upon whether the patient is haemodynamically stable (Figure 12.2). If the patient is haemodynamically unstable consequent upon the fast AF, a suitable option may be a quick general anaesthetic and urgent cardioversion to sinus rhythm using synchronised DC shock. In these instances, pharmacological cardioversion may take too long, and there is the risk of proarrhythmia and worsening cardiac impairment, especially since some antiarrhythmic drugs are negatively inotropic (Figure 12.3)

Patients admitted in acute AF should be started on intravenous heparin. This should reduce the risk of thrombus formation, and if the duration of AF is clearly 48 h or less, cardioversion may be done without the need for long-term anticoagulation afterwards. However one problem is that many patients do not know precisely when their episode of AF started. In a transoesophageal echocardiography study by Stoddard and colleagues (1995), 15% of patients admitted with acute AF of 48 h or less had left atrial appendage thrombi. In cases where the duration of AF is more than 48 h, anticoagulation with warfarin (INR 2–3) should be started for a minimum of 3 weeks, and if appropriate, cardioversion should be attempted and anticoagulation continued for at least 4 weeks.

Most patients with acute AF do not require immediate control of heart rate. Patients can usually be managed by rate control using digoxin, rate-limiting calcium antagonists (verapamil and diltiazem), or beta-blockers, whilst assessment is made of underlying comorbidity and appropriateness of the management strategy. Initial treatment directed at slowing the ventricular rate will usually improve or resolve mild to moderate symptoms. The drug selected for rate control and the route of administration (that is, oral *vs* intravenous) will be dictated by the clinical presentation. For example, digoxin is the preferred drug in

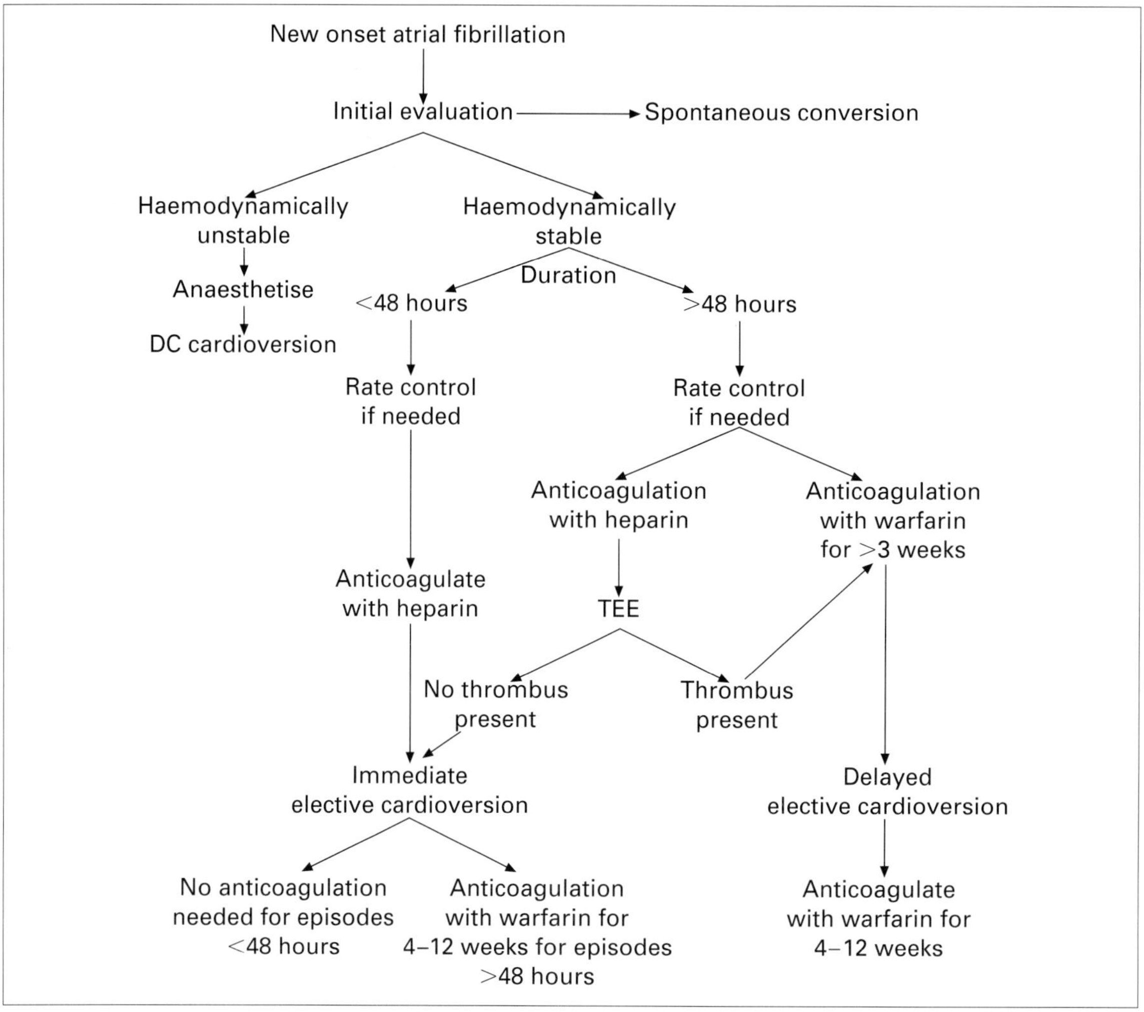

Figure 12.2
Algorithm for management of new onset AF. DC = direct current; TEE = transoesophageal echocardiogram. Reproduced from Jung and DiMarco (1998), with permission from Excerpta Medica Inc.

patients with AF due to congestive heart failure. Whilst digoxin can be administered both orally and intravenously in acute AF, there is little advantage of giving digoxin intravenously except in instances when the patient is unable to take oral tablets (for example, post-operatively), because malabsorption is likely. When AF occurs in the setting of acute myocardial infarction, it usually occurs in the first 24 h and is self-limiting in the absence of heart failure or a prior history of AF. Nevertheless, the development of AF in patients with acute myocardial infarction is associated with significant cardiac impairment and a poor outcome.

In the absence of contraindications, intra-

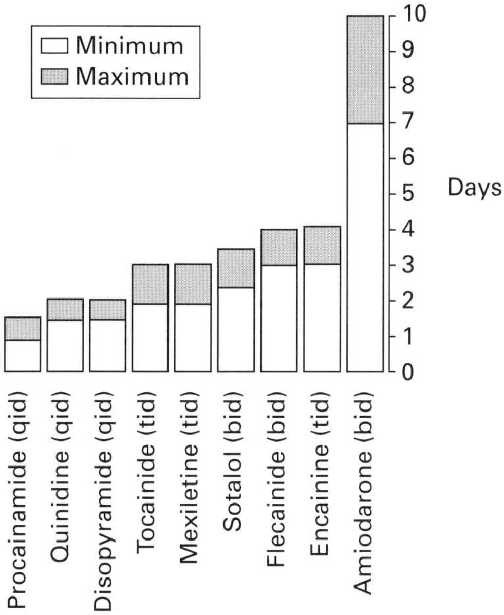

Figure 12.3
Time from initiation of therapy to possible determination of effectiveness. qid = 4 times a day; tid = three times a day; bid = twice a day.

venous administration of a beta-blocker such as esmolol or metoprolol, or a calcium antagonist acting at the atrioventricular node such as verapamil or diltiazem, may be useful (and possibly more effective) alternative to digoxin. Esmolol is a relatively cardioselective beta-adrenoceptor blocker, which has the advantage of a rapid action and short half-life. Thus an infusion of esmolol would rapidly control the ventricular response in fast AF and on cessation of the infusion the effects would wear off rapidly. Esmolol would therefore be useful in a postoperative setting and after myocardial infarction, when there is uncertainty over the use of prolonged beta-blockade in the acute stage (Schwartz et al, 1988). Intravenous diltiazem, which is available in the USA, is another useful option for control of the ventricular rate in fast AF, although verapamil may also be used with caution given its negative inotropic effects. In cases in which fast AF is present in association with heart failure or cardiac impairment, digoxin or intravenous amiodarone may be sensible choices for heart-rate control. In patients with an underlying Wolff-Parkinson-White syndrome, the use of atrioventricular node blocking agents such as verapamil may accelerate conduction in the accessory pathway, leading to an increase in AF rate, which may degenerate into ventricular arrhythmias (Strasberg et al, 1989).

After achieving control of the ventricular rate in patients with mild to moderate symptoms, assessment of the patient, and correction of precipitants such as thyrotoxicosis or febrile illness, a decision is required about whether the acute episode of AF should be cardioverted to sinus rhythm. The role of cardioversion depends upon the duration of the arrhythmias as well as the presence of a reversible aetiological factor.

Sustained AF

Amongst the more chronic forms of AF, clinical classification also assists management strategies. In paroxysmal (recurrent) AF episodes are generally self-terminating. Thus, the main objective of management is the prevention of paroxysms and long-term maintenance of sinus rhythm. In sustained AF, the management objective is either cardioversion to sinus rhythm (persistent AF) or heart-rate control with appropriate antithrombotic therapy (permanent AF). The term "permanent" also implies that AF has been present for a long time and that cardioversion has not been indicated, or that one or several attempts of

		Sustained	
	Paroxysmal	*Persistent*	*Permanent*
Objective	Prevention of paroxysms and maintenance of sinus rhythm	Cardioversion to sinus rhythm	Heart-rate control and reduction of thromboembolism
Cardioversion?	If AF becomes persistent	Yes	No [± previous unsuccessful attempts at cardioversion]
Heart-rate control	Class I or III agent	Not main objective of management	Yes (see text)
Antithrombotic therapy	Anticoagulation, especially if age >75 years and structural heart disease	Anticoagulation for 3 weeks before and 4 weeks after cardioversion	Warfarin for high risk patients; aspirin for others

Table 12.2
Aims of intervention in AF – summary.

cardioversion has failed to restore sinus rhythm. If cardioversion is the management objective for patients with persistent AF, appropriate use of antiarrhythmic therapy to maintain sinus rhythm, and anticoagulation to reduce the risk of thromboembolism, should be considered (Table 12.2).

References

Friedman HZ, Weber-Bornstein N, Deboe SF et al. CCU admission criteria for suspected acute myocardial infarction in new onset atrial fibrillation. *Am J Cardiol* 1987; **59:** 866.

Jung F and DiMarco JP. Treatment strategies for atrial fibrillation. *Am J Med* 1998; **104:** 272–86.

Lip GYH. How would I manage a 60-year-old woman presenting with atrial fibrillation? *Proc R Coll Physicians Edinb* 1999; **29:** 301–6.

Schwartz M, Michelson EL, Sawin HS, MacVaugh H 3rd. Esmolol: safety and efficacy in postoperative cardiothoracic patients with supraventricular tachyarrhythmias. *Chest* 1988; **93:** 705–11.

Shlofmitz RA, Hirsch BE, Meyer BR. New onset atrial fibrillation. Is there a need for emergent hospitalization? *J Gen Intern Med* 1986; **1:** 139.

Stoddard ME, Dawkins PR, Prince CR, Ammash NM. Left atrial appendage thrombus is not uncommon in patients with acute atrial fibrillation and a recent embolic event: a transesophageal echocardiographic study. *J Am Coll Cardiol* 1995; **25:** 452–9.

Strasberg B, Sagie A, Rechavia E et al. Sclarovsky S, Agmon J. Deleterious effects of intravenous verapamil in Wolff-Parkinson-White patients and atrial fibrillation. *Cardiovasc Drugs Ther* 1989; **2:** 801–6.

13

Paroxysmal atrial fibrillation

Introduction

Epidemiology

Paroxysmal atrial fibrillation (PAF) is reported to comprise between 25% and 62% of cases of AF seen by practitioners in hospital and primary care settings (Peterson and Godtfredsen, 1986; Godtfredsen, 1975; Takahashi et al, 1981; Kannel et al, 1983; Phillips et al, 1990). The reported prevalence varies widely because of differences in definitions and population studied, and many episodes are symptom-free. In addition, many patients with PAF ultimately develop chronic and sustained arrhythmia. For example, Takahashi and colleagues (1981) described a consecutive hospital-based series of 234 patients with AF, and found that 94 (40.2%) patients had a paroxysmal form of AF (Figure 13.1a and 13.1b). Of the 1212 patients with AF admitted to hospital in Denmark, Godtfredsen and colleagues (Peterson and Godtfredsen, 1986; Godtfredsen, 1975) found that 426 (35%) patients had PAF, and 786 (65%) patients had sustained AF. Our survey of 7451 emergency medical admissions to a city centre hospital found that of 245 patients with AF, 44% had newly diagnosed AF, 45% had previous chronic AF, and 8% had PAF, with no information for seven patients (Zarifis et al, 1997). Nevertheless, hospital-based surveys may misrepresent the true picture of the clinical epidemiology of AF (Lip et al, 1997b). The Stroke Prevention in Atrial Fibrillation (SPAF) I and II investigators (Flaker, 1995) defined PAF as the presence of sinus rhythm at either 1-month or 3-month follow-up visit after enrolment. Using such criteria, 486 (27.8%) of recruited patients had intermittent AF and 1263 patients had chronic AF.

The prevalence of PAF is probably underestimated in population and epidemiological studies, since it is known that symptom-free PAF is common on Holter monitoring (Page et al, 1994) (Figure 13.2). Page et al (1994) estimated, for example, that symptom-free episodes of PAF are 12 times more frequent than episodes with symptoms. The prevalence of PAF was 25% in the Framingham study, but this was defined as AF not present on routine biennial examination after being present at a previous hospital admission (Kannel et al, 1983). By contrast, the Minnesota study showed that 62% of all AF cases were intermittent (Phillips et al, 1990). In the west Birmingham Atrial Fibrillation study, in which patients with known AF in two general practices were surveyed (total practice population aged >50 years = 4542), 73% of the 111 patients with AF had chronic AF, and 27% had PAF (Lip et al, 1997b).

There may be age and sex influences on rate and duration of PAF. For example, Hnatkova

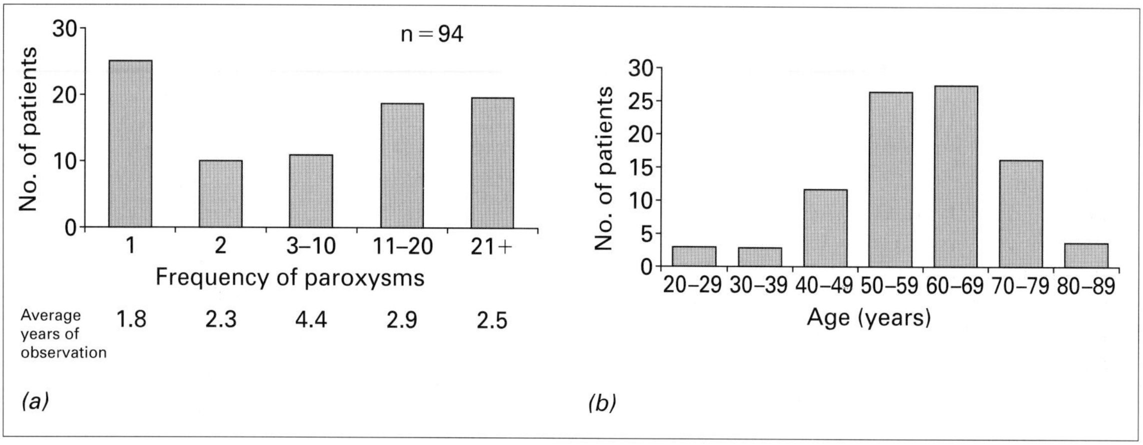

Figure 13.1
(a) Frequency of paroxysmal AF. (b) Age distribution for paroxysmal AF. Adapted from Takahashi et al (1981).

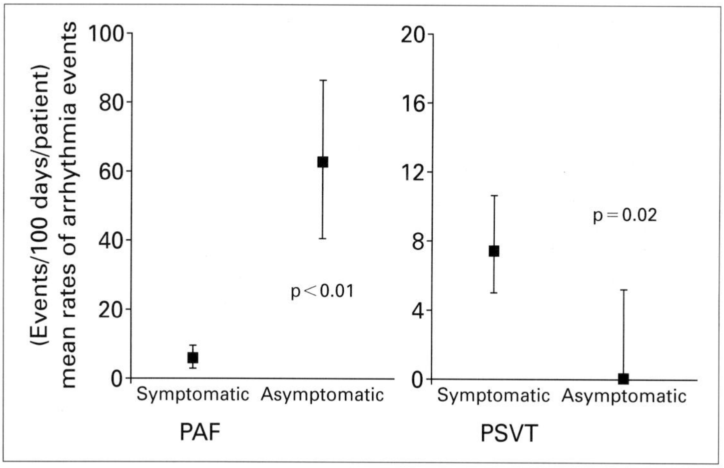

Figure 13.2
Asymptomatic and symptomatic supraventricular arrhythmias. Reproduced with permission from Page et al (1994).

and colleagues (1998) studied heart rate during 236 episodes of PAF in 32 patients receiving placebo or antiarrhythmic therapy. Women had a higher mean heart rate at AF onset (mean 123 beats/min *vs* 115 beats/min, p = 0.02) and during the remainder of the episode (120 beats/min *vs* 112 beats/min at the start, p = 0.01; 116 beats/min *vs* 108 beats/min subsequently, p = 0.01). Paroxysms also lasted longer in women (mean 89.8 min *vs* 50.5 min, p = NS) and in the aged (mean 83.8 min *vs* 46.9 min, p = NS), which may reflect differing autonomic responses to AF. The slower ventricular rate during PAF in older patients probably reflected an increasing prevalence of impaired atrioventricular con-

	PAF No. (%)		
	Takahashi et al 1981 (n = 94)	Suttorp et al 1993 (n = 124)	Clementy et al 1992 (n = 944)
Hypertension	15 (16.0)	42 (34)	262 (27.8)
Coronary disease	13 (13.8)	31 (25)	55 (5.8)
Hypertension & coronary disease	23 (24.5)	NA	NA
Rheumatic disease	3 (3.2)	10 (8)	128 (13.6)
Hyperthyroidism	2 (2.1)	3 (2)	NA
Miscellaneous	15 (16.0)	14(12)	151 (15.9)
Idiopathic	23 (24.5)	53 (43)	435 (46)

*NA indicates not available

Table 13.1
Underlying cause of paroxysmal atrial fibrillation (PAF).*

Cardiovascular Causes	Noncardiovascular Causes
Hypertension	Hypoxia and respiratory failure
Coronary artery disease	Diabetes
Cardiomyopathy	Drugs (cocaine, theophylline, alcohol, caffeine)
Mitral valve disease	Hyperthyroidism
Pericarditis	Postoperative thoracotomy
	Electrolyte abnormalities (low K^{2+} and Mg^{2+}, high Ca^{2+})

*PAF indicates paroxysmal atrial fibrillation: CAF, chronic atrial fibrillation

Table 13.2
Common causes of PAF and CAF.*

duction. In patients with frequent paroxysms of AF, the same investigators also reported a circadian variation (Sopher et al, 1998) with nocturnal episodes tending to be shorter (median = 1.15 min) than diurnal episodes (median = 1.5 min). The mean heart rate before AF onset was also lower at night. Thus, in patients with frequent symptomatic PAF, autonomic influences affect the duration of episodes of AF, with possible pathophysiological and therapeutic implications.

The underlying causes of PAF and chronic AF are usually similar, and include common cardiovascular disorders such as hypertension (16–34%), coronary artery disease (6–24%), and rheumatic heart disease (3–14%) (Tables 13.1 and 13.2). As opposed to chronic AF, no underlying cause can be shown in nearly 50%

of patients with PAF (Phillips and Levine, 1949; Suttorp et al, 1993; Clementy et al, 1992). Compared with patients with chronic AF, patients with PAF are usually younger, with less heart disease (Flaker et al, 1995).

Natural history

The natural history of PAF is unclear, largely because of uncertainty about its actual incidence, the high frequency of symptom-free episodes, and because many studies involve only those patients with symptoms from the arrhythmia. Analysis of the cardiac rhythm preceding episodes of PAF (Hnatkova et al, 1998) showed no consistent mode of PAF onset. There was a highly significant increase in ectopic beats, but heart rate did not significantly change. In more than half of the cases, PAF was initiated by a solitary ectopic beat. Thus, the mode of onset of AF is inconsistent, both across a population with PAF and within individual patients.

The recurrence rate is generally high in patients who present with PAF. Nevertheless, the reported incidence of recurrence is highly variable, ranging from 70% at 1 year without antiarrhythmic therapy (Coplen et al, 1990) to 90% at 4 years (Rostagno et al, 1995). In a cohort of 341 patients with intermittent AF who were followed for 26 months in the SPAF trial (Flaker et al, 1995), 49% had recurrent AF on at least one ECG, and 104 additional patients underwent cardioversion (electrical or pharmacological). In the cardioversion group, the recurrence rate during the follow-up period was 54%.

As many as one third of patients with PAF may develop sustained AF (Petersen and Godtfredsen, 1986). The transition from PAF to chronic AF usually depends upon underlying aetiology (Aboaf and Wolf, 1996), with the highest progression (nearly two thirds) in patients with rheumatic mitral stenosis, compared with 40% among those with hypertension and 27% among those with ischaemic heart disease. There is also a relation to the duration of paroxysms. For example, when PAF lasts less than 2 days, progression to chronic AF occurs in 31% of patients, but when PAF lasts longer than 2 days, chronic AF occurs in 46%.

The data from SPAF (Flaker et al, 1995) suggested that compared with patients without a recurrence of AF, patients with AF recurrences were usually older (64 *vs* 60 years), were more likely to have congestive heart failure (17 *vs* 8%), and more likely to have had a prior myocardial infarction (15 *vs* 5%), and had larger left atrial diameters (4.4 *vs* 4.0) or significant left ventricular wall motion abnormalities. Moderate to severe left ventricular dysfunction was present in 12% of those with recurrent AF, compared with only 3% of those without recurrences. On transoesophageal echocardiography, Verhorst and colleagues (1997) reported that a left atrial annulus size greater than 3.9 cm and greater atrial stasis, with left atrial appendage flow velocity less than 30 cm/sec, and left atrial spontaneous contrast, were significantly associated with AF recurrence.

The transition from paroxysmal AF to chronic or sustained AF can be predictable. Compared with patients with chronic AF, those with PAF are more likely to have new onset or recent onset AF, and to have less hypertension or heart failure (Flaker et al, 1995). On echocardiography, patients with PAF have a smaller left atrial diameters and less left ventricular dysfunction. The P-wave triggered signal averaged ECG is another predictor of the transition from paroxysmal AF to chronic or sustained AF (Abe et al, 1997).

Autonomic influences in PAF

The electrophysiological characteristics of atrial cells (action potential duration and refractoriness, conduction speed) can be profoundly influenced by vagal and adrenergic influences. The former tend to favour macroreentry phenomena, whereas the latter favour abnormal automaticity and triggered activity. In normal hearts, vagal influences usually predominate, thus explaining why the clinical pattern of vagally mediated paroxysmal AF is usually seen in the absence of detectable heart disease in young male adults, commonly with an ECG pattern of common flutter alternating with fibrillation. By contrast, adrenergic-mediated paroxysmal AF is observed in the presence of any heart disease, which provokes a vagal withdrawal. Thus, the clinical history may be a guide to determine which autonomic predominance contributes to destabilisation of the arrhythmogenic substrate, although no clear distinction between the two subtypes may be made in many cases. Simply observing the behaviour of sinus rate variability just before the onset of the arrhythmia allows some documentation of the mechanism, but the role of autonomic influences should perhaps be taken into consideration every time conventional antiarrhythmic treatment is inadequate (Coumel, 1994).

Management

In PAF, the objective of management is the suppression of paroxysms, heart rate control during paroxysms, and the long-term maintenance of sinus rhythm. In view of this, an appropriate drug such as class I or class III agent should be chosen, as well as appropriate use of antithrombotic therapy (Table 13.3).

If a patient has only mild and infrequent symptoms, it is advisable to avoid antiarrhythmic drug therapy if at all possible (Figure 13.3). This management stratagem is justified by evidence of substantial morbidity associated with antiarrhythmic therapy, and the concern over worsened long-term prognosis,

Source, y	*Agent*	*No. of Patients*	*No. (%) Converting*	*P*
Noc et al, 1990	Amiodarone	13	10 (77)	<.001
	Verapamil	11	0 (0)	NS
Suttorp et al, 1989	Flecainide	17	14 (82)	<.001
	Verapamil	17	1 (6)	NS
Pietersen and Hellemann, 1991	Flecainide	39	18 (46)	NA
Reimold et al, 1993	Propafenone	25	. . . (42)	NA
	Sotalol	22	. . . (48)	NA

*Criteria for PAF and duration of follow-up variable among studies.
NS indicates not significant. NA: not available.

Table 13.3
Antiarrhythmic efficacy in paroxysmal atrial fibrillation (PAF).*

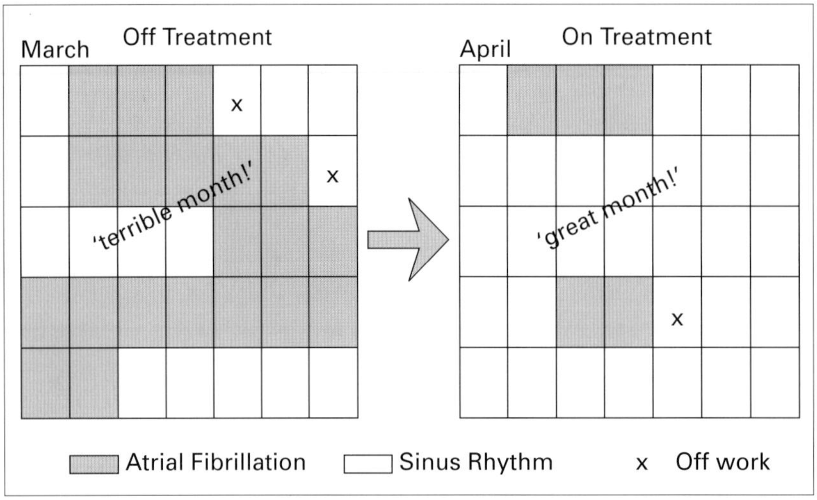

Figure 13.3
Diary of a patient with paroxysmal AF indicating the value of therapy that reduces but does not abolish episodes. Reproduced from Sopher and Camm (1996), with permission from Excerpta Medica Inc.

particularly with Class I agents, especially in the presence of poor cardiac function and severe ischaemic heart disease. General measures should always be considered, such as withdrawal of caffeine or alcohol, or stress counselling, especially if paroxysms of AF can be related to these. Occasionally, PAF may be related to conditions that may benefit from atrial pacing, such as the sick sinus syndrome. It is also important to distinguish between AF and atrial flutter, since there are important management differences between these two conditions. For example, the use of a class I agent (for example, quinidine, disopyramide, flecainide) in patients with atrial flutter may accelerate the ventricular response with a 1:1 atrioventricular conduction (Figure 13.4). This may be due in part to the slowing in atrial rate and the anticholinergic effects (especially with disopyramide and quinidine) that result in an increase in atrioventricular conduction. Young patients with paroxysmal AF and intact atrioventricular conduction may potentially be at risk of 1:1 conduction. In these patients, it is therefore advisable to co-administer class I agents with digoxin, beta-blocker, or verapamil, to avoid the potential for accelerated atrioventricular conduction.

Digoxin

Digoxin should be avoided in paroxysmal AF, since evidence suggests that this drug makes paroxysmal AF worse. In fact, clinical evidence has shown that paroxysms of AF occur more frequently and for significantly longer in patients receiving digoxin (Galun et al, 1991; Rawles et al, 1990). Moreover, during an episode of paroxysmal AF, the initial heart rate appears no better controlled whether or not digoxin is being taken (Galun et al, 1991; Rawles et al, 1990). The mechanism for this is unclear, but digoxin increases vagal tone, moderating the speed of atrioventricular conduction, and also reduces the atrial refractory period. This latter property may paradoxically render the atrium more susceptible to AF, and may reduce or even prevent the chance of reversion to sinus rhythm (Rawles et al, 1990).

However in the CRAFT study (Murgatroyd et al, 1999), 43 representative patients with

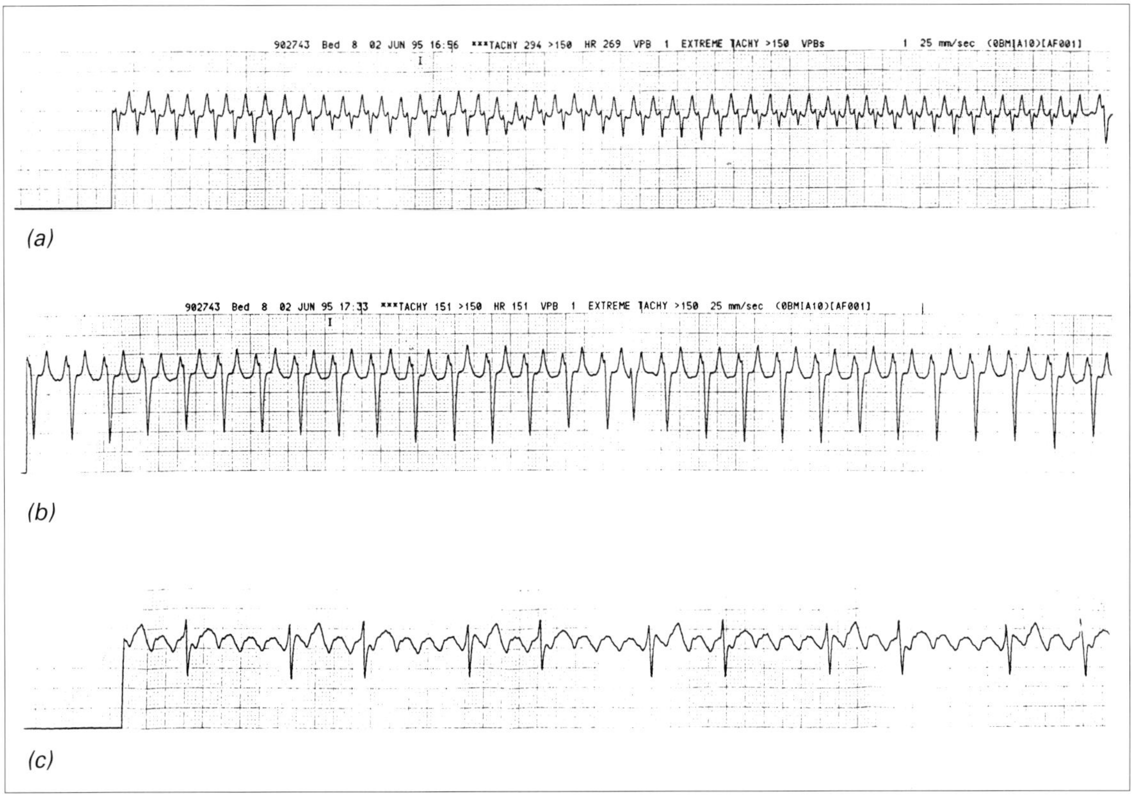

Figure 13.4
ECG monitor traces. (a) Atrial flutter with 1:1 conduction. (b) Same patient with atrial flutter with 2:1 block (after i.v. adenosine). (c) Atrial flutter with variable block (in different patient).

frequent symptomatic AF episodes were recruited into a randomised, double-blind crossover comparison of digoxin and placebo: the median time to two episodes was 13.5 days on placebo and 18.7 days on digoxin ($p < 0.05$), whilst the relative risk of two episodes (placebo: digoxin) was 2.19 (95% CI 1.07–4.50). A similar effect was shown for the median time to one episode, which was increased from 3.5 to 5.4 days (relative risk 1.69 [0.88–3.24], $p < 0.05$). In this study, 24 ambulatory ECG recordings did not show significant differences in the frequency or duration of AF or in ventricular rate. Thus digoxin reduced the frequency of symptomatic AF episodes, but the effect was small and may be due to a reduction in the ventricular rate or irregularity rather than an antiarrhythmic action.

Digoxin is also ineffective for the long-term maintenance of sinus rhythm or cardioversion of AF.

Verapamil

Verapamil is relatively ineffective in controlling paroxysmal AF, and its administration to

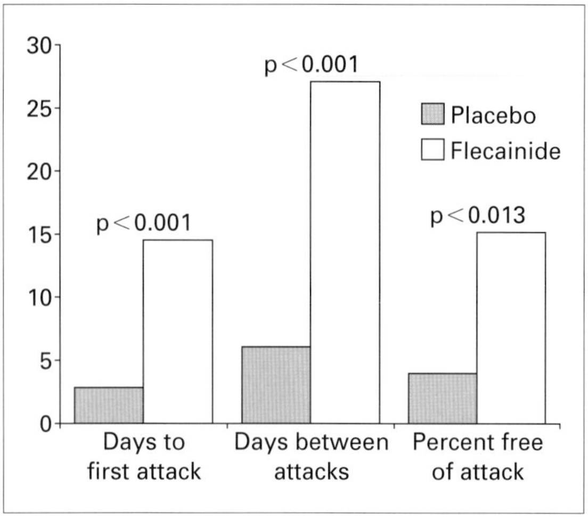

Figure 13.5
Flecainide used to maintain sinus rhythm in paroxysmal AF. Reproduced with permission from Anderson et al (1989).

patients with underlying Wolf-Parkinson-White syndrome who present with paroxysmal AF may occasionally lead to serious adverse effects, including ventricular fibrillation and severe haemodynamic impairment.

Class I antiarrhythmics

Class I antiarrhythmics nevertheless remain popular drugs for use in paroxysmal AF. Quinidine remains a frequently used class Ia drug, especially in the USA, for maintaining sinus rhythm after cardioversion or for reducing the number of paroxysms of AF.

Class Ic antiarrhythmics such as flecainide are effective in preventing recurrences of PAF in up to 60% of patients, but the drug does not limit the ventricular response. Studies of flecainide have also confirmed a significant increase in the median time to first recurrence of AF (Anderson et al, 1989) (Figures 13.5 and 13.6). Propafenone, another class Ic compound, may also be effective in paroxysmal AF (Pritchett et al, 1991; UK propafenone study group, 1995). This is particularly pertinent in view of its inherent rate-limiting (class II) properties, allowing potentially greater ventricular rate control. Nevertheless, doubts about the safety of class I agents have been raised by the Cardiac Arrhythmia Suppression Trial, in which patients after myocardial infarction who were given flecainide for ven-

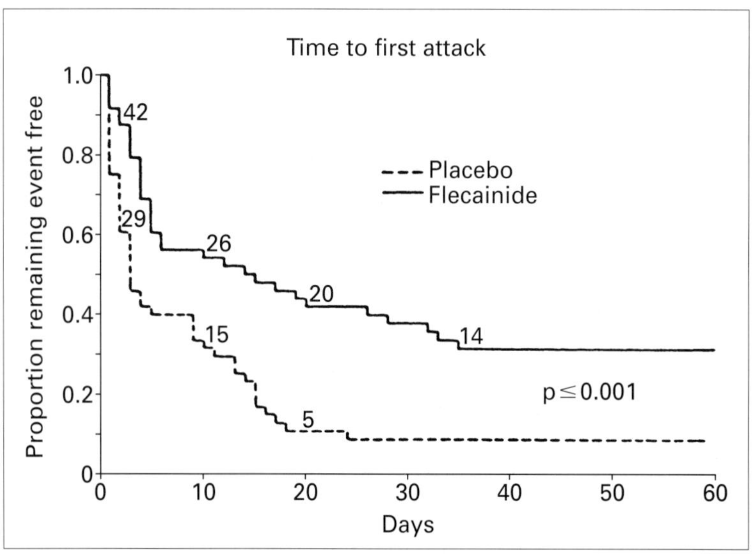

Figure 13.6
Line graph showing life-table analysis of time to first attack of paroxysmal AF in 48 patients, given as fraction of patients without attacks (ordinate) versus time (abscissa) from beginning therapy. The graph shows a product-time estimate. Time to first attack for patients who went the entire treatment period without having an attack was estimated as days on treatment +1, and the observation was classified as censored. Reproduced with permission from Anderson et al (1989).

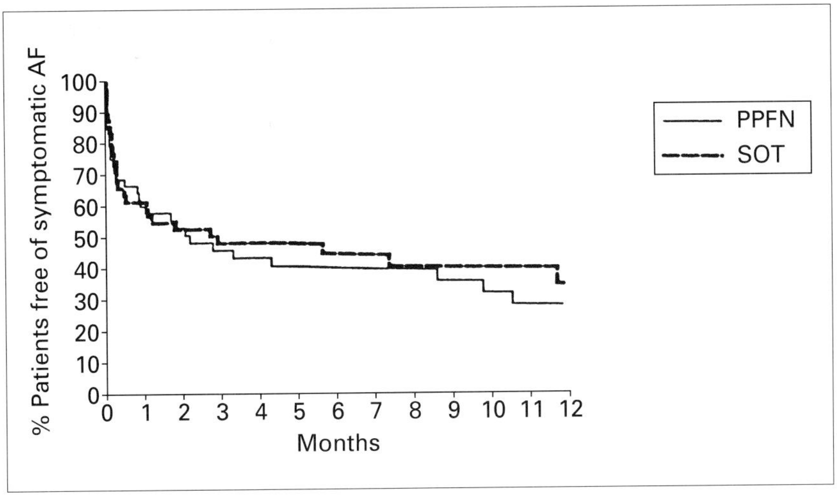

Figure 13.7
Proportion of patients remaining in sinus rhythm is depicted for patients randomised to propafenone (PPFN) and sotalol (SOT). Recurrence rate was greatest for both drugs during the first 3 months after cardioversion, and decreased thereafter. There was no significant difference between the effect of sotalol or propafenone (P = 0.72). Reproduced from Reimold et al (1993), with permission from Excerpta Medica Inc.

tricular arrhythmias had a worsened prognosis (Echt et al, 1991). The risks to patients with supraventricular arrhythmias, however, are less certain, but these drugs should be avoided in patients with evidence of heart failure or structural heart disease. Indeed, flecainide-induced ventricular arrhythmias have been reported in patients treated for AF (Falk, 1989).

Class III antiarrhythmic agents

Sotalol, another commonly prescribed drug, combines both class II (beta blockade) and class III (prolongation of repolarisation) antiarrhythmic effects and is effective in paroxysmal AF (Reimold et al, 1993) (Figure 13.7). There is little evidence, however, substantiating the efficacy of sotalol as a class III antiarrhythmic, specifically when used at conventional doses in paroxysmal AF, over and above its beta-blocking effects.

Amiodarone, another class III drug, is effective for the treatment of PAF but its use has to be moderated by its potentially serious, albeit relatively rare, side-effects. Nevertheless, amiodarone is of particular value in PAF for treating patients refractory to other measures, and low doses (usually much less than those required for the control of ventricular arrhythmias) may be effective with little risk of side-effects. The drug can be used both orally and intravenously, and unlike oral administration (which has a slow onset of action due to the long half-life of the drug), intravenous amiodarone may act relatively rapidly. However, there are seldom indications for the use of a rapid loading regimen using intravenous amiodarone in the suppression of PAF. Care should also be taken when using amiodarone since it can significantly increase the plasma concentrations of digoxin and lead to potential toxicity. It can also lead to overanticoagulation in patients taking warfarin, perhaps by a hepatic interaction.

Antithrombotic therapy

Antithrombotic therapy should be considered in patients with PAF in two circumstances: before cardioversion; and as long-term therapy for thromboprophylaxis against stroke and thromboembolism.

In patients with recurrent episodes of self-limited PAF, or in whom normal sinus rhythm is to be reestablished chemically or electrically, there is a significant risk of thromboembolism, and prophylactic anticoagulation with warfarin is needed for a minimum of 3 weeks before cardioversion. In patients with AF of less than 48 h duration who do not have a prior history of stroke or thromboembolism, left ventricular dysfunction, or rheumatic heart disease, there is a low risk of clinical thromboembolism if converted early, even without screening TOE (Weigner et al, 1997).

The precise role of long-term antithrombotic therapy in paroxysmal AF remains uncertain. In a clinicopathological study, Yamanouchi and colleagues (1997) reported that symptomatic cerebral infarctions were present in 54% of PAF patients compared with 22% of controls ($p < 0.001$). Symptomatic brain infarction was 2.4 times more common in PAF cases than in PAF-free controls, and about 60% of the infarctions in the PAF cases were judged to be cardioembolic in origin. Data from the placebo-controlled trials that included patients with paroxysmal AF, such as the BAATAF and SPAF studies, suggest that patients with PAF in placebo groups had a similar annual stroke rate to patients with chronic AF (Table 13.4). Among patients not on anticoagulation in SPAF, the yearly stroke rate was the same in PAF and chronic AF (5.6% *vs* 5.9%, SPAF 1991). In the Boston Area Anticoagulation Trial in Atrial Fibrillation (BAATAF, 1990) there was also a similar incidence of stroke in the two groups (13% *vs* 17%) with a yearly incidence of 2.5% and 2%, respectively. As with chronic AF, the presence of underlying heart disease showed the best correlation with stroke probability. Pooled analysis from the AF Investigators (1994) of the five initial randomised controlled trials showed that on univariate analysis the type of AF (PAF or chronic) and the length of time the patient was in AF had no effect on the annual stroke event rate (5.7%).

However, data from Petersen and Godtfredsen (1986) and the Framingham study (Abaof, 1996) suggest that patients with PAF may be at intermediate risk of stroke (annual incidence 1–2%) compared with patients with chronic AF and sinus rhythm. In the retrospective study by Wiener (1987) of 426 patients, the incidence of thromboembolism in patients with PAF was 2%, compared with 5% amongst those with chronic AF.

Antithrombotic therapy of paroxysmal AF should be considered, since evidence from the AF Investigators' meta-analysis suggests that patients with PAF have a similar stroke rate to patients with chronic AF (AF Investigators, 1994).

Nevertheless, the range of thromboembolic risk in such patients are likely to be wide. The patient with one short paroxysm once a year is likely to be at less risk than a patient with PAF who is having long daily paroxysms (Lip, 1997a). Therefore all patients with PAF may not be the same. Factors to be considered should include the presence of underlying structural heart disease and the patient's age. There have been no definitive trials of the benefits of antithrombotic therapy in patients with PAF per se, but it would seem reasonable to consider antithrombotic therapy based on patients' comorbidity, age, and the presence of

Source, y	No. of patients	No Warfarin % y		Warfarin % y		Warfarin % y, PAF + CAF
		PAF	CAF	PAF	CAF	
BAATAF, 1990	420	2.5	2.8	NA	NA	0.41
SPAF Study, 1991	1330	5.6	5.9	NA	NA	2.3
Peterson and Godtfredsen, 1986	426	2.0	5.1	NA	NA	NA
Roy et al, 1986	254	5.33	5.93	1.06	0.0	NA

*PAF Paroxysmal Atrial Fibrillation
CAF Chronic Atrial Fibrillation
BAATAF Boston Area Anticoagulation Trial for Atrial Fibrillation Investigators
SPAF Stroke Prevention in Atrial Fibrillation.
NA Not Available

Table 13.4
Stroke rates in PAF and CAF.*

structural heart disease. Thus, in patients aged over 75 years, in those with clinical risk factors for stroke and structural heart disease warfarin would be a more sensible choice.

Pacemakers

The role of pacemaker therapy and other non-pharmacological interventions in patients with AF (Table 11.5) has been addressed in detail in Chapter 11. Essentially, pacemakers are occasionally required in patients with PAF, especially in association with the sick sinus syndrome, to avoid associated bradycardias or in an attempt to prevent recurrent episodes of AF.

Nevertheless, the use of dual chamber pacemakers in patients with paroxysmal AF may result in tracking of (fast) atrial rates to the upper rate limit of the pacemaker, which is overcome by the use of a pacemaker with mode switching capability (Brignole et al, 1997; Kamalvand et al, 1997). Such a sophisticated pacemaker changes from DDDR (or DDD) to a non-tracking but atrial sensing mode (DDIR, DDI, VDIR, or VDI), in the presence of a fast atrial tachyarrhythmia. When the arrhythmia terminates, the pacemaker resumes normal DDD or DDDR function.

	Clinical evidence grade	Prevention of paroxysms	Other benefits	Disadvantages
Atrial pacing in sick sinus syndrome	**A**	Yes	Reduction in mortality, heart failure, thromboembolism	• Small risk of undergoing procedure and progression of atrioventricular block
AV nodal ablation and mode-switching dual chamber pacemaker	**B**	Potential	Effective	• Pacemaker dependence • May not maintain atrial function
New pacing methods, including dual-site pacing, new algorithms, etc	**C**	Potential	—	• Unproven
Maze procedure (surgery or radiofrequency ablation)	**C**	Potentially curative	—	• Major procedures • Postoperative sinus node dysfunction • Risk of thromboembolism
Atrial defibrillator	**C**	Potential	Effective	• Discomfort during defibrillation • Limited evidence

Table 13.5
Non-pharmacological interventions for PAF.

References

Abe Y, Fukunami M, Yamaha T et al. Prediction of transition to chronic atrial fibrillation in patients with paroxysmal atrial fibrillation by signal averaged electrocardiography. A prospective study. *Circulation* 1997; **96:** 2612.

Aboaf AP, Wolf PA. Paroxysmal atrial fibrillation. A common but neglected entity. *Arch Intern Med* 1996; **156:** 362.

Anderson JL, Gilbert EM, Alpert BL et al. Prevention of symptomatic recurrences of paroxysmal atrial fibrillation in patients initially tolerating anti-arrhythmic therapy: a multicenter, double-blind, cross-over study of flecainide and placebo with transtelephonic monitoring. *Circulation* 1989; **80:** 1557–70.

Atrial Fibrillation Investigators. Risk factors for stroke and efficacy of antithrombotic therapy in atrial fibrillation: Analysis of pooled data from five randomized controlled trials. *Arch Intern Med* 1994; **154:** 1449.

Boston Area Anticoagulation Trial for Atrial Fibrillation Investigators. The effect of low dose warfarin on the risk of stroke in patients with nonrheumatic atrial fibrillation. *N Engl J Med* 1990; **323:** 1505–11.

Brignole M, Gianfranchi L, Menozzi C et al. Assessment of atrioventricular junction ablation and DDDR mode-switching pacemaker versus pharmacologic treatment in patients with severely symptomatic paroxysmal atrial fibrillation. A randomized controlled study. *Circulation* 1997; **96:** 2617.

Clementy J, Dulhoste MN, Laiter C et al. Flecainide acetate in the prevention of paroxysmal atrial fibrillation: a nine-month followup of more than 500 patients. *Am J Cardiol* 1992; **70(suppl):** 44A.

Coplen SE, Antman EM, Berlin JA et al. Efficacy and safety of quinidine therapy for maintenance of sinus rhythm after cardioversion. *Circulation* 1990; **82:** 1106.

Coumel P. Paroxysmal atrial fibrillation: a disorder of autonomic tone? *Eur Heart J* 1994; **15(suppl A):** 9–16.

Davidson E, Weinberger I, Rotenberg Z et al. Atrial fibrillation: cause and time of onset. *Arch Intern Med* 1989; **149:** 457.

Echt DS, Liebson PR, Mitchell LB et al. Mortality and morbidity in patients receiving encainide, flecainide, or placebo. The Cardiac Arrhythmia Suppression Trial. *N Engl J Med* 1991; **324:** 781–8.

Falk RH. Flecainide-induced ventricular tachycardia and fibrillation in patients treated for atrial fibrillation. *Ann Intern Med* 1989; **111:** 107–11.

Flaker GC, Fletcher KA, Rothbart RM et al. Clinical and echocardiographic features of intermittent atrial fibrillation that predict recurrent atrial fibrillation. Stroke Prevention in Atrial Fibrillation (SPAF) Investigators. *Am J Cardiol* 1995; **76:** 355–8.

Galun E, Flugelman MY, Glickson M, Eliakim M. Failure of long-term digitalization to prevent rapid ventricular response in patients with paroxysmal atrial fibrillation. *Chest* 1991; **99:** 1038–40.

Godtfredsen J. Atrial fibrillation, etiology, course, and prognosis: a follow-up of 1212 cases. Copenhagen, Denmark: University of Copenhagen; 1975. Thesis.

Hnatkova K, Waktare JE, Murgatroyd FD et al. Analysis of the cardiac rhythm preceding episodes of paroxysmal atrial fibrillation. *Am Heart J* 1998; **135:** 1010–49.

Hnatkova K, Waktare JE, Murgatroyd FD et al. Age and gender influences on rate and duration of paroxysmal atrial fibrillation. *Pacing Clin Electrophysiol* 1998; **21:** 2455–8.

Kamalvand K, Tan K, Kotsaki A et al. Is mode switching beneficial? A randomized study in patients with paroxysmal atrial tachyarrhythmias. *J Am Cardiol* 1997; **30:** 496.

Kannel WB, Abbott RD, Savage DD. Coronary heart disease and atrial fibrillation: the Framingham Study. *Am Heart J* 1983; **106:** 389–96.

Lip GYH, Beevers DG. Interpretation of IST and CAST stroke trials. International Stroke Trial.

Chinese Acute Stroke Trial. *Lancet* 1997a; **350:** 443–4.

Lip GYH, Golding DJ, Nazir M et al. A survey of atrial fibrillation in general practice: the West Birmingham Atrial Fibrillation Project. *Br J Gen Pract* 1997b; **47:** 285–9.

Murgatroyd FD, Gibson SM, Baiyan X et al. Double-blind placebo-controlled trial of digoxin in symptomatic paroxysmal atrial fibrillation. *Circulation* 1999; **99:** 2765–70.

Noc M, Stajer D, Horvat M. Intravenous amiodarone versus verapamil for acute conversion of paroxysmal atrial fibrillation to sinus rhythm. *Am J Cardiol* 1990; **65:** 679–80.

Page RL, Wilkinson WE, Clair WK et al. Asymptomatic arrhythmias in patients with symptomatic paroxysmal atrial fibrillation and paroxysmal supraventricular tachycardia. *Circulation* 1994; **89:** 224–7.

Petersen P, Godtfredsen J. Embolic complications in paroxysmal atrial fibrillation. *Stroke* 1986; **17:** 622–5.

Phillips SJ, Whisnant JP, O'Fallon WM, Frye RL. Prevalence of cardiovascular disease and diabetes mellitus in residents of Rochester, Minnesota. *Mayo Clin Proc* 1990; **65:** 344–59.

Phillips E, Levine SA, Auricular fibrillation without other evidence of heart disease. *Am J Med* 1949; **7:** 478.

Pietersen AH, Hellemann H. Usefulness of flecainide for prevention of paroxysmal atrial fibrillation and flutter. *Am J Cardiol* 1991; **67:** 713–17.

Pritchett EL, McCarthy EA, Wilkinson WE. Propafenone treatment of symptomatic paroxysmal supraventricular arrhythmias. *Ann Intern Med* 1991; **114:** 539–44.

Rawles JM, Metcalfe MJ, Jennings K. Time of occurrence, duration, and ventricular rate of paroxysmal atrial fibrillation: the effect of digoxin. *Br Heart J* 1990; **63:** 225–7.

Reimold SC, Cantillon CO, Friedman PL, Antman EM. Propafenone versus sotalol for suppression of recurrent symptomatic atrial fibrillation. *Am J Cardiol* 1993; **71:** 558–63.

Rostagno C, Bacci F, Martelli M et al. Clinical course of lone atrial fibrillation since first symptomatic arrhythmic episode. *Am J Cardiol* 1995; **76:** 837.

Roy D, Marchand E, Gagne P et al. Usefulness of anticoagulant therapy in the prevention of embolic complications of atrial fibrillation. *Am Heart J* 1986; **112:** 1039–43.

Sopher SM, Camm AJ. Atrial fibrillation: maintenance of sinus rhythm versus rate control. *Am J Cardiol* 1996; **77:** 24A–37A.

Sopher SM, Hnatkova K, Waktare JE et al. Circadian variation in atrial fibrillation in patients with frequent paroxysms. *Pacing Clin Electrophysiol* 1998; **21:** 2445–9.

Stroke Prevention in Atrial Fibrillation Investigators. Stroke Prevention in Atrial Fibrillation study: final results. *Circulation* 1991; **84:** 527.

Suttorp MJ, Kingma JH, Koomen EM et al. Recurrence of paroxysmal atrial fibrillation or flutter after successful cardioversion in patients with normal left ventricular function. *Am J Cardiol* 1993; **71:** 710–13.

Suttorp MJ, Kingma JH, Lie-A-Huen L, Mast EG. Intravenous flecainide versus verapamil for acute conversion of paroxysmal atrial fibrillation or flutter to sinus rhythm. *Am J Cardiol* 1989; **63:** 693–6.

Takahashi N, Seki A, Imataka K, Fujii J. Clinical features of paroxysmal atrial fibrillation. *Jpn Heart J* 1981; **22:** 143–9.

Verhorst PMJ, Kamp O, Welling RC et al. Transesophageal echocardiographic predictors for maintenance of sinus rhythm after electrical cardioversion of atrial fibrillation. *Am J Cardiol* 1997; **79:** 1355.

Weigner MJ, Caulfield TA, Danias PG et al. Risk for clinical thromboembolism associated with conversion to sinus rhythm in patients with atrial fibrillation lasting less than 48 hours. *Ann Intern Med* 1997; **126:** 615.

Wiener I. Clinical and echocardiographic correlates of systemic embolization in nonrheumatic atrial fibrillation. *Am J Cardiol* 1987; **59:** 177.

Yamanouchi H, Mizutani T, Matsushita S, Esaki Y. Paroxysmal atrial fibrillation: high frequency of embolic brain infarction in elderly autopsy patients. *Neurology* 1997; **49:** 1691–4.

Zarifis J, Beevers DG, Lip GYH. Acute admissions with atrial fibrillation in a British multiracial hospital population. *Br J Clin Pract* 1997; **51:** 91–6.

14

Persistent atrial fibrillation and cardioversion

In patients with persistent atrial fibrillation (AF), the objective of management is cardioversion from AF to sinus rhythm. Aspects of management which should be considered include anticoagulation therapy to reduce the risk of thromboembolism, and antiarrhythmic therapy to maintain sinus rhythm. In hospital, it is recommended to start heparin therapy immediately upon admission of a patient with recent onset AF, since the duration of the arrhythmia cannot be predicted. Cardioversion can be done pharmacologically using class I or class III agents, or electrically using a standard transthoracic method or internal cardioversion (Tables 14.1 and 14.2). Spontaneous conversion of sinus rhythm can be observed in up to 48% of patients with paroxysmal AF and patients with recent onset AF (within 24 h).

Benefits of cardioversion

The potential benefits of a return to sinus rhythm include an improvement in the patient's well-being, improved haemodynamic status and exercise capability (secondary to the return of atrial filling, and consequent improved cardiac output), the avoidance of (potentially dangerous) drug therapy, and perhaps a reduction in stroke and thromboembolic risk. Many studies have shown an improvement in exercise capacity and left ventricular function by a return to sinus rhythm (Van Gelder et al, 1993; Gosselink et al, 1994; Upshaw, 1997; Alam and Thorstand, 1992) (Figure 14.1). The return of atrial systole as demonstrated by return of the A wave on Doppler Echocardiography (Manning et al, 1994) (Figure 14.2) can contribute as much as 30% of the stroke volume, especially in the elderly and in patients with evidence of diastolic dysfunction. The return of atrial transport also reduces atrial size and stasis within the atria, thus potentially reducing the risk of stroke and thromboembolism (Gosselink et al, 1993; Manning et al, 1989).

Assessment for cardioversion

Full assessment of the patient with persistent AF for cardioversion should include an assessment of underlying aetiological factor(s). Patients with specific pathology (such as mitral stenosis and poor left ventricular function) are unlikely to successfully cardiovert. By contrast, a patient with AF secondary to thyrotoxicosis or a chest infection that has since been treated would have a high success rate if cardioversion was attempted. If the underlying aetiology and triggering factor(s) continue to exert an effect, attempts at cardioversion may be unsuccessful.

A careful history of previous attempts at cardioversion, reactions to antiarrhythmic

- Arrange admission to hospital for ECG monitoring (e.g. Coronary Care Unit).
- Ensure electrolytes (especially potassium) are normal.
- Ensure anticoagulation adequate, with an INR of 2.0 to 3.0.
- If the patient is normally taking digoxin, with no evidence of digitoxicity, the drug can be taken to the day before the procedure.
  If digitoxicity is present, serum digoxin levels should be checked and the procedure delayed.

Table 14.1
How to cardiovert a patient with AF.

Pharmacological

- Start infusion of drug (e.g. flecainide, amiodarone) under continuous ECG monitoring.

Electrical

- Patient to be fasted.
- Short general anaesthesia to eliminate discomfort associated with the transthoracic shock.
- Synchronised DC shock, start at 200 Joules, with intermediate 'step-ups', eventually to 360 Joules.
- After the procedure, the patient is monitored for at least 1 hour to ensure stability of rhythm and blood pressure.

Table 14.2
How to cardiovert a patient with AF (2).

drugs (if used), and toleration of general anaesthetic (in patients for electrical cardioversion) should be obtained. Serum electrolytes should be checked in view of potential interactions with some antiarrhythmic agents — for example, the increased risk of *torsades des pointes* with hypokalaemia if class I agents are used. In elective cardioversion, patients should have adequate anticoagulation (target INR 2–3) for a minimum of 3 weeks before the procedure. Patients taking digoxin do not need routine measurement of serum digoxin levels, unless there is evidence of toxicity. Patients should be instructed to stop taking their digoxin tablets on the day of their procedure.

Proper selection of patients suitable for the procedure, and the use of antiarrhythmic therapy to prevent recurrences of arrhythmia, usually permit a successful outcome (Table 14.3). Nevertheless there are still many uncertainties and differences in management strategies (Mead et al, 1999; Schlicht et al, 1996; Lip et al, 1996).

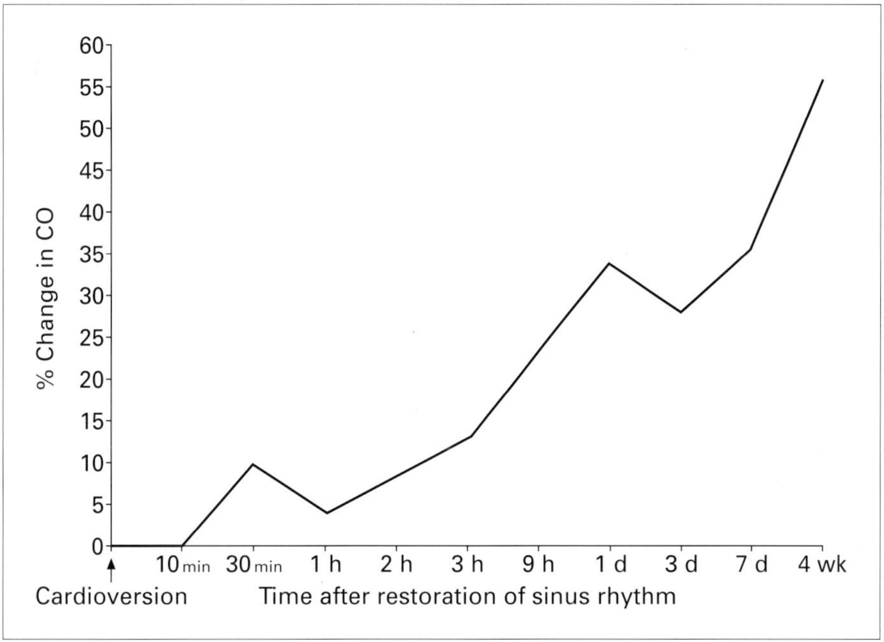

Figure 14.1
Time course of cardiac output (CO) after restoration of sinus rhythm in patients with heart disease. Note the gradual increase in CO during the 4 weeks after cardioversion. Adapted from Upshaw (1997).

Methods of cardioversion

Cardioversion of AF can be done by pharmacological or electrical methods. Electrical cardioversion was first introduced by Lown (1967) and is commonly used. However, recent developments in the use of antiarrhythmic drugs have identified suitable drugs, especially class I and III antiarrhythmic agents, that are effective for cardioversion of AF and the maintenance of sinus rhythm. Internal cardioversion is now a useful technique for patients resistant to transthoracic cardioversion, although the procedure is still limited to specialised centres (Levy et al, 1992).

Although cardioversion of AF has been generally regarded as a "classical" therapeutic option and an essentially straightforward procedure, there remain unanswered questions, especially with regard to patient selection, the routine use and selection of antiarrhythmic therapy, the optimal reduction in thromboembolic risk, and whether cardioversion of atrial flutter should be treated similarly. Indeed there remains considerable management variation, even amongst consultant physicians, in performing cardioversion, in the use of antiarrhythmic therapy (Lip et al, 1996), and in the choice of anticoagulation regimes (Chang et al, 1990).

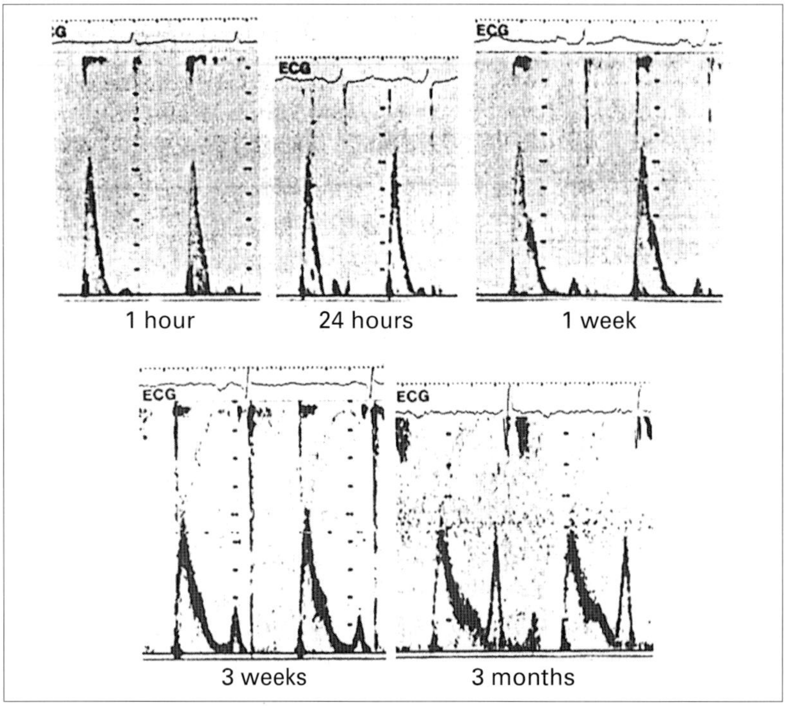

Figure 14.2
Serial transmitral pulsed Doppler inflow velocity profiles from an individual patient. Note the progressive increase in peak A wave velocity and percent A wave filling over the observation period. For each spectrum, the vertical calibration markings indicate 0.2 m/s flow velocity; horizontal distances between calibration markings indicate 1 s. Adapted from Manning et al (1994).

Predictors of refractoriness to cardioversion or unsuccessful maintenance of sinus rhythm

Predictors of refractoriness to cardioversion or unsuccessful maintenance of sinus rhythm include the following: age, duration of arrhythmia, the presence of uncontrolled hypertension, structural heart disease (dilated impaired left ventricles, valve disease, etc), and other organic heart disease (Brodsky et al, 1989; Van Gelder et al, 1991b; Dethy et al, 1988). Older age, in combination with a large number of previous episodes of arrhythmia and a long previous duration of arrhythmia, is predictive of the unsuccessful maintenance of sinus rhythm (Crijns et al, 1991; Van Gelder et al, 1991b). In addition, the presence of coronary artery disease, significant chronic obstructive pulmonary disease, hypertension, and organic heart disease (such as heart failure, pericarditis, mitral valve disease, aortic stenosis, and cardiomyopathy) are adverse factors for successful cardioversion and long-term maintenance of sinus rhythm (Mancini and Goldberger, 1982; Van Gelder et al, 1991b). In addition, if a precipitant (such as pyrexia, thyrotoxicosis, etc) is identified when the patient develops AF, correction of the precipitating factor allows a high chance of successful cardioversion. Indeed, if AF is secondary to hyperthyroidism cardioversion should be delayed until thyroid function has returned to normal. AF complicating cardiac surgery is common and tends to be self-limiting.

The effects of left atrial size are less certain. In a small study (50 patients), a left atrial dimension of 45 mm or more was important, and had a positive predictive value of 66% for

	Intravenous Therapy for Acute Conversion	Oral Therapy for Cardioversion and Prevention of Recurrences
Class Ia		
Procainamide	15 m/kg over 60 minutes	500–750 mg every 6–8 hours
Quinidine gluconate		324–648 mg every 8–12 hours
Disopyramide		150 mg every 6–8 hours or 150–300 mg twice a day
Class Ic		
Flecainide	2 mg/kg IV*	50–150 mg every 12 hours
Propafenone	2 mg/kg IV*	150–300 mg every 8 hours
Class III		
Ibutilide	1–2 mg/kg IV	
Amiodarone	5–7 mg/kg IV up to 1,500 mg/24 hrs	400–800 mg daily for 3–4 weeks followed by 100–400 mg daily
Sotalol		80–240 mg every 12 hours
Expected rate of conversion to sinus rhythm		
Procainamide	40%–80%	
Quinidine	40%–86%	
Flecainide	67%–96%	
Amiodarone	37%–73%	
Sotalol	8%–54%	
Ibutilide	33%–63%	

*Not available in United States
IV = intravenous

Table 14.3
Drug loading and maintenance doses for pharmacological cardioversion and prevention of recurrences to atrial fibrillation, and expected success rates. Reproduced from Jung and DiMarco (1998), with permission from Excerpta Medica Inc.

recurrence of AF (Brodsky et al, 1989). However, recent studies have, by contrast, shown the converse — that is, left atrial size does not appear to influence outcome after cardioversion (Dittrich et al, 1989; Van Gelder et al, 1991b; Brodsky et al, 1989). Therefore, atrial size does not strongly influence outcome of cardioversion, and absolute left atrial size should not preclude attempt at cardioversion, especially if this is the initial episode of AF and the duration of AF is relatively brief (weeks). An increase in left atrial size may also be consequent upon the presence of AF, which may explain why it does not necessarily predict outcome after cardioversion. Even in the presence of a dilated left atrium, long term sinus rhythm (79% at 12 months) is possible with the use of antiarrhythmic drugs (Brodsky et al, 1989).

The series by Dalzell and colleagues (1991) in 80 patients showed that sex, left atrial enlargement, electrode pad positions, aetiology of AF, presence of left ventricular failure,

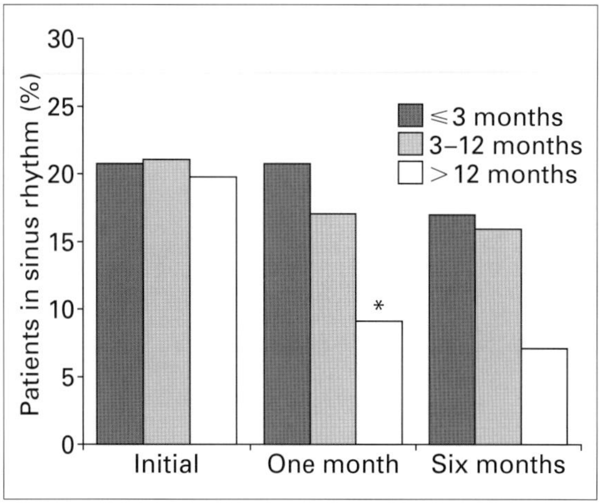

Figure 14.3
*Percentages of patients in sinus rhythm at the time of cardioversion and at 1- and 6-months follow-up are shown according to duration of AF (<3 months, 3 to 12 months and >12 months) before cardioversion. *p < 0.02. Reproduced from Dittrich et al (1989), with permission from Excerpta Medica Inc.*

and prior treatment with verapamil or beta-adrenergic blockers were not significant determinants of cardioversion success or success of low energy shocks. However, prior treatment with digoxin was significant, both for cardioversion success and success at low energies. In patients with transthoracic impedance of 70 ohms or less, low energy shocks were more often successful than in patients with transthoracic impedance of more than 70 ohms. On univariate analysis, however, cardioversion success with low energy shocks was significantly associated with prior treatment with digoxin and also with the duration of AF, and, for shocks of 100 joules or less, with prior treatment with amiodarone. On multifactorial linear regression analysis, only duration of AF of 24 h to less than 1 month, and of 1 month to 3 years were significant predictors of cardioversion success irrespective of shock strength, and of success of low energy shocks.

In general, AF duration is probably the most important predictor of successful conversion to sinus rhythm, with a decreasing tendency to spontaneous conversion with an increased duration of AF (Dittrich et al, 1989; Van Gelder et al, 1991b; Brodsky et al, 1989) (Figure 14.3). There is a twofold increase in the proportion remaining in sinus rhythm after cardioversion in patients with a short duration AF (less than 3 months), compared with those in whom AF has been present for more than 12 months (Dittrich et al, 1989). However, the duration of AF alone should not be the sole basis for exclusion of such patients from cardioversion, and many other factors, such as the clinical state and the presence of structural heart disease, should be considered. Indeed, patients who have been in AF for a long time are less likely to successfully cardiovert, although there have been case reports of successful cardioversion in patients who had been in AF for as long as 10 years (Lip and Hogg, 1993). Selection of patients is therefore important, and suitable patients for cardioversion should include the following: those with recent onset AF; those without structural heart disease (for example: mitral valve disease, poor left ventricular function, left atrium not dilated); and those in whom a precipitating cause for AF, if present, has been treated (for example: thyrotoxicosis, chest infection). The relation to the duration of AF is a reflection of electrical and structural remodelling, resulting in persistence of AF and increasing resistance to cardioversion. This is illustrated by the experimental goat model of AF by Wijfells and colleagues (1995) in which prolongation of artificially induced AF leads to persistence of the arrhythmia ("AF begets AF"). Morphological changes in atrial myocardium are also evident in chronic AF, compared with recent onset AF, with greater fibrosis, myocyte loss, and degener-

Author	n	Age	AF duration	LA size	LVdys	Valve
Dethy et al, 1988	50	n	y	y	?	n
Dittrich et al, 1989	65	n	y	n	n	n
Brodsky et al, 1989	43	n	y	y	n	y
Van Gelder et al, 1991b	246	y	y	n	?	y
Crijns et al, 1991	127	y	y	?	n	y
Tebbe et al, 1995	1152	n	y	y	y	n

Some uncertainty — probably duration of AF most important

Table 14.4
Predictors of refractoriness to cardioversion of AF or unsuccessful maintenance of sinus rhythm.

ation of the endoplasmic reticulum (Ausma et al, 1997).

Overall, the data available have some inconsistencies, with some but not all studies confirming one factor or another as important in predicting success of cardioversion or long-term maintenance of sinus rhythm (Table 14.4). Patients with sinus or atrioventricular (AV) node dysfunction, as in bradycardia-tachycardia syndrome, are also relatively unfavourable candidates for cardioversion, which may unmask the underlying bradycardia and conduction abnormality, although a pacemaker may help management.

Thromboembolism after cardioversion of AF

Thromboembolism may complicate cardioversion of AF of 48 hours' duration or more in 5–7% of cases in which anticoagulation is not used, but this is reduced to 1% with anticoagulation (Tables 14.5 and 14.6). The highest risk appears to be in the first week after cardioversion, although this is based on observational case series (Bjerkelund and Orning, 1969).

The role of prophylactic anticoagulation has been clinically examined in several large series. Bjerkelund and Orning (1969) reported a series of 437 patients with atrial arrhythmias in whom electrical cardioversion was attempted on 572 occasions: 228 patients were on long-term anticoagulant therapy, whilst 209 were not given anticoagulants. In this series 13 (3%) patients had thromboembolic events, including 2 (1.1%) of the 186 patients in the anticoagulant group, compared with 11 (6.8%) of the 162 patients who were not on anticoagulants and were successfully cardioverted. These results show that prior anticoagulant therapy was beneficial in attempted cardioversion. Furthermore, an advantageous effect of warfarin was shown despite more patients with congestive heart failure, mitral valve disease, and hypertension (factors that increase the risk for thromboembolism) being present in the anticoagulated group. The thromboembolic events that did occur were predominantly noted 1–6 days after cardioversion, suggesting a "high-risk" period after cardioversion. However, this study was not randomised, and since patients were on chronic anticoagulant therapy, the value of short term anticoagulant therapy could not be defined. The study also included

Study	*n*	*% thromboembolism no warfarin*
Morris 1964	66	4.5
Bjerkelund 1969	162	6.8
Weinberg 1989	28	7.1
Arnold 1992	115	6.3
Roy 1986	42	4.8

Patients with AF ≥2 days are subject to a 5–7% risk of cardioversion-related thromboembolism without warfarin.

Table 14.5
Cardioversion-related thromboembolism without warfarin. Adapted with permission from Silverman and Manning (1998).

Study	*n*	*% thromboembolism on warfarin*
Rokseth 1963	274	1.6
Bjerkelund 1969	186	1.1
Weinberg 1989	51	0
Arnold 1992	52	0
Klein 1997	54	1.6

Use of 2 to 4 weeks warfarin before cardioversion of patients with AF ≥2 days reduces thromboembolic risk to ~1.2%.

Table 14.6
Cardioversion-related thromboembolism with warfarin. Adapted with permission from Silverman and Manning (1998).

patients with atrial flutter and atrial tachycardia (in addition to AF), but the risk of thromboembolism in these subgroups was not specifically defined.

In another retrospective study of 79 patients by Weinberg and Mancini (1989) who underwent cardioversion, none of the 51 patients who received anticoagulant therapy has an embolic event, whilst two (7%) of 28 who were not anticoagulated had an embolic stroke. Although these numbers are small, the results do support short-term anticoagulant treatment, especially in high-risk patients, defined in this study as patients aged over 55 years, those with duration of AF of more than 1 year, with coronary artery disease, cardiomyopathy, or hypertension.

Arnold and colleagues (1992) retrospectively assessed 454 elective direct current cardioversions done for AF or atrial flutter over 7 years. The incidence of embolic complications was 1.32% (six patients in total). Of these six

- Mechanical — resumption of mechanical atrial systolic function may result in the embolisation of any pre-existing clot.
- Transient atrial dysfunction post-cardioversion ("stunning").
- Duration of AF — recently formed, poorly adherent thrombus more likely to dislodge compared to older thrombus (more firmly adherent).
- Abnormalities in haemorheological function and prothrombotic markers intrinsic to AF.

Table 14.7
Factors contributing to thromboembolism following cardioversion of AF.

patients, all had AF, none were on anticoagulants, and the duration of AF was less than 1 week in five of them. None of the patients with atrial flutter had thromboembolic events, confirming the low thromboembolic risk for cardioversion in this subgroup of patients.

In patients with acute onset AF of less than 48 h, current clinical practice suggests that postcardioversion anticoagulation may not be necessary, since there is insufficient time for intra-atrial thrombus to form. However, a recent study by Stoddard and colleagues (1995) suggested that even in patients with acute onset AF (<48 h), over 14% had left atrial or left atrial appendage thrombus, compared with a prevalence of 27% in patients with chronic AF. Furthermore, in the patients with acute AF, 17% had systemic embolisation after cardioversion, compared with 30% of patients with chronic AF. Thus, although the prevalence of thrombus and embolisation is much lower in acute-onset AF than in patients with chronic AF, the proportions are not inconsequential and can in fact cause devastating strokes. In the study by Stoddard and colleagues (1995), independent predictors of thrombus formation included the presence of mitral stenosis and those with left ventricular ejection fractions of less than 40%. Systemic thromboembolism, however, was predicted by the presence of a mobile left atrial thrombus, chronic heart failure, coronary artery disease, and impaired left ventricular function (ejection fraction less than 40%).

Whilst the above-mentioned studies were not randomised trials, the evidence in favour of anticoagulant therapy before cardioversion of AF is very persuasive. Indeed, various possibilities have been suggested for the mechanisms and factors contributing to thromboembolism after cardioversion of AF (Table 14.7).

Mechanical explanation — The sudden resumption of mechanical and atrial systolic function may result in the embolisation of any pre-existing clot formed within the left atrium. The time for the return of atrial systole is variable, and can take up to 3 weeks after cardioversion (Manning et al, 1989; 1994).

Duration of AF — Recently formed, poorly adherent thrombus is more likely to dislodge at the time of cardioversion, whereas older thrombus is likely to be more firmly adherent by fibroblastic infiltration. One estimate of the time required for the latter is about 14 days, so adequate anticoagulation for this time period might prevent new clot formation and allow the most recently formed thrombi to adhere sufficiently. However, this time period cannot be precisely defined, and is very likely to vary according to haemodynamic status, atrial size, and underlying atrial pathology, together with the effectiveness of anticoagulation. Manning and colleagues (1994) also reported that the return of atrial systole was slower in patients with a longer duration of prior AF.

Transient atrial dysfunction after cardioversion — Cardioversion may actually promote new thrombus formation due to transient atrial dysfunction ("stunning") in the postcardioversion period (Fatkin et al, 1994b; Grimm et al, 1997). This is shown by the new development of spontaneous echocontrast on transoesophageal echocardiography after cardioversion and thromboembolic complications, even in the absence of demonstrable left atrial thrombi. Even in atrial flutter, atrial function is still reduced in the first 24 h after cardioversion, with 18% in complete atrial standstill (Jordaens et al, 1993).

Abnormalities in haemorheological function and prothrombotic markers — The presence of AF is associated with abnormalities of haemostasis, blood rheology, and endothelial dysfunction, which confer a hypercoagulable state that appears to rise transiently in the immediate period after cardioversion (Lip, 1995; Oltrona et al, 1997). At 2 weeks after cardioversion there may be a reduction in thrombogenesis as evident by a reduction in fibrin D-dimer levels (Lip et al, 1996). AF is also associated with raised levels of atrial natriuretic peptide, which may contribute to haemoconcentration, a raised haematocrit, and subsequent thromboembolism and stroke (Peterson et al, 1988). Abnormalities in haemorheological function and prothrombotic markers have been linked to the presence of spontaneous echocontrast, which is a marker of intra-atrial stasis, thrombogenesis, and subsequent thromboembolism (Daniel et al, 1988; Fatkin et al, 1997).

Left atrial size — Left atrial enlargement is associated with increased spontaneous echocontrast on transoesophageal echocardiography, indicating stasis or slow, sluggish blood flow within the enlarged atrial cavity. The rheological mechanism for spontaneous echocontrast is thought to involve the presence of fibrinogen, or its products, and red cell aggregation or rouleau formation (Fatkin et al, 1994; Merino et al, 1992), thus providing a link between haemorheological abnormalities and visual demonstration of flow abnormalities with the left atrium.

Abnormalities in cerebral blood flow — There appears to be increased cerebral blood flow after cardioversion from AF to normal sinus rhythm, and this may predispose to cerebral embolism in the distribution of the middle cerebral artery (Petersen, 1990).

Electrical cardioversion

Most clinicians would be familiar with electrical cardioversion using externally placed electrodes at the apex and sternum and applying a synchronised direct current (DC) shock under general anaesthetic to depolarise the myocardial cells, after which sinus node activity resumes. Other methods of electrical cardioversion, which are used less often, include transoesophageal cardioversion and internal cardioversion.

External DC cardioversion was first described in 1967 by Lown, and has since had widespread use in the management of arrhythmias. Electrical cardioversion works by allowing uniform repolarisation and restoring ordered conduction. After the initial asystolic period, the sino-atrial node rapidly resumes its role as cardiac pacemaker, allowing synchronised atrial electrical activity.

Energy requirements for successful DC cardioversion vary according to many factors, such as the duration of AF, transthoracic impedance (thickness of chest wall), prior use of antiarrhythmic agents, and appropriate placement of electrodes. Energy requirements for cardioversion have also been related to the size of the fibrillatory waves; for example, recent onset AF is associated with coarser (greater than 2 mm) fibrillatory waves and lower cardioversion energy requirements (Lown, 1967). AF also shortens the atrial effective refractory period (ERP) and predisposes to further episodes of AF. There has also been recent experimental and clinical evidence that calcium sparing agents such as verapamil and diltiazem result in lower energy requirements and a greater success rate of electrical cardioversion (Tieleman et al, 1997; 1998; Daoud et al, 1997; 1999).

Daoud and colleagues (1999) showed that even several minutes of AF may be enough to induce atrial contractile dysfunction after cardioversion. This is attenuated by the administration of verapamil, suggesting that postcardioversion atrial dysfunction may be at least partially mediated by cellular calcium overload. Similarly, pretreatment with verapamil, but not with the sodium channel antagonist procainamide, markedly attenuated the acute AF-induced changes in atrial electrophysiological properties, suggesting that calcium loading during AF may be at least partially responsible for AF-induced electrical remodelling (Daoud et al, 1997).

External cardioversion

External or transthoracic electrical cardioversion works by repolarising the errant atrial conduction, restoring ordered conduction. During the initial asystolic period, the sinoatrial node rapidly resumes its role as cardiac pacemaker. External electrical cardioversion is effective in restoring sinus rhythm, but is efficacy can range from 20% to 90%, being highly influenced by the underlying aetiology. The highest recorded success rates for cardioversion are seen in patients with AF secondary to hyperthyroidism, whilst the lowest rates are seen in patients with severe mitral regurgitation.

Attention to proper technique for external cardioversion will greatly improve efficacy (Ewy, 1994; Yapa and Green, 1990). R-wave synchronisation is necessary to avoid shock-induced ventricular arrhythmias. Technical aspects that have to be considered include electrode size, position of electrodes (antero-apical compared to anteroposterior), transthoracic impedance (influenced by pressure on electrode, electrode gel, and previous shocks), output wave form, and stored energy. Previous enthusiasm for the superiority of anteroposterior electrode pad positions for cardioversion has been dampened by the recent randomised trial by Mathew and colleagues (1999) in which cardioversion success rate and energy requirements were similar in the anteroanterior and anteroposterior positions.

The recommended initial energy for electrical cardioversion is 200 joules and 75% of patients or more are successfully cardioverted with this energy. High energies (360 joules) are needed if 200-joule shocks do not restore sinus rhythm. There is limited evidence on the effect of antiarrhythmic agents on energy requirements and the success rate of cardioversion. However, in cases of resistant AF, a 4-week loading of amiodarone before cardioversion (at a daily dose of 600 mg) and a low-dose maintenance regime after successful cardioversion (on average 200 mg daily) appears to be effective in achieving cardioversion and sustaining sinus rhythm (Gosselink et al, 1992). In one study of 127 patients undergoing cardioversion, the sequential use of different types of antiarrhythmic drugs also improved arrhythmia prognosis in chronic AF or flutter after successful cardioversion (Crijns

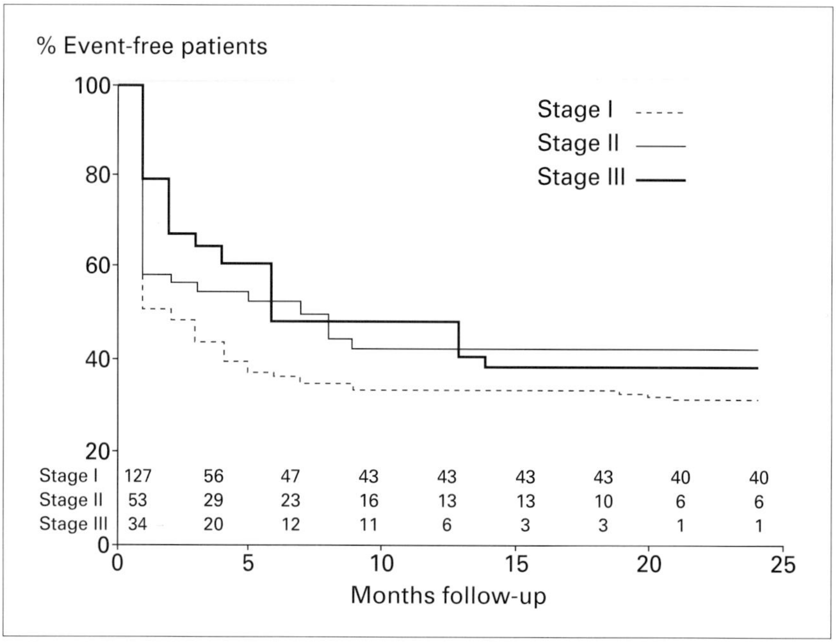

Figure 14.4
Actuarial 2-year arrhythmia-free episodes during the separate treatment stages. The figures below the curves indicate the number of patients at risk. Adapted from Crijns et al (1999).

et al, 1991). Serial drug treatment in that study, initially with flecainide (stage I), followed by quinidine or sotalol if recurrence occurred (stage II), and eventually with amiodarone (stage III), increased the 2-year proportion of arrhythmia-free patients from 31% at stage I to 63% at the end of serial treatment (Figure 14.4). Complications of external cardioversion are rare but include systemic thromboembolism, ventricular arrhythmia, sinus bradycardia, hypotension, pulmonary oedema, and transient ST and T-wave segment elevation.

In the management of AF, external DC cardioversion should be considered in the acute stage, for a patient initially presenting with acute onset fast AF who is becoming haemodynamically unstable, in whom cardioversion to sinus rhythm may be life-saving. Cardioversion should also be considered as an elective procedure for suitable patients, due to its probable haemodynamic benefits and possible reduction in long-term stroke risk. Careful patient selection would ensure successful electrical cardioversion in over 90% of cases. As previously discussed, patients with a high success rate of initial cardioversion and maintenance of sinus rhythm include younger patients (aged <60 years), with short duration of AF (<1 year), no structural heart disease (that is, no valve disease, dilated atria or ventricles, preserved left ventricular function) and an identifiable precipitant (such as pyrexia, thyroid disease, etc).

There is no evidence that electrical cardioversion of AF results in damage to the myocardium. Muscle enzymes such as creatine kinase are released during skeletal muscle injury, but cardiac isoenzyme MB subfractions are not significantly raised. In an elegant study using radionuclide scanning with labelled pyrophosphate, Metcalfe and colleagues (1988) showed that damage to the myocardium, if any, was minimal.

Internal cardioversion

High-energy direct current internal cardioversion (200–300 joules) is useful in patients who fail both external and pharmacological cardioversion. In patients who fail external cardioversion, internal cardioversion (using electric shocks delivered within the right atrium) is a useful technique with no more occurrences over long-term follow-up (Levy et al, 1992). In one randomised comparison of external and internal cardioversion of chronic AF, the efficacy of internal cardioversion was significantly greater than that of external cardioversion (91% *vs* 67%, respectively; Levy et al, 1992). The effectiveness of internal cardioversion was confirmed in the recent report of The Multicenter Low Energy Transvenous Atrial Defibrillation (XAD) trial (Levy et al, 1997).

Internal cardioversion seems to be particularly useful in obese patients and in those with chronic lung disease. Even in patients with AF lasting more than 1 year, internal low energy atrial cardioversion also seems to be highly effective in restoring sinus rhythm, although additional antiarrhythmic treatment may often be required particularly in the first days after conversion (Boriani et al, 1999b). The use of intravenous flecainide may help, by reducing the AF threshold in patients treated with low-energy internal atrial cardioversion, resulting in lower shock-induced discomfort (Boriani et al, 1999a). Furthermore, in patients with chronic persistent AF, flecainide may increase the procedure success rate.

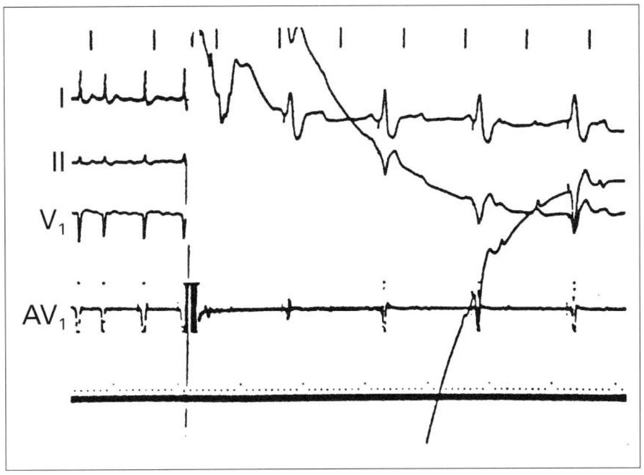

Figure 14.5
Recording during shock delivery in internal cardioversion for AF. On the left side, the patient is in AF. Following internal shock sinus rhythm is restored and transient AV block is seen with ventricular pacing.

Low energy (less than 20 joules) cardioversion of AF using biphasic shocks and two electrode catheters positioned in the right atrium (cathode) and the coronary sinus (anode), or in the left pulmonary artery as an alternative, is another technique (Figures 14.5 and 14.6). Low energy cardioversion restored sinus rhythm in 70–89% of patients, even including patients with failed external cardioversion and AF complicating diagnostic or ablation procedures. The technique does not require general anaesthesia and is currently under intensive evaluation.

The principle of internal cardioversion has been extended to the development of implantable atrial defibrillator, for patients with paroxysmal AF, where paroxysms of AF are detected by the device and low-energy conversion to sinus rhythm is performed. Preliminary reports suggest that these devices are effective and well-tolerated (see chapter 11). At present, internal cardioversion is only avail-

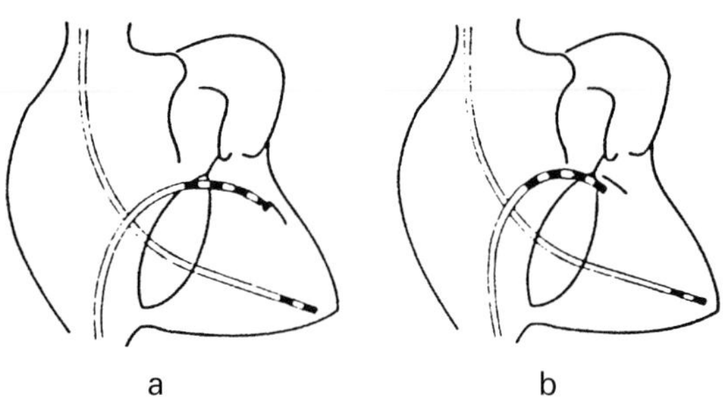

Figure 14.6
Technique of transcatheter cardioversion. (a) Position of the catheter (6F USCI, quadripolar) in the His bundle area. (b) Position in which the shock is delivered. Note that the proximal electrode used as a cathode is in the right atrial cavity.

able in specialist electrophysiological centres that are offering this technique to cases resistant to cardioversion.

Pharmacological cardioversion

An alternative to electrical cardioversion is pharmacological (or chemical) cardioversion, especially in patients with recent onset AF (Table 14.3). In general, drugs that are usually used to maintain sinus rhythm after electrical cardioversion, such as class I and class III antiarrhythmic drugs, are also effective for pharmacological cardioversion. The calcium antagonists are generally effective for rate control, but not cardioversion (Tisdale et al, 1998). A meta-analysis of trials comparing flecainide, amiodarone, and quinidine showed the following proportions of patients to be in normal sinus rhythm at 12 months after cardioversion for AF: amiodarone 59.8%; quinidine 50%, and flecainide 34% (Zarembski, 1995).

There are relatively few direct comparisons between multiple (≥3) drug regimens for cardioversion. Boriani and colleagues (1998a) undertook a study of a population of 417 patients with recent onset AF, which compared attempted cardioversion with placebo, intravenous amiodarone (5 mg/kg bolus, followed by 1.8 g/24 h), intravenous propafenone (2 mg/kg bolus, followed by 0.0078 mg/kg/min), oral propafenone (single 600 mg dose) and oral flecainide (single 300 mg dose). They showed that intravenous propafenone resulted in a higher conversion rate within 1 h compared with the oral loading regimens of propafenone or flecainide, but the conversion rates at 3 h and 8 h were similar (about 75%). However, intravenous amiodarone was not different from placebo until 8 h, when cardioversion had occurred in 57%. Importantly, placebo achieved conversion to sinus rhythm in 37% of patients at 8 h.

Class Ia agents

There are no placebo-controlled trials to show the safety and efficacy of intravenous or oral quinidine, procainamide, or disopyrimide in restoring sinus rhythm in recent onset AF. Nevertheless, quinidine is still a frequently used class Ia drug for cardioversion and the maintenance of sinus rhythm after cardioversion.

Class I drugs should not be used in patients with heart failure, low ejection fractions, or major conduction problems. Amiodarone is the drug of choice if heart failure is present. The concerns about the use of class I agents is primarily the result of the Cardiac Arrhythmia Suppression Trial (CAST), which showed that flecainide and encainide increased the number of deaths amongst patients with ventricular arrhythmias after myocardial infarction (Echt et al, 1991). One study showed no excess mortality when flecainide was given for supraventricular arrhythmias, but this cannot be equated with proof or safety (Pritchett et al, 1991).

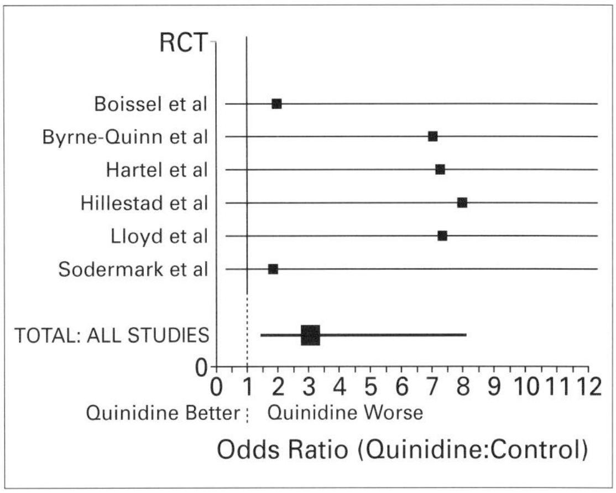

Figure 14.7
Odds ratio (Quinidine: Control) for total mortality in full-exposure groups of six randomized control trials (RCT) are depicted along with pooled ('typical' odds ratio) result from all trials. Horizontal lines depict 95% confidence interval. Pooled odds ratio and its 95% confidence interval fall to the right of the vertical line, indicating a significant increase in total mortality in quinidine-treated group as compared with control group (p < 0.05). Adapted with permission from Coplen et al (1990).

Quinidine, for example, is effective for cardioversion in patients with lone AF, but adverse effects can occur in 22%, requiring drug discontinuation in 15%. The efficacy of quinidine is supported by a meta-analysis of six controlled trials that have shown that patients treated with quinidine are less likely to have a recurrence of AF. Quinidine suppressed the recurrence of AF in about 50% of patients at 1 year, compared with half that in the untreated group (Coplen et al, 1990) (Figures 14.7 and 14.8). Importantly, however, this analysis also showed a three-fold higher total mortality in the quinidine group, with six deaths (3 sudden) from cardiovascular causes in the quinidine group and only two (0 sudden) in the control group. The incidence of sudden death, presumably due to *torsade des pointes*, is similar to the known risk of quinidine previously reported by others (Figure 14.9). In an overview by Reimold and colleagues (1992) of 2415 patients in 21 studies (some uncontrolled), quinidine was more effective than placebo in maintaining sinus rhythm up to 1 year after cardioversion, but the crude mortality rate at 1 year was 2% in the quinidine group compared with 0.6% in the placebo group. Data from the more recent Stroke Prevention in Atrial Fibrillation (SPAF) trial also showed an increase in mortality in patients with AF who also had congestive heart failure and were being treated with antiarrhythmic drugs, (primarily quinidine), with the relative risk of cardiac death being 3.3 and that of arrhythmic death being 5.8 (Flaker et al, 1992) (Figure 14.10). Other similar drugs used in cardioversion and the maintenance of sinus rhythm include disopyramide and procainamide, although the efficacy of these drugs is lower.

Class Ic agents

Both flecainide and propafenone are effective drugs in the cardioversion of AF, with a success rate of between 25–55% when given orally, and of nearly 90% when used intravenously. Oral flecainide or propafenone have also been useful in the acute termination of recent onset of AF in selected patients with paroxysmal AF ("pill in the pocket" approach) and in long-term therapy to maintain sinus rhythm. Single oral loading doses of propafenone 600 mg or flecainide 300 mg have success rates of 50% at 3 h and 80% at

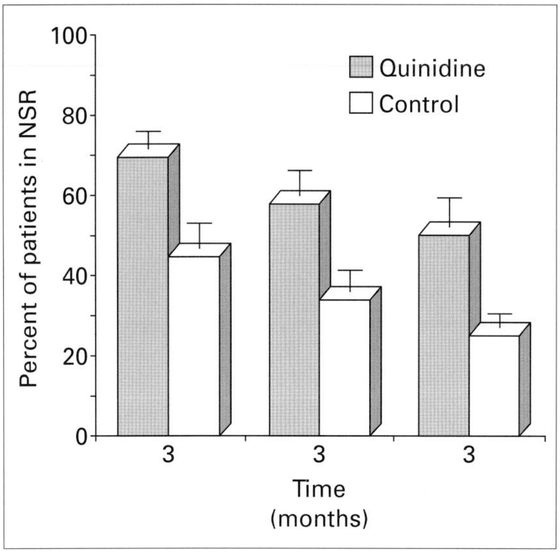

Figure 14.8
Proportion of patients remaining in normal sinus rhythm (NSR) at 3, 6 and 12 months after cardioversion was greater at all time intervals in quinidine-treated group as compared with control group (p < 0.001).

8 h for both drugs (Capucci et al, 1994; Boriani, 1997).

Open studies and placebo-controlled studies using intravenous flecainide or propafenone has shown these agents to be highly effective for cardioversion AF within hours (Donovan et al, 1991; Suttorp et al, 1990; Kondili et al, 1990). Several studies of flecainide have shown its efficacy in cardioversion (in up to 92% of patients, if given intravenously) and in preventing recurrence of the arrhythmia. However, the drug has no rate-limiting properties, and caused adverse effects in 74% of patients, although these were mostly tolerable. Propafenone, another class Ic compound, may potentially be more useful than flecainide, since it has inherent rate-limiting (class II) properties, thus allowing greater ventricular rate control. A single-blind, placebo-controlled study of propafenone as a single oral loading dose (600 mg) in converting recent-onset AF in 240 hospital patients showed that propafenone as a single oral loading dose was effective, especially in elderly patients, with most conversions occurring within 8 h (Boriani et al, 1998b). In the study by Suttorp and colleagues (1990), however, flecainide was more effective than propafenone in converting patients to sinus rhythm (90% *vs* 55% conversion rate to sinus rhythm, respectively).

Nevertheless, treatment of AF with class Ic antiarrhythmia agents is occasionally complicated by conversion of AF into atrial flutter or atrial tachycardia, which may lead to a fast ventricular response (2:1 or 1:1 atrioventricular conduction). This is a particular problem (up to 5% of patients on long-term treatment) in young patients with intact atrioventricular conduction. Combination therapy with beta-blockers, rate-limiting calcium antagonist, or

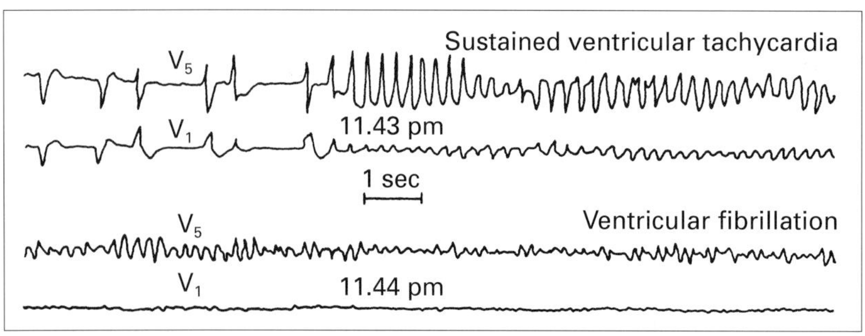

Figure 14.9
Torsade des pointes leading to ventricular fibrillation.

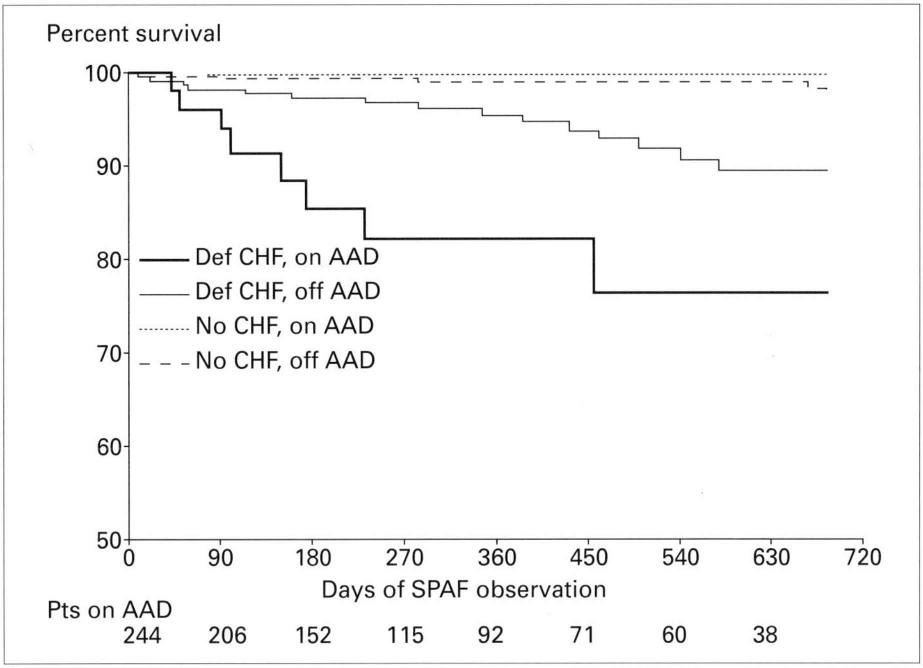

Figure 14.10
Survival to cardiac-related death in patients with and without heart failure (CHF) at entry. AAD = antiarrhythmic drug therapy; Def = definite history of; Pts = patients; SPAF = stroke prevention in AF. Adapted with permission from Flaker et al (1992).

digoxin is therefore advised to protect the ventricle from this effect.

Class III agents

Amiodarone is highly effective in the cardioversion of AF, even in previously refractory cases; and in maintaining this effect long-term (Noc et al, 1990; Horner, 1992; Blevins et al, 1987). The drug can be used both orally and intravenously, and unlike oral administration (which has a slow onset of action due to the long half-life of the drug), intravenous amiodarone may act relatively rapidly.

When compared with class I agents, amiodarone is less likely to revert AF and restore sinus rhythm, but is more effective in preventing recurrent AF once sinus rhythm has been restored (Donovan et al, 1995). Intravenous amiodarone restores sinus rhythm in up to 83% of patients in whom its efficacy is similar to electrical cardioversion (Horner, 1992; Donovan et al, 1995). In the study by Horner (1992) conversion to sinus rhythm was achieved in 29% of the group treated with oral amiodarone, 42% of the group treated with DC cardioversion, and 64% of the group given intravenous amiodarone. However, when only first attempts at cardioversion were analysed there was no difference between intravenous amiodarone and DC cardioversion. In addition, non-randomised studies have shown that amiodarone maintained sinus rhythm in up to

79% of cases during a 15 to 27 month follow-up (Brodsky et al, 1987; Skoularigis et al, 1993). However, one placebo-control study suggests that intravenous amiodarone may be no better than placebo, although all patients had also been treated with digoxin (Galve et al, 1996). In that study, only 68% in the amiodarone group and 60% in the control group had returned to sinus rhythm at 24 h. Among patients who did not convert to sinus rhythm, treatment with amiodarone was associated with a slower ventricular rate. Recurrence of AF during 15-day follow-up was 12% in the amiodarone group and 10% in controls. A recent prospective controlled study of 67 consecutive patients with AF randomised to amiodarone or placebo resulted in conversion to sinus rhythm in 48.5% who received amiodarone and in none of the placebo group (Kochiadakis et al, 1999). Those who converted had smaller atria than those who did not, and sex, age, baseline heart rate, left ventricular ejection fraction, and duration of AF did not suffer significantly between patients who converted and those who did not.

A bolus of oral amiodarone is frequently used for acute termination of recent onset AF, although placebo-controlled trials are limited. Oral amiodarone 600 mg daily converted about 18% of patients who had failed serial cardioversion and alternative drugs with no adverse effects (Tieleman et al, 1987). In the Veterans Affairs Congestive Heart Failure Survival Trial of Antiarrhythmic Therapy (Deedwania et al, 1998) there was a high spontaneous conversion rate and maintenance of sinus rhythm by amiodarone in patients with heart failure and AF, with patients who converted having a lower mortality rate than those who did not. The drug also prevented the development of new-onset AF and significantly reduced the ventricular rate in those with persistent AF.

Ibutilide, a class III antiarrhythmic agent, has been approved in the USA for intravenous termination of AF or flutter, although ventricular proarrhythmia occurred in up to 4% of patients (Ellenbogen et al, 1996; Stambler et al, 1996). The study by Ellenbogen and colleagues (1996) reported rates of successful arrhythmia termination of 3% for placebo and 12%, 33%, 45%, and 46% respectively, for 0.005, 0.010, 0.015 and 0.025 mg/kg ibutilide. Mean time to termination of arrhythmia was 19 min (range 3–70) from the start of infusion. Importantly, successful arrhythmia termination was not affected by enlarged left atrial diameter, decreased ejection fraction, presence of valvular heart disease, or the use of concomitant medications. Stambler and colleagues (1996) showed that cardioversion efficacy was higher in atrial flutter than fibrillation (63% *vs* 31%, $p < 0.0001$), but in AF and not in flutter, conversion rates were higher in patients with a shorter duration of arrhythmia or a normal left atrial size. Of the 180 ibutilide-treated patients, 8.3% developed polymorphic ventricular tachycardia during or soon after the infusion.

Dofetilide, a class III antiarrhythmic agent, selectively inhibits the rapid component of the delayed rectifier potassium current, thus prolonging the effective refractory period and duration of the action potential. Dofetilide can be administered intravenously, with a rapid onset of electrophysiological action, and has showed good efficacy in the termination of AF, although efficacy of conversion was higher in patients with atrial flutter (Falk et al, 1997; Sedgwick et al, 1995; Norgaard et al, 1999). In the recent study by Norgaard and colleagues (1999) the conversion rate was 30.3% after dofetilide and 3.3% after placebo; conversion rate was higher in atrial flutter than in AF (64% *vs* 24%). *Torsade des pointes* ventricular tachycardia developed in two (3%) patients.

Digoxin

Older studies have suggested that digoxin is useful for cardioversion of AF in patients with congestive cardiac failure, but the drug may have restored sinus rhythm indirectly by improving the haemodynamic status through its positive inotropic effects rather than through direct electrophysiological effects. Three recent randomised trials have confirmed that digoxin is no better than placebo in cardioversion of recent onset AF (Falk et al, 1987; Jordaens et al, 1997; DAAF 1997) (Figure 14.11).

The DAAF trial (1997) was a randomised, double-blind placebo-controlled multicentre trial designed to investigate whether digoxin increased the rate of conversion to sinus rhythm in 239 patients with acute AF. 46% of the placebo group and only 51% of the digoxin group had converted to sinus rhythm at 16 h but this difference was not significant. Digoxin had a pronounced and rapid effect on heart rate and a (non-significant) shorter time to sinus rhythm. Jordaens and colleagues (1997) undertook a randomised, double-blind study with high-dose intravenous digoxin 1.25 mg or placebo in 40 patients with recent onset (<1 week) AF. Cardioversion occurred in nine of 19 patients on digoxin and eight of 20 on placebo (p = NS). The mean time to conversion tended to be shorter only for digoxin. Thus, intravenous digoxin offered no substantial advantage over placebo in recent onset AF with respect to cardioversion, and provided only weak rate control.

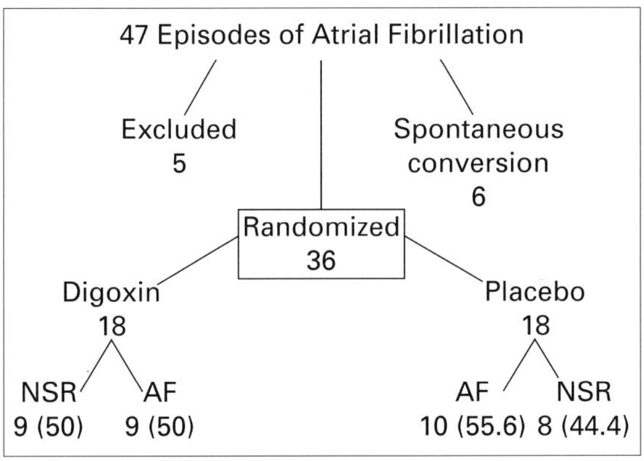

Figure 14.11
Course of 47 episodes of AF initially considered to meet entrance criteria for the study. Numbers in parentheses represent percentages of patients on either digoxin or placebo. NSR = normal sinus rhythm. Adapted from Falk et al (1987).

Is pharmacological cardioversion safer than electrical cardioversion?

There are limited data on thromboembolism after pharmacological cardioversion. The proportion of thromboembolic events in chemical and electrical cardioversion are nearly the same (1.5% *vs* 1.7%) but the older studies are small and uncontrolled.

However in a non-randomised comparison of pharmacological versus electrical cardioversion of AF, Manning and colleagues (1995) undertook serial assessment of left atrial function by doppler peak A wave velocities and showed that atrial function diminished more in patients who underwent electrical cardioversion rather than pharmacological cardioversion. In addition, Manning and colleagues (1994) reported that in patients with longer duration of AF, there was a slow return of the A wave, and hence a longer period was required for the return of atrial haemodynamics. There may also be some differences between pharmacological agents with respect to the degree of atrial dysfunction after cardioversion (Pollak and Falk, 1995). The study by Pollak and Falk (1995) suggested that there may be aggravation of atrial dysfunction by sotalol after cardioversion. In a randomised, double-blind study of sotalol for maintenance of sinus rhythm, peak A wave velocity and A wave time-velocity integral in the 20 patients receiving placebo were reduced compared with normal values, but in the 17 patients receiving sotalol (median dose 320 mg twice daily) these variables were further reduced. Thus, after electrical cardioversion, when atrial stunning is prominent, sotalol may have a negative atrial inotropic effect, but this resolves at 1 month.

Pharmacological cardioversion entails the same thromboembolic risks as electrical cardioversion, and thus should be managed in a similar way. Investigations into atrial function with pharmacological cardioversion have also shown a significant degree of atrial stunning or dysfunction in the immediate period after cardioversion, suggesting that intra-atrial stasis and thrombogenesis are likely to continue.

Is cardioversion of atrial flutter free of thromboembolic risk?

Until recently, cardioversion of atrial flutter was considered not to require anticoagulation. Nevertheless recent data have suggested that atrial flutter also confers an increased risk, and should be managed similarly to AF (Seidl et al, 1998). In a study of thromboembolism associated with atrial flutter, risk indicators for an embolic event in an univariate analysis were organic heart disease ($p = 0.037$), depressed left ventricular function ($p = 0.02$), history of systemic hypertension ($p = 0.004$), and diabetes mellitus ($p = 0.0038$); (Seidl et al, 1998). Grimm and colleagues (1997) showed that left atrial appendage stunning after cardioversion also occurred in patients with atrial flutter, although to a lesser degree than in those with AF. New or increased spontaneous echocontrast occurred in 21% with atrial flutter, compared with 50% of patients with AF. In a transoesophageal echocardiography study in 47 consecutive, non-anticoagulated patients scheduled for elective cardioversion of atrial flutter, atrial thrombus, spontaneous echocontrast, or both were found in 34%. After successful cardioversion, atrial mechanical activity was absent in 28% immediately after restoration of sinus rhythm (Irani et al, 1997).

These findings suggest that contrary to traditional teaching, atrial thrombus and spontaneous echocontrast are not uncommon in patients with atrial flutter, and thus cardioversion of this arrhythmia may be associated with increased risk of thromboembolism.

Management after cardioversion

Following successful cardioversion to sinus rhythm, it is important to continue with oral anticoagulants and possibly antiarrhythmic therapy, the latter to maintain sinus rhythm and prevent arrhythmia recurrence.

Antithrombotic therapy

Recommendations by the American College of Chest Physicians (Lampacis et al, 1998) on anticoagulation for the prevention of thromboembolism during cardioversion of AF are as follows:

- the administration of warfarin for 3 weeks before elective cardioversion of AF of 2 days' duration or more
- continuation of warfarin therapy for a minimum of 4 weeks after cardioversion
- administration of intravenous heparin followed by warfarin if cardioversion cannot be postponed for 3 weeks
- atrial flutter should be treated similarly to AF
- no anticoagulant therapy for AF of less than 2 days' duration or for cardioversion of supraventricular tachycardia.

These recommendations are not based upon any

- Delay in cardioversion: AF begats AF!
- Bleeding: Major (requiring hospitalisation, blood transfusion or surgery) in 1–2%; Minor (epistaxis, haematuria, menorrhagia) in 6–18%
- 25–50% may not receive full 1 month of prophylactic warfarin pre-cardioversion
- Need for regular INR checks — transient subtherapeutic INRs common

Adapted from Klein et al, 1997
Schlicht et al, 1996
Carlsson et al, 1996

Table 14.8
Problems with current anticoagulation regime for cardioversion.

Study	*n*	*% with LA thrombi*	*% successful cardioversion**	*% post CV T-E**
Manning et al, 1995	233	15	95	0
Stoddard et al, 1995	206	18		0
Klein et al, 1997	62	13	84	0
Corrado et al, 1999	123	9		

*of patients without atrial thrombi on TOE
i.e. ~15% of pts with AF ≥48 hrs will have atrial thrombi on TOE; TOE-guided CV is safe and feasible

Table 14.9
TOE-guided cardioversion.

randomised controlled trial evidence and are dependent upon information from case series.

The guidelines have been subject to recent debate (Table 14.8), especially with the increased use of transoesophageal echocardiography-guided cardioversion (Manning et al, 1993; 1995) (Table 14.9). The recommendation that anticoagulation with warfarin should be done for 3 weeks before elective cardioversion is based upon the estimated time needed for mural thrombus to endothelise. Nevertheless, the main danger-period is actually after cardioversion, during increased intra-atrial stasis and thrombogenesis during the slow return of atrial systolic function. The latter can take up to 3 weeks to fully return, although this is likely to vary (Manning et al, 1989; O'Neill et al, 1990; Upshaw, 1997) (Figure 14.12). In cases in which patients are at high risk of reverting back to AF, anticoagulation should be considered for much longer than the suggested 4 weeks.

In emergency situations or urgent cases in which AF has been present for 48 h or more, but it is not possible to wait for 3 weeks of anticoagulation, the recommendations suggest

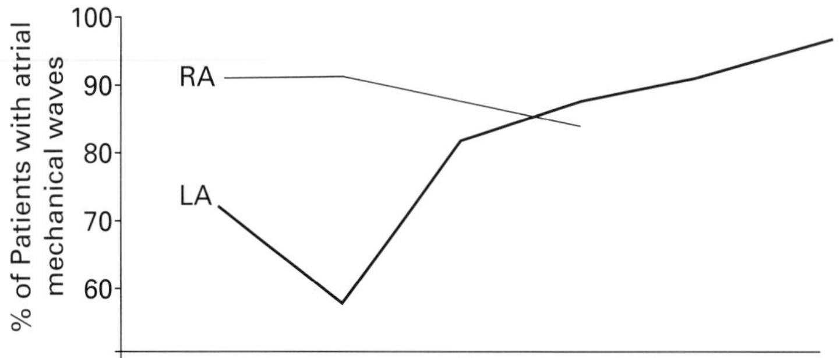

		≤30 min	1 h	6 h	1 d	4½ d	3 wk
LA	No. Studied	67	12	59	92	12	38
	No. with LA waves	49	7	49	82	11	37
	% of Total	73	58	83	89	92	97
RA	No. Studied	64	12	...	39	...	...
	No. with RA waves	59	11	...	33	...	...
	% of Total	92	92	...	85	...	...
	% of Total	30, 33–35, 39	31, 32, 34	25, 34, 36	31, 34, 35, 37–39	33	25, 33, 38

0 ↑ Cardioversion — Time after restoration of sinus rhythm

Figure 14.12
Time course for resumption of atrial contraction after restoration of sinus rhythm from chronic AF. Note the presence of left atrial (LA) mechanical waves in only 73% of patients 30 min after cardioversion and the gradual increase to nearly 100% 3 weeks after cardioversion; there were more right atrial (RA) than mechanical waves for nearly a day after cardioversion. For times after restoration of sinus rhythm, ≤30 min includes studies from immediate to 40 min after cardioversion; 1 h, from 30 min to 1 h; 6 h, from 4 to 8 h; 4½ d, from 3 to 6 d; and 3 weeks, from 2 to 4 weeks. Adapted with permission from Upshaw (1997).

initiation of intravenous heparin and echocardiography (preferably transoesophageal echocardiography), cardioversion, and anticoagulation with warfarin after cardioversion for a minimum of 4 weeks. The safety and reliability of such a strategy is being investigated in the ACUTE study (Klein et al, 1997) (Figure 14.13).

Indeed, there are problems with the current ACCP anticoagulation regime for cardioversion. These include:

- delays in cardioversion — since "AF begets AF", prolongation of the duration in AF results in less likelihood of successful reversion to sinus rhythm
- bleeding: in some series, major bleeding (requiring hospital admission, blood transfusion, or surgery) occurred in 1–2%, and minor bleeding (epistaxis, haematuria, menorrhagia) occurred in 6–18% of patients who were anticoagulated and awaiting cardioversion
- 25–50% of patients may not receive a full month of prophylactic warfarin pre-cardioversion.

Regular INR checks are needed, especially

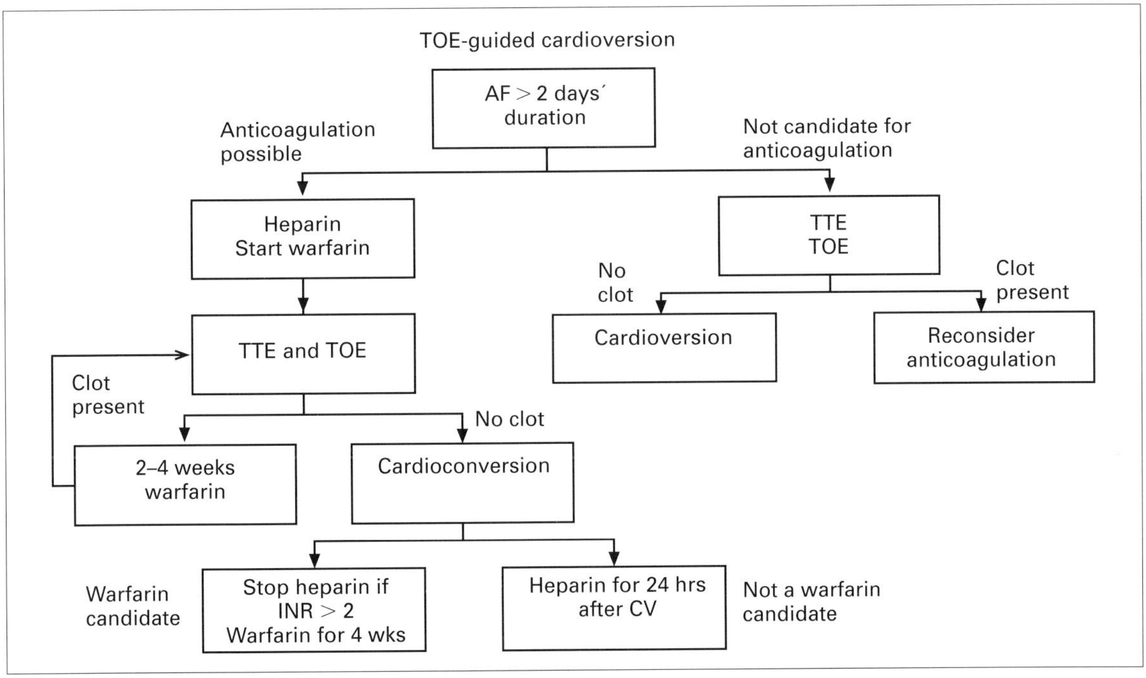

Figure 14.13
TOE-guided cardioversion.

since transient subtherapeutic INR is common. However, in patients at high risk of recurrent AF, it may be prudent to continue anticoagulation for longer, although the finding that left atrial appendage thrombus is relatively common, even in acute-onset AF of less than 3 days' duration, gives further impetus for early, full anticoagulation, starting with intravenous heparin (followed by warfarin) pending cardioversion (Stoddard et al, 1995).

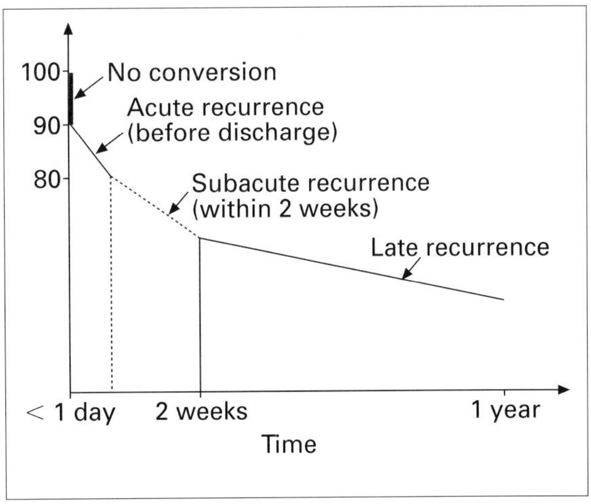

Figure 14.14
Recurrence post-cardioversion of atrial fibrillation.

Antiarrhythmic therapy

After elective electrical cardioversion, it is our practice to continue with antiarrhythmic drugs to help maintain sinus rhythm, unless an obvious precipitant such as an infection, pyrexia, or thyrotoxicosis is present. Without antiarrhythmic drugs, the risk of relapse of AF is high (Figure 14.14), with the proportion

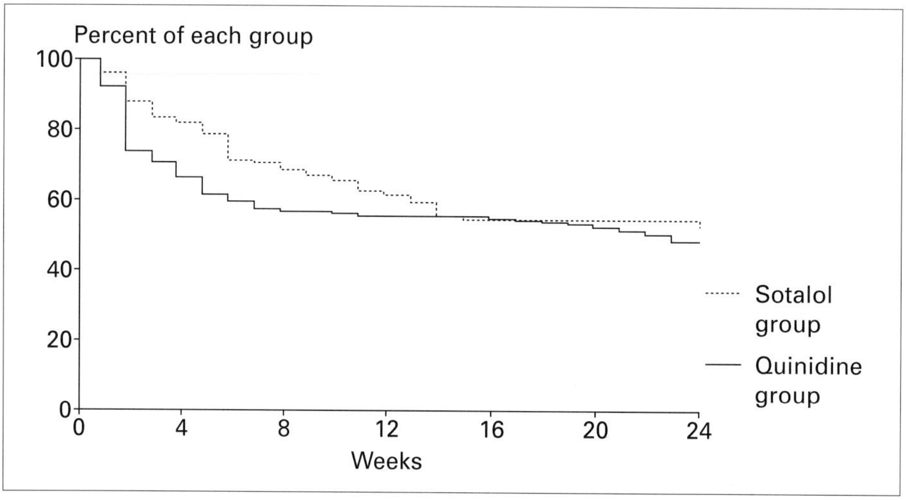

Figure 14.15
Graph showing percentage of each treatment group still in sinus rhythm. There are a significantly higher number of discontinuations in the quinidine group of patients, most of them appearing early. Reproduced from Juul-Moller et al (1986).

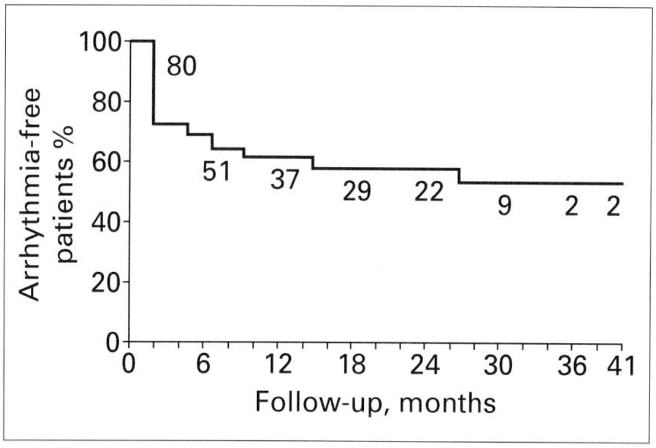

Figure 14.16
Arrhythmia free episodes after cardioversion to sinus rhythm during low dose amiodarone. Reproduced with permission from Gosselink et al (1992).

remaining in sinus rhythm ranging from 69% at 1 month to 58% at 6 months, 23% at 1 year, and 16% at 2 years (Dittrich et al, 1989). In general, suitable agents are the class I or III antiarrhythmic drugs, with which the proportion remaining in sinus rhythm at 1 year is significantly increased twofold, compared with no drugs used (Juul Moller et al, 1990; Gosselink et al, 1992; Gold et al, 1986; Roy et al, 2000) (Figures 14.15–14.17). Even then, the best results with drug prophylaxis only allow around 50% of patients to maintain sinus rhythm at 1 year.

The optimal duration of antiarrhythmic drug use after cardioversion remains controversial. A recent survey of consultant physicians showed wide variation in use of antiarrhythmic drugs after cardioversion, with differences between cardiologists and non-cardiologists (Lip et al, 1996). If antiarrhythmic drugs are used, they are probably most useful during the 3 months after successful cardioversion, especially if an identifiable precipitating cause of AF (for example, thyrotoxicosis) is present. However, if patients have adverse features for possible recurrence of AF, antiarrhythmic therapy should perhaps be continued for a longer period.

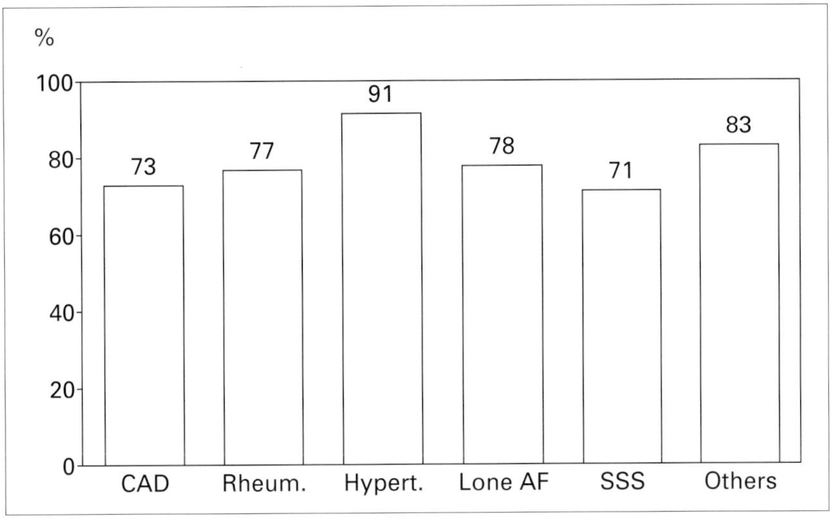

Figure 14.17
Success of amiodarone therapy in maintaining sinus rhythm in patients with atrial fibrillation with respect to the underlying cardiac or non-cardiac disorder. The differences were statistically not significant. CAD = coronary artery disease, Rheum. = rheumatic heart disease, Hypert. = systemic hypertension, SSS = sick sinus syndrome. Adapted from Gold et al (1996), with permission from Excerpta Medica Inc.

However, use of such drugs is complicated by negative inotropic effects and safety concerns, especially proarrhythmic properties. In a meta-analysis of the use of quinidine after cardioversion for the maintenance of sinus rhythm, a greater proportion of patients using quinidine were in sinus rhythm at 1 year, but there was a larger number of deaths in the quinidine group (Coplen et al, 1990). However, careful examination of this report reveals that there were only a small number of events, and if the analysis was simply confined to cardiovascular events, including sudden cardiac death, the differences between the two groups are less marked. Antiarrhythmic drugs should thus be considered after cardioversion in patients at risk of recurrence of AF. It is, nevertheless, still uncertain whether a strategy of aggressive cardioversion and maintenance of sinus rhythm is superior to the strategy of heart-rate control and antithrombotic therapy, with respect to long-term mortality and morbidity in AF. To address the long term morbidity and mortality aspects of a strategy of aggressive cardioversion compared with heart-rate control and anticoagulation, large studies such as the AFFIRM, PIAF, and RACE are underway in the USA, Germany, and the Netherlands, respectively (AFFIRM Investigators, 1997; Hohnloser and Kuck, 1997). Results from the PIAF (Pharmacological Intervention in Atrial Fibrillation) Study, presented by Dr Hohnloser at the European Society of Cardiology meeting in Barcelona in August 1999 are summarised in Table 14.10.

Transoesophageal echocardiography guided cardioversion

Transoesophageal echocardiography (TOE) has a high sensitivity and specificity in detecting left

- Prospective pilot study of patients with AF aged 18–75 years with documented AF for 7–365 days, followed up over a 12 month period
- Patients (n=252) randomised to heart rate (HR) control (using diltiazem 2–4 × 90 mg) OR cardioversion and maintenance of sinus rhythm (using amiodarone 600 mg/day [weeks 1–3] and 200 mg/day [weeks 4–52]

Results

- No significant difference between rate versus rhythm control with respect to change in symptoms
- Pharmacological conversion using amiodarone was achieved in 23% of patients, and sinus rhythm maintained for over 1 year in 60%
- Exercise tolerance was (as expected) better with sinus rhythm control compared to AF rate control

Table 14.10
Pharmacological Intervention in Atrial Fibrillation (PIAF) study.

atrial thrombus (Hwang et al, 1993; Silverman and Manning, 1998). In TOE-guided cardioversion, the patient is heparinised and warfarin is initiated (target INR 2.0 to 3.0). A biplane or multiplane TOE is done to assess left atrial size and to check for the presence of atrial thrombi or possible mitral stenosis. If a thrombus is seen, the patient is anticoagulated for a minimum of 4 weeks and a follow-up TOE done to document thrombus resolution before attempted cardioversion. If severe spontaneous echocontrast is present, or the left atrial appendage cannot be adequately evaluated for technical reasons, or TOE is contraindicated, patients should receive 4 weeks' warfarin before elective cardioversion, as per conventional management (see above). Anticoagulation with warfarin should be continued for at least 4 weeks after cardioversion in all patients, irrespective of the cardioversion method.

Several small studies to date show TOE-guided cardioversion resulted in no clinical thromboembolism (95% CI 0–1). For example, the ACUTE pilot study, which compared conventional therapy (4 weeks warfarin before cardioversion) with TOE-guided cardioversion, showed that TOE-guided strategy was safe and effective, with fewer anticoagulation management or complications (Klein, 1997). Early studies by Manning and colleagues (1993) also suggested that TOE could be used satisfactorily before cardioversion in combination with intravenous heparin to avoid episodes of systemic thromboembolism, hence reducing the risks from long-term anticoagulant therapy.

However, a recent meta-analysis suggests that despite the use of TOE, there is a 1.3% risk of thromboembolism without anticoagulation use, compared with a risk of thromboembolism of 2% without the use of TOE and with no anticoagulation, and a risk of only 0.3% without TOE and warfarinisation ($p = 0.039$). This meta-analysis definitely suggests that TOE is not predictive of risk of thromboembolism, and as such use of TOE does not reduce the risk of thromboembolism after cardioversion.

What are the reasons for this? Firstly, TOE

- Conventional therapy [n=603] vs transoesophageal echocardiography [TOE]-guided [n=619] cardioversion
- Primary end point of stroke, TIA, or peripheral embolism no different (0.81% in TOE arm vs 0.5% in conventional therapy group p=0.501).
- More major and minor bleeding events with conventional therapy (major –1.5% vs 0.81%; p=0.261; minor –4% vs 2.3%; p=0.084),
- Higher all-cause mortality in the TOE arm (2.42% vs 1%; p=0.055)
- Cardiac mortality not different (1.29% in TOE arm; 0.66% in conventional group; p=0.265).
- At 8 weeks, similar rates of sinus rhythm (52.7% in TOE arm, 50.4% in conventional Rx; p=0.431).

Table 14.11
Assessment of cardioversion using transesophageal echocardiography (ACUTE 1) multicentre study.

may not be able to predict thromboembolic events, because, occasionally, the clot is too small and not easily seen. This is due to the power resolution of TOE and is unavoidable. Furthermore, in patients undergoing cardioversion before and after TOE, there is an increase in spontaneous echocontrast in the left atrium, suggesting an increase in intra-atrial stasis after cardioversion. The latter is in keeping with the presumed return of atrial systolic function only 3–4 weeks after cardioversion (Manning et al, 1989). The study by Manning and colleagues (1989) used doppler E to A velocities to determine the return of atrial systolic function (as indicated by return of the A wave), but there are many confounding factors for such measurements, including heart rate, age, ventricular compliance, preload and afterload, and the doppler sampling volume.

TOE-guided cardioversion is probably best for patients at increased risk for warfarin morbidity; and those with short (<1 month) duration of AF at presentation (Silverman and Manning, 1998). The TOE-guided approach has a similar safety profile to conventional management, and has the advantages of a simplified anticoagulation regime and a shorter duration of sustained AF. The procedure is also cost-effective. The large, multicentre ACUTE (Assessment of Cardioversion Using TOE) study results which were presented at the American College of Cardiology meeting in March 2000 are summarised in Table 14.11 (Klein et al, 1997).

References

AFFIRM Investigators. Atrial Fibrillation Follow up Investigation of Rhythm Management – The AFFIRM Study Design. *Am J Cardiol* 1997; **79:** 1198–202.

Alam M, Thorstand C. Left ventricular function in patients with atrial fibrillation before and after cardioversion. *Am J Cardiol* 1992; **69:** 694–6.

Arnold AZ, Mick MJ, Mazurek RP et al. Role of prophylactic anticoagulation for direct current cardioversion in patients with atrial fibrillation or atrial flutter. *J Am Coll Cardiol* 1992; **19:** 851–5.

Ausma J, Wijffels M, Thone F et al. Structural changes of atrial myocardium due to sustained atrial fibrillation in the goat. *Circulation* 1997; **96:** 3157–63.

Bjerkelund CJ, Orning OM. The efficacy of anticoagulant therapy in preventing embolism related to D.C. electrical cardioversion of atrial fibrillation. *Am J Cardiol* 1969; **23:** 208–16.

Blevins RD, Kerin NZ, Benaderet D et al. Amiodarone in the management of refractory atrial fibrillation. *Arch Intern Med* 1987; **147:** 1401–4.

Boriani G, Biffi M, Capucci A et al. Oral propafenone to convert recent-onset atrial fibrillation in patients with and without underlying heart disease. A randomized, controlled trial. *Ann Intern Med* 1997; **126:** 621–5.

Boriani G, Biffi M, Capucci A et al. Conversion of recent-onset atrial fibrillation to sinus rhythm: effects of differing drug protocols. *Pacing Clin Electrophysiol* 1998a; **21:** 2470–4.

Boriani G, Biffi M, Capucci A et al. Oral loading with propafenone: a placebo-controlled study in elderly and nonelderly patients with recent onset atrial fibrillation. *Pacing Clin Electrophysiol* 1998b; **21:** 2465–9.

Boriani G, Biffi M, Capucci A et al. Favorable effects of flecainide in transvenous internal cardioversion of atrial fibrillation. *J Am Coll Cardiol* 1999a; **33:** 333–41.

Boriani G, Biffi M, Pergolini F et al. Low energy internal atrial cardioversion in atrial fibrillation lasting more than a year. *Pacing Clin Electrophysiol* 1999b; **22:** 243–6.

Brodsky MA, Allen BJ, Capparelli EV et al. Factors determining maintenance of sinus rhythm after chronic atrial fibrillation with left atrial dilatation. *Am J Cardiol* 1989; **63:** 1065–8.

Brodsky MA, Allen BJ, Waler CJ et al. Amiodarone for maintenance of sinus rhythm after conversion of atrial fibrillation in the setting of a dilated left atrium. *Am J Cardiol* 1987; **60:** 572.

Capucci A, Boriani G, Botto GL et al. Conversion of recent-onset atrial fibrillation by a single oral loading dose of propafenone or flecainide. *Am J Cardiol* 1994; **74:** 503–5.

Carlsson J, Tebbe U, Rox J et al. Cardioversion of atrial fibrillation in the elderly. ALKK-Study Group. Arbeitsgemeinschaft Leitender Kardiologisscher Krankenhausaertze. *Am J Cardiol* 1996; **78:** 1380–4.

Chang HJ, Bell JR, Deroo DB et al. Physician variation in anticoagulating patients with atrial fibrillation. *Arch Intern Med* 1990; **150:** 83–6.

Coplen SE, Antman EM, Berlin JA et al. Efficacy and safety of quinidine therapy for maintenance of sinus rhythm after cardioversion. A meta-analysis of randomized control trials. *Circulation* 1990; **82:** 1106–16.

Corrado G, Tadeo G, Beretta S et al. Atrial thrombi resolution after prolonged anticoagulation in patients with atrial fibrillation. *Chest* 1999; **115:** 140–3.

Crijns JH, Van Gelder IC, Van Gilst WH et al. Serial antiarrhythmic drug treatment to maintain sinus rhythm after electrical cardioversion for chronic atrial fibrillation or atrial flutter. *Am J Cardiol* 1991; **68:** 335–41.

The Digitalis in Acute Atrial Fibrillation (DAAF) Trial Group. Intravenous digoxin in acute atrial fibrillation. Results of a randomized, placebo-controlled multicentre trial in 239 patients. *Eur Heart J* 1997; **18:** 649–54.

Dalzell GW, Anderson J, Adgey AA. Factors determining success and energy requirements for cardioversion of atrial fibrillation. *Q J Med* 1991; **78:** 85–95.

Daniel WG, Nellessen U, Schroder E et al. Left atrial spontaneous echo contrast in mitral valve disease: an indicator for an increased thromboembolic risk. *J Am Coll Cardiol* 1988; **11:** 1204.

Daoud EG, Knight BP, Weiss R et al. Effect of verapamil and procainamide on atrial fibrillation-induced electrical remodeling in humans. *Circulation* 1997; **96:** 1542–50.

Daoud EG, Marcovitz P, Knight BP et al. Short-term effect of atrial fibrillation on trial contractile function in humans. *Circulation* 1999; **99:** 3024–7.

Deedwania PC, Singh BN, Ellenbogen K et al. Spontaneous conversion and maintenance of sinus rhythm by amiodarone in patients with heart failure and atrial fibrillation: observations from the Veterans Affairs Congestive Heart Failure Survival Trial of Antiarrhythmic Therapy (CHF-STAT). The Department of Veterans Affairs CHF-STAT Investigators. *Circulation* 1998; **98:** 2574–9.

Dethy M, Chassat C, Roy D, Mercier LA. Doppler echocardiographic predictors of recurrence of atrial fibrillation after cardioversion. *Am J Cardiol* 1988; **62:** 723–6.

Dittrich HC, Erickson JS, Schneidermen T et al. Echocardiographic and clinical predictors for outcome of elective cardioversion of atrial fibrillation. *Am J Cardiol* 1989; **63:** 193–7.

Donovan KD, Dobb GJ, Coombs et al. Reversion of recent onset atrial fibrillation to sinus rhythm by intravenous flecainide. *Am J Cardiol* 1991; **67:** 137–41.

Donovan KD, Power BM, Hockings BE et al. Intravenous flecainide versus amiodarone for recent-onset atrial fibrillation. *Am J Cardiol* 1995; **75:** 693.

Echt DS, Liebson PR, Mitchell LB et al. Mortality and morbidity in patients receiving encainide, flecainide or placebo. *N Engl J Med* 1991; **324:** 781–8.

Ellenbogen KA, Stambler BS, Wood MA et al. Efficacy of intravenous ibutilide for rapid termination of atrial fibrillation and atrial flutter: a dose-response study. *J Am Coll Cardiol* 1996; **28:** 130–6.

Ewy GA. The optimal technique for electrical cardioversion of atrial fibrillation. *Clin Cardiol* 1994; **17:** 79–84.

Falk RH, Knowlton AA, Bernard SA et al. Digoxin for converting recent-onset atrial fibrillation to sinus rhythm. A randomised, double-blinded trial. *Ann Intern Med* 1987; **106:** 503–5.

Falk RH, Pollak A, Singh SN, Friedrich T. Intravenous dofetilide, a class III antiarrhythmic agent, for the termination of sustained atrial fibrillation or flutter. Intravenous Dofetilide Investigators. *J Am Coll Cardiol* 1997; **29:** 385–90.

Fatkin D, Herbert E, Feneley MP. Hematologic correlates of spontaneous echo contrast in patients with atrial fibrillation and implications for thromboembolic risk. *Am J Cardiol* 1994a; **73:** 672–6.

Fatkin D, Kuchar DL, Thorburn CW, Feneley MP. Transesophageal echocardiography before and during direct current cardioversion of atrial fibrillation: evidence for "atrial stunning" as a mechanism of thromboembolic complications. *J Am Coll Cardiol* 1994b; **23:** 307–16.

Fatkin D, Loupas T, Low J et al. Inhibition of red cell aggregation prevents spontaneous echocardiographic contrast formation in human blood. *Circulation* 1997; **96:** 889.

Flaker GC, Blackshear JL, McBride R et al. Antiarrhythmic drug therapy and cardiac mortality in atrial fibrillation. *J Am Coll Cardiol* 1992; **20:** 527.

Galve E, Rius T, Ballester R et al. Intravenous amiodarone in treatment of recent-onset atrial fibrillation: results of a randomized, controlled study. *J Am Coll Cardiol* 1996; **27:** 1079–82.

Gold RL, Haffajee CI, Charos G et al. Amiodarone for refractory atrial fibrillation. *Am J Cardiol* 1986; **57:** 124–7.

Gosselink AT, Crijns HJ, Hamer HP et al. Changes in left and right atrial size after cardioversion of atrial fibrillation: role of mitral valve disease. *J Am Coll Cardiol* 1993; **22:** 1666–72.

Gosselink AT, Crijns HJ, Van Gelder IC et al. Low-dose amiodarone for maintenance of sinus rhythm after cardioversion of atrial fibrillation or flutter. *JAMA* 1992; **267:** 3289–93.

Gosselink ATM, Crijns HJGM, Van Den Berg MP et al. Functional capacity before and after cardioversion of atrial fibrillation: a controlled study. *Br Heart J* 1994; **72:** 161–6.

Grimm RA, Leung DY, Black IW et al. Left atrial appendage "stunning" after spontaneous conversion of atrial fibrillation demonstrated by transesophageal Doppler echocardiography. *Am Heart J* 1995; **130:** 174–6.

Grimm RA, Stewart WJ, Arheart K et al. Left atrial appendage "stunning" after electrical cardioversion of atrial flutter: an attenuated response compared with atrial fibrillation as the mechanism for lower susceptibility to thromboembolic events. *J Am Coll Cardiol* 1997; **29:** 582–9.

Hohnloser SH, Kuck KH. Atrial fibrillation: maintaining stability of sinus rhythm or ventricular rate control? The need for prospective data: the PIAF trial. *Pacing Clin Electrophysiol* 1997; **20:** 1989–92.

Horner SM. A comparison of cardioversion of atrial fibrillation using oral amiodarone, intravenous amiodarone and DC cardioversion. *Acta Cardiol* 1992; **47:** 473–80.

Hwang JJ, Chen JJ, Lin SC et al. Diagnostic accuracy of transesophageal echocardiography for detecting left atrial thrombi in patients with rheumatic heart disease having undergone mitral valve operation. *Am J Cardiol* 1993; **72:** 677.

Irani WN, Grayburn PA, Afridi I. Prevalence of thrombus, spontaneous echo contrast, and atrial stunning in patients undergoing cardioversion of atrial flutter. A prospective study using transesophageal echocardiography. *Circulation* 1997; **95:** 962–6.

Jordaens L, Missault L, Geomonpre E et al. Delayed restoration of atrial function after conversion of atrial flutter by pacing or electrical cardioversion. *Am J Cardiol* 1993; **71:** 63–7.

Jordaens L, Trouerbach J, Calle P et al. Conversion of atrial fibrillation to sinus rhythm and rate control by digoxin in comparison to placebo. *Eur Heart J* 1997; **18:** 643–8.

Juul-Moller S, Edvardsson N, Rehnqvist-Ahlberg N. Sotalol versus quinidine for the maintenance of sinus rhythm after direct current conversion of atrial fibrillation. *Circulation* 1990; **82:** 1932–9.

Jung F and DiMarco JP. Treatment strategies for atrial fibrillation. *Am J Med* 1998; **104:** 272–86.

Klein AL, Grimm RA, Black IW et al. Cardioversion guided by transesophageal echocardiography: the ACUTE Pilot Study. A randomized, controlled trial. Assessment of Cardioversion Using Transesophageal Echocardiography. *Ann Intern Med* 1997; **126:** 200–9.

Kochiadakis GE, Igoumenidis NE, Solomou MC et al. Efficacy of amiodarone for the termination of persistent atrial fibrillation. *Am J Cardiol* 1999; **83:** 58–61.

Kondili A, Kastrati A, Popa Y. Comparative evaluation of verapamil, flecainide and propafenone for the acute conversion of atrial fibrillation to sinus rhythm. *Wien Klin Wochenschr* 1990; **102:** 510–13.

Laupacis A, Albers G, Dalen J et al. Anthithrombotic therapy in atrial fibrillation. *Chest* 1998; **114:** 5795–895.

Levy S, Lauribe P, Dolla E et al. A randomized comparison of external and internal cardioversion of chronic atrial fibrillation. *Circulation* 1992; **86:** 1415–20.

Levy S, Ricard P, Lau CP et al. Multicenter low energy transvenous atrial defibrillation (XAD) trial results in different subsets of atrial fibrillation. *J Am Coll Cardiol* 1997; **29:** 750–5.

Lip GYH, Rumley A, Dunn FG, Lowe GD. Plasma fibrinogen and fibrin D-dimer levels in atrial fibrillation: effect of cardioversion to sinus rhythm. *Int J Cardiol* 1995; **51:** 245–53.

Lip GYH, Zarifis J, Watson RD, Beevers DG. Physician variation in the management of patients with atrial fibrillation. *Heart* 1996; **7:** 200–5.

Lip GYH. Cardioversion of atrial fibrillation. *Postgrad Med J* 1995; **71:** 457–65.

Lip GYH. Does atrial fibrillation confer a hypercoagulable state? *Lancet* 1995; **346:** 1313–14.

Lip GYH and Hogg KJ. Cardioversion of atrial fibrillation – how important is a long arrhythmia duration? *Scot Med J* 1993; **39:** 78–9.

Lown B. Electrical reversion of cardiac arrhythmias. *Br Heart J* 1967; **29:** 469–89.

Mancini GBJ, Goldberger AL. Cardioversion of atrial fibrillation: consideration of embolization, anticoagulation, prophylactic pacemaker and long term success. *Am Heart J* 1982; **104:** 617–21.

Manning WJ, Leeman DE, Gotch PJ, Come PC. Pulsed Doppler evaluation of atrial mechanical function after electrical cardioversion of atrial fibrillation. *J Am Coll Cardiol* 1989; **13:** 617–23.

Manning WJ, Silverman DI, Katz SE et al. Impaired left atrial mechanical function after cardioversion: relation to the duration of atrial fibrillation. *J Am Coll Cardiol* 1994; **23:** 1535–40.

Manning WJ, Silverman DI, Gordon SPF et al. Cardioversion from atrial fibrillation without prolonged anticoagulation with use of transesophageal echocardiography to exclude the presence of atrial thrombi. *N Engl J Med* 1993; **328:** 750.

Manning WJ, Silverman DI, Keighley CS et al. Transesophageal echocardiographically facilitated early cardioversion from atrial fibrillation using short-term anticoagulation: final results of a prospective 4.5 year study. *J Am Coll Cardiol* 1995; **25:** 1354.

Mathew TP, Moore A, McIntyre M et al. Randomised comparison of electrode positions for cardioversion of atrial fibrillation. *Heart* 1999; **81:** 576–9.

Mead GE, Elder AT, Faulkner S, Flapan AD. Cardioversion for atrial fibrillation: the views of consultant physicians, geriatricians and cardiologists. *Age Ageing* 1999; **28:** 73–5.

Merino A, Hauptman P, Badimon L et al. Echocardiographic 'smoke' is produced by an interaction of erythrocytes and plasma proteins modulated by shear forces. *J Am Coll Cardiol* 1992; **20:** 1661–8.

Metcalfe MJ, Smith F, Jennings K, Paterson M. Does cardioversion of atrial fibrillation result in myocardial damage? *BMJ* 1988; **296:** 1364.

Noc M, Stajer D, Horvat M. Intravenous amiodarone versus verapamil for acute conversion of paroxysmal atrial fibrillation to sinus rhythm. *Am J Cardiol* 1990; **65:** 679–80.

Norgaard BL, Wachtell K, Christensen PD et al. Efficacy and safety of intravenously administered dofetilide in acute termination of atrial fibrillation and flutter: a multicenter, randomized, double-blind, placebo-controlled trial. *Am Heart J* 1999; **137:** 1062–9.

Oltrona L, Broccolino M, Merlini PA et al. Activation of the hemostatic mechanism after pharmacological cardioversion of acute nonvalvular atrial fibrillation. *Circulation* 1997; **95:** 2003–6.

O'Neill PG, Puleo PR, Bolli R, Rokey R. Return of atrial mechanical function following electrical cardioversion of atrial arrhythmias. *Am Heart J* 1990; **120:** 353–9.

Petersen P, Kastrup J, Wilhelmsen R, Schutten HJ. Atrial natriuretic peptide in atrial fibrillation before and after electrical cardioversion therapy. *Eur Heart J* 1988; **9:** 639–41.

Petersen P. Thromboembolic complications in atrial fibrillation. *Stroke* 1990; **21:** 4–13.

Pollak A, Falk RH. Aggravation of postcardioversion atrial dysfunction by sotalol. *J Am Coll Cardiol* 1995; **25:** 665–71.

Pritchett ELC, Wilkinson WE. Mortality in patients treated with flecainide and encainide for supraventricular arrhythmias. *Am J Cardiol* 1991; **67:** 976–80.

Reimold SC, Chalmers TC. Berlin JA, Antman EM. Assessment of the efficacy and safety of antiarrhythmic therapy for chronic atrial fibrillation: observations on the role of trial design and implications of drug-related mortality. *Am Heart J* 1992; **124:** 924.

Roy D, Talajic M, Dorian P et al. Amiodarone to prevent recurrence of atrial fibrillation. *N Engl J Med* 2000; **342:** 913–20.

Schlicht JR, Davis RC, Naqi K, Cooper W. Rao BV. Physician practices regarding anticoagulation and cardioversion of atrial fibrillation. *Arch Intern Med* 1996; **156:** 290–4.

Sedgwick ML, Lip GYH, Rae AP, Cobbe SM. Chemical cardioversion of atrial fibrillation with intravenous dofetilide. *Int J Cardiol* 1995; **49:** 159–66.

Seidl K, Hauer B, Schwick NG et al. Risk of thromboembolic events in patients with atrial flutter. *Am J Cardiol* 1998; **82 (5):** 580–3.

Silverman DI, Manning WJ. Role of echocardiography in patients undergoing elective cardioversion of atrial fibrillation. *Circulation* 1998; **98:** 479–86.

Skoularigis J, Rothlisberger C, Skudicky D et al. Effectiveness of amiodarone and electrical cardioversion for chronic rheumatic atrial fibrillation after mitral valve surgery. *Am J Cardiol* 1993; **72:** 423.

Stambler BS, Wood MA, Ellenbogen KA et al. Efficacy and safety of repeated intravenous doses of ibutilide for rapid conversion of atrial flutter or fibrillation. Ibutilide Repeat Dose Study Investigators. *Circulation* 1996; **94** (7): 1613–21.

Stoddard MF, Dawkins PR, Prince CR, Ammash NM. Left atrial appendage thrombus is not uncommon in patients with acute atrial fibrillation and a recent embolic event: a transesophageal echocardiographic study. *J Am Coll Cardiol* 1995; **25:** 452–9.

Suttorp MJ, Kingma JH, Jessurun ER et al. The value of class IC antiarrhythmic drugs for acute conversion of paroxysmal atrial fibrillation or flutter to sinus rhythm. *J Am Coll Cardiol* 1990; **16:** 1722–7.

Tebbe U, Carlsson J, Seidl K et al. Cardioversion in atrial fibrillation. Results and complications in 1,152 prospective patients. Study Group of the Working Society of Leading Cardiologic Hospital Physicians. *Med Klin* 1995; **90:** 681–7

Tieleman RG, De Langen C, Van Gelder IC et al. Verapamil reduces tachycardia-induced electrical remodeling of the atrial. *Circulation* 1997; **95:** 1945–53.

Tieleman RG, Van Gelder IC, Crijns HJ et al. Early recurrences of atrial fibrillation after electrical cardioversion: a result of fibrillation-induced electrical remodeling of the atria? *J Am Coll Cardiol* 1998; **31:** 167–73.

Tieleman RG, Gosselink AT, Crijns HJ et al. Efficacy, safety and determinants of conversion of atrial fibrillation and flutter with oral amiodarone. *Am J Cardiol* 1997; **79:** 53–7.

Tisdale JE, Padhi ID, Goldberg AD et al. A randomized, double-blind comparison of intravenous diltiazem and digoxin for atrial fibrillation after coronary artery bypass surgery. *Am Heart J* 1998; **135:** 739–47.

Upshaw CB Jr. Hemodynamic changes after cardioversion of chronic atrial fibrillation. *Arch Intern Med* 1997; **157:** 1070–6.

Van Gelder IC, Crijns HJ, Blanksma PK et al. Time course of hemodynamic changes and improvement of exercise tolerance after cardioversion of chronic atrial fibrillation unassociated with cardiac valve disease. *Am J Cardiol* 1993; **72:** 560–6.

Van Gelder IC, Crijns HJ, Van der Laarse A et al. Incidence and clinical significance of ST segment elevation after electrical cardioversion of atrial fibrillation and atrial flutter. *Am Heart J* 1991a; **121:** 51–6.

Van Gelder IC, Crijns HJ, Van Gilst WH et al. Prediction of uneventful cardioversion and maintenance of sinus rhythm from direct-current electrical cardioversion of chronic atrial fibrillation and flutter. *Am J Cardiol* 1991b; **68:** 41–6.

Weinberg D, Mancini J. Anticoagulation for cardioversion of atrial fibrillation. *Am J Cardiol* 1989; **63:** 745–6.

Wijffels MCEF, Kirchhof CJHJ, Dorland R et al. Atrial fibrillation begets atrial fibrillation. A study in awake chronically instrumented goats. *Circulation* 1995; **92:** 1954.

Yapa RSS, Green GJ. Embolic stroke following cardioversion of atrial fibrillation to sinus rhythm with oral amiodarone therapy. *Postgrad Med J* 1990; **66:** 410.

Zarembski DG, Nolan PE Jr, Slack MK, Caruso AC. Treatment of resistant atrial fibrillation. A meta-analysis comparing amiodarone and flecainide. *Arch Intern Med* 1995; **155:** 1885.

15

Permanent atrial fibrillation and heart rate control

Introduction

In permanent atrial fibrillation (AF), the effective management strategy should be heart rate control and appropriate rate of antithrombotic therapy. Heart rate control can be achieved using pharmacological and non-pharmacological methods (Table 15.1). The latter has seen many advances in the fields of electrophysiology and pacemakers. Non-pharmacological strategies for rate control are discussed in Chapter 11, with or without permanent pacemaker therapy (in permanent AF, this would essentially be a VVIR pacemaker), or surgery for AF. These methods tend to be reserved for cases of AF resistant or intolerant of drug therapy. Whilst ablation and VVIR pacing may be effective for heart rate control, there may be little effect on exercise capacity (Buys et al, 1997).

Antithrombotic therapy has also gained a lot of attention in the last decade, following publication of the initial trials of warfarin and aspirin as thromboprophylaxis in AF. Subsequent trials of low-intensity anticoagulation (INR <1.5) and aspirin-warfarin combination therapy have been disappointing, and thus efforts have been directed towards refining risk stratification in AF and development of new antithrombotic strategies. Antithrombotic therapy for AF will be discussed in chapter 16.

Rate control in AF

The definition of what is adequate heart rate control in AF is still subject to much debate. Optimal heart-rate control during AF is probably that level of heart rate at which cardiac output is best. One definition for heart-rate control in AF is when the ventricular response rate ranges from 60–80 bpm at rest and 90–115 bpm during moderate exercise. However, the recent Royal College of Physicians of Edinburgh Consensus Conference on Atrial Fibrillation suggested that for adequate heart rate control, the ventricular rate needs to be under 90 bpm at rest and 180 bpm during exercise (RCPEdin, 1998). In some patients in AF, however, inappropriate fast paroxysms can occur with relatively minor exertion, even when resting heart rate is "controlled". Thus 24 h Holter monitoring may occasionally be needed to assess circadian heart-rate control, as well as exercise testing to assess maximal heart rates during exercise.

Uncontrolled heart rates in AF may have significant effects on symptoms (such as palpitations, dyspnoea, reduced exercise tolerance, etc), which usually relate the haemodynamic effects of AF, and complications such as rate-related cardiac ischaemia and heart failure. Heart failure may also be an untoward effect of fast heart rates on cardiac function, resulting in a "tachycardia-induced cardiomyopathy",

	Control of resting heart rate	*Control of exercise heart rate*	*Thromboembolic risk still present?*	*Symptomatic benefit*	*Haemodynamic benefit*
Digoxin monotherapy	Yes	No	Yes	+	+
Digoxin + beta-blocker or calcium antagonist	Yes	Yes	Yes	++	+
Radiofrequency ablation + pacemaker	Yes	Yes	Yes	++	++
Radiofrequency modification	Yes	Yes	Yes	+++	+++

+ slight benefit
++ some benefit
+++ good benefit

Table 15.1
Strategies for heart-rate control in AF.

in which ultrastructural and morphological changes occur, resulting in a dilated left ventricle with poorly contractile function (Gallagher et al, 1997). The loss of atrial contribution to ventricular filling as well as the irregularity of the ventricular response may add to the haemodynamic changes taking place in AF.

Rate control can be achieved by non-pharmacological and pharmacological means. Non-pharmacological methods have been discussed in chapter 11, and essentially consist of atrioventricular node modification or ablation, with or without permanent pacemaker therapy (in permanent AF, this would essentially be a VVIR pacemaker), or surgery for AF. These methods tend to be reserved for cases of AF resistant or intolerant of drug therapy. Whilst ablation and VVIR pacing may be effective for heart rate control, there may be little effect on exercise capacity (Buys et al, 1997).

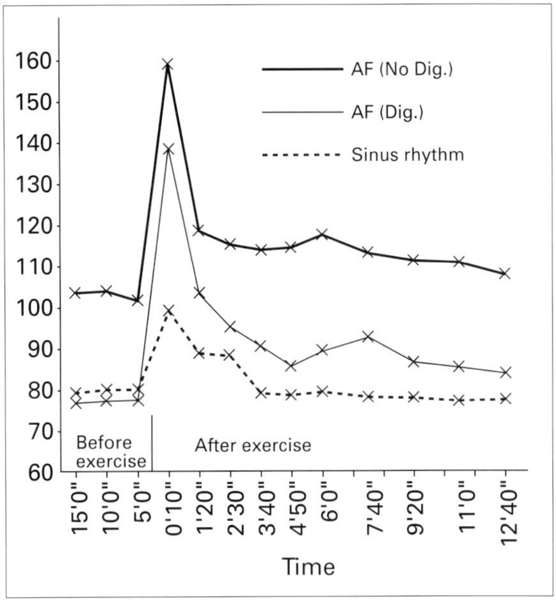

Figure 15.1
Heart rate changes with exercise (AF vs sinus rhythm): effects of digoxin.

Pharmacological heart rate control

Digoxin — Digoxin is the commonest drug for heart rate control in AF, acting primarily by vagotonic inhibition of atrioventricular nodal conduction. However, digoxin is less effective for rate control than the beta blockers or rate-limiting calcium channel blockers, and is less likely to control the ventricular rate during pyrexia, stress, or exercise, when vagal tone is low and sympathetic tone is high (Li Saw Hee and Lip, 1998) (Figure 15.1). Digoxin is generally effective for rate control at rest. In heart failure, the increase in cardiac contractility and improvement in haemodynamics with digoxin will also reduce symptoms of low output and reflex sympathetic activation. Digoxin has little or no ability to terminate the arrhythmia, and often does not slow the heart rate with recurrent AF (Rawles et al, 1990; Galun et al, 1991).

Digoxin can be administered orally, intravenously, or intramuscularly, but the absorption from intramuscular injection is unreliable. The speed of heart-rate control with digoxin is not impressive, taking about 6–12 h to achieve heart rates less than 100 bpm after its initiation. Intravenous digoxin begins to act faster, within 15 to 30 min, with a peak effect attained in 1–6 h. This relatively slow onset of action may be undesirable in some situations. The correlation between serum digoxin levels and heart rate control is also poor (Botker et al, 1991), but the presence of low serum digoxin levels indicates that a higher dose could be administered (Figure 15.2).

Apparent resistance to digoxin can be present in AF secondary to thyrotoxicosis, chest disease, congestive cardiac failure, and pyrexia. Large doses of digoxin are often required for monotherapy, and patients

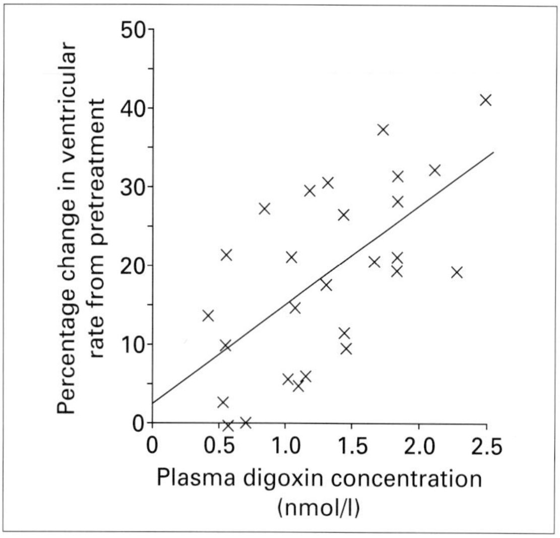

Figure 15.2
Correlation between percentage change in ventricular rate in atrial fibrillation and plasma digoxin concentration.

frequently require the addition of a beta-blocker or rate-limiting calcium channel blocker for optimal rate control (David et al, 1979; Tommaso et al, 1983; Farshi et al, 1999) (Table 15.2).

Farshi and colleagues (1999) compared the effects of five pharmacological regimens (0.25 mg digoxin, 240 mg diltiazem-CD, 50 mg atenolol, 0.25 mg digoxin plus 240 mg diltiazem-CD, 0.25 mg digoxin plus 50 mg atenolol) on the circadian rhythm and exercise-induced changes of ventricular rate (VR) in patients with chronic AF, they found that digoxin and diltiazem, as single agents at the doses tested, were least effective for controlling ventricular rate in AF during daily activity. By contrast, digoxin plus atenolol produced the most effective rate control, reflecting a synergistic effect on the AV node (Figures 15.3 and 15.4).

Many drugs have potentially important pharmacokinetic interactions with digoxin. Many of these drugs, such as verapamil, quinidine, and amiodarone, are commonly administered with digoxin, and dosing of the cardiac glycoside must be adjusted accordingly. These interactions can be regarded as those influencing drug absorption, metabolism and excretion (Table 15.3).

Beta-blockers — Beta-blockers such as propranolol, atenolol, metoprolol, or esmolol can be valuable for heart-rate control for AF in specific settings. In permanent AF, beta-blockers prevent the effects of sympathetic tone, decrease the resting heart rate, and blunt the heart rate response to exercise, but may also reduce exercise tolerance. However, in one comparison of sotalol, propafenone, and procainamide, sotalol (a beta-blocker with class III properties) actually increased the exercise

Think of:
- Patient not taking tablets.
- Accessory pathway present e.g. Wolff-Parkinson-White syndrome.
- Thyrotoxicosis.
- Poor left ventricular function.
- Respiratory or thoracic disease (including cor pulmonale, pleural effusion and lung cancer).
- Metabolic and electrolyte abnormalities, hypoxia.

Table 15.2
Digoxin-resistant AF.

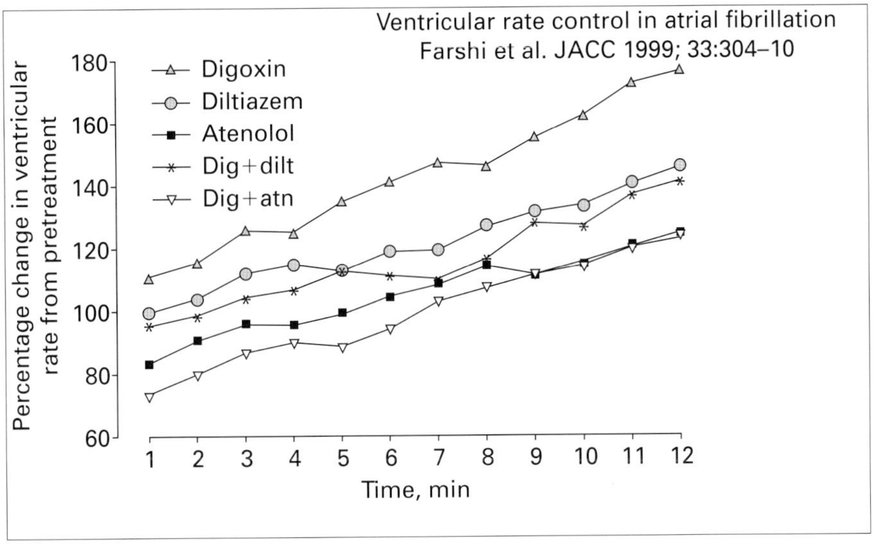

Figure 15.3
Effect of various pharmacologic regimens on exercise-induced ventricular rate (VR) patients with CAF. Reproduced with permission of Farshi et al (1999).

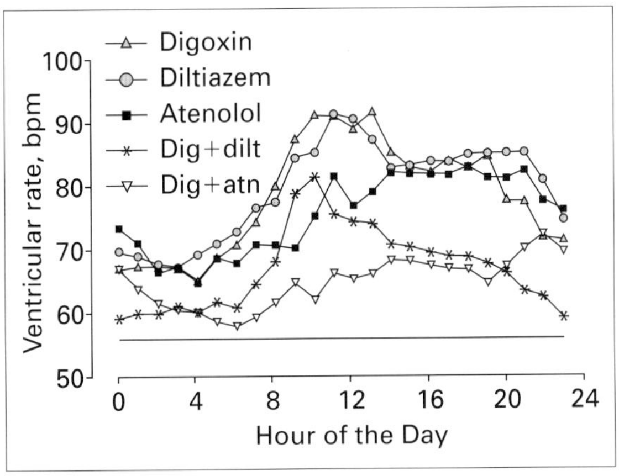

Figure 15.4
Circadian distribution of hourly mean ventricular rate (VR) in patients with CAF as influenced by various treatment regimens. All regimens exhibited significant circadian variation of VR ($p < 0.001$). Adapted from Farshi et al (1999).

performance in patients who had chronic AF and who also had symptomatic ventricular arrhythmias (Hsieh et al, 1998). As discussed in chapter 13, beta-blockers are useful in those patients with underlying adrenergic-induced AF, but the use of beta-blockers in bradycardia-dependent or vagally-mediated AF may actually increase the propensity to AF by inducing sinus bradycardia (Coumel et al, 1994).

Beta-blockers are superior to the use of digoxin alone, but may be used in combination with digoxin and calcium channel blockers (not verapamil) in chronic AF. Esmolol, a short-acting and rapidly-acting intravenous beta-blocker, is used for heart-rate control in acute AF, either alone or with digoxin; its quick onset and short half-life makes it useful in patients in whom there is uncertainty whether an oral (longer acting) beta-blocker can be safely or conveniently used, for example, in postoperative patients (Shettigar et al, 1993; Schwartz et al, 1988). Esmolol is also synergistic with digoxin, with a rapid control of heart rate at a mean interval of 21 min (Shettigar et al, 1993). One comparison between esmolol and verapamil in controlling

Decreased renal excretion
Concurrent cardiac drugs (quinidine, verapamil, amiodarone)
Depressed renal blood flow (beta-blockers)
Increased renal clearance
Thyroxine
Decreased non-renal clearance
Anti-arrhythmic drugs (quinidine, verapamil, amiodarone, propafenone)
Calcium antagonists (verapamil, and possibly others)
Decreased gut absorption
Cholestyramine, sulphasalazine
Decreased conversion in gut to digoxin reduction products
Erythromycin, tetracycline (in some patients)

Table 15.3
Drug interactions with digoxin.

ventricular response in 45 patients with AF or atrial flutter showed that esmolol compared favourably with verapamil in respect of efficacy and safety in acutely decreasing the ventricular response during AF or flutter (Platia et al, 1989) (Figure 15.5). Importantly, cardioversion to sinus rhythm was significantly more likely with esmolol. In patients in whom a conventional beta-blocker controls exercise-induced heart rate at the expense of inappropriately slow resting heart rates, using pindolol and xamoterol may avoid the latter.

Beta-blockers may benefit particular subgroups of patients with AF. For example, a non-selective beta-blocker such as propranolol may be used to treat both thyrotoxicosis and associated AF, if present. Recent randomised trials have shown the benefits of beta-blockers

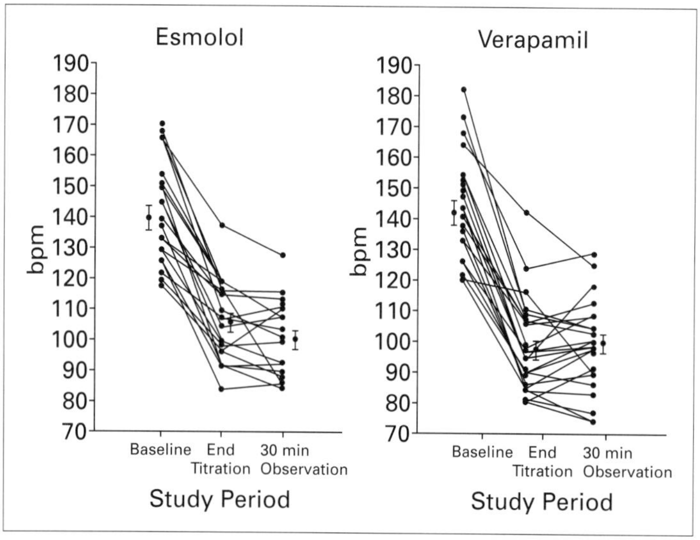

Figure 15.5
Heart rate during the 3 study periods. Values are for individual patients. Bpm = beats per minute. Adapted with permission from Platia et al (1989).

in improving outcome in patients with stable heart failure secondary to left ventricular systolic dysfunction (CIBIS-II, 1999; MERIT-HF, 1999; Packer et al, 1999). Although there are no trials in patients with AF and heart failure, it would seem reasonable to try beta-blockers for heart-rate control in these patients. Similarly, the cardioprotective benefits of beta-blockers makes these agents the drug of choice in patients after myocardial infarction. Beta-blockers and the rate-limiting calcium antagonists are suitable for rate control in AF associated with hypertension or hypertrophic cardiomyopathy.

Rate-limiting calcium channel blockers — Non-dihydropyridine calcium antagonists such as verapamil or diltiazem, both of which increase refractoriness and slow conduction in the AV node, are effective agents for heart-rate control. These can be administered intravenously in the emergency setting, but negative inotropic effects, particularly with verapamil, require their cautious use in heart failure.

Intravenous verapamil can be given in acute AF (5 to 10 mg over 2–3 min, repeated every 15 to 30 min as necessary), with a maintenance infusion rate of about 0.125 mg/min. It acts rapidly (within 2 min) and the peak effect occurs in 10–15 min. Oral verapamil is used in chronic AF, and increased from 40 mg 3–4 times daily to 480 mg daily, dependent on the patient (e.g. hepatic function and heart rate response). The Diltiazem Atrial Fibrillation/ Atrial Flutter Study Group regimen consists of an intravenous bolus of diltiazem 20 mg alone or followed in 15 min by another 25 mg, followed by a continuous infusion at a rate of 10–15 mg/h (Salerno et al, 1989), which controls ventricular rate in 83% of patients, usually within 4 min. One study in patients with AF after coronary artery bypass graft surgery showed that ventricular rate control occurred far more rapidly in patients treated with intravenous diltiazem rather than digoxin, although the (relatively low) rate of conversion to sinus rhythm was actually higher in the digoxin group (Tisdale et al, 1998). Oral therapy with verapamil or diltiazem is also effective for chronic AF rate control, and is often used in combination with digoxin (Klein and Kaplinsky, 1982) (Figure 15.6). Exercise capacity can improve when verapamil or diltiazem are used to control the heart rate in AF. In the study by Lundstrom and Ryden (1990), the use of diltiazem (270 mg/day) or verapamil (240 mg/day), in patients with chronic AF gave good rate control at rest and exercise, in addition to improvements in symptom-limited exercise tolerance and respiratory gas exchange anaerobic threshold.

Although they slow the ventricular rate, both verapamil and diltiazem rarely cardiovert AF to sinus rhythm (Tisdale et al, 1998). Calcium channel blockers might also potentially prolong paroxysms of AF in patients with paroxysmal AF, although electrical remodelling appears to be prevented by calcium channel blockers, improving the potential for successful cardioversion (Daoud et al, 1997). However, these drugs may paradoxically increase the ventricular response in patients with AF and pre-excitation, by impairing conduction via the normal AV node-His-Purkinje system and by increasing antegrade conduction over the accessory pathway. Both agents have a negative inotropic effect (more so with verapamil) and should be used with some caution in patients with heart failure and hypotension.

Clonidine — Clonidine (having anti-adrenergic properties) is an alternative for hypertensive patients since it reduces standing heart rates in AF by 15–20% (Scardi et al, 1993; Roth et al, 1992). In a randomised trial

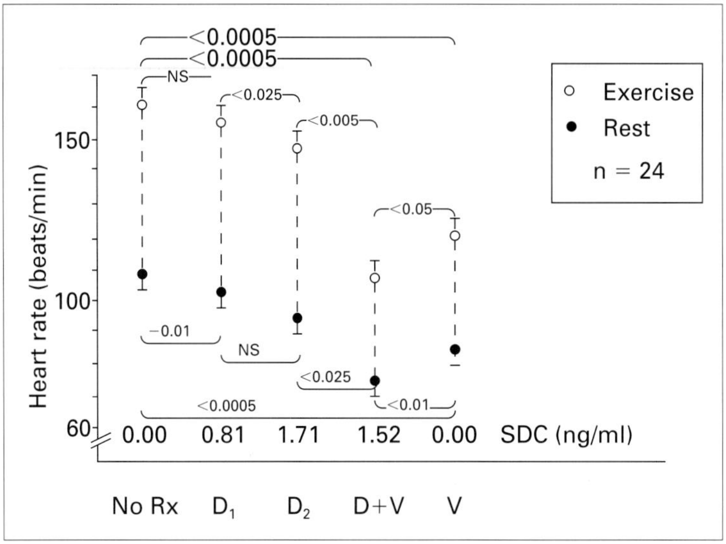

Figure 15.6
Ventricular rate of 24 patients with chronic atrial fibrillation at rest and after mild exercise (300 kpm for 3 min) before therapy (No Rx); during treatment with digoxin, 0.25 mg daily (D_1) or 0.50 mg daily (D_2); during combined therapy of digoxin, 0.25 mg, and verapamil, 240 mg daily (D + V); and during treatment of verapamil, 240 mg daily (V). The p value was <0.001 for the entire comparison analysed by one-way analysis of variance for multiple comparisons; p values are also shown for comparison among treatment phases. SDC = mean serum digoxin concentration during each treatment. Adapted from Klein and Kaplinsky (1982), with permission from Excerpta Medica Inc.

of clonidine (0.075 mg orally at baseline and after 2 h if heart rate did not decrease by at least 20%) or control, heart rate decreased to below 100 bpm in eight of nine patients receiving clonidine compared with two of nine patients in the control group (Roth et al, 1992). The difference in the mean decrease in heart rate was 38 bpm (95% CI, 20–56 bpm). Thus low-dose clonidine may be an easy, efficient, and effective treatment for patients with rapid AF who are haemodynamically stable, although larger trials are still needed with this agent.

Other antiarrhythmic agents for rate control — Amiodarone is effective in controlling the ventricular rate in AF and flutter, and should be considered especially in patients intolerant of other agents (Galve et al, 1996; Blevins et al, 1987). Amiodarone is also quite effective in the prevention of paroxysms of AF and in the long-term maintenance of sinus rhythm after successful cardioversion. Rate control is achieved with amiodarone via its sympatholytic and calcium antagonist properties, which depress atrioventricular conduction. It should not, however, be used as a first-line agent for heart-rate control in AF, in view of its potential side-effects, although these are minimal at low doses (200 mg/day). This drug would thus be useful when other atrioventricular nodal blocking agents fail to slow the ventricular rate adequately or when these agents are not well tolerated.

Class I agents are not usually advocated for

	Acute Intravenous Therapy (Loading Dose)	Chronic Oral Therapy
Beta-blockers		
Metoprolol	5 mg IV every 5 minutes up to 15 mg	50–100 mg twice daily
Propranolol	1–8 mg IV (1 mg every 2 minutes)	10–120 mg three times daily; long-acting preparation: 80–320 mg once daily
Esmolol	0.05–0.2 mg/kg/min IV	
Pindolol		2.5–20 mg twice to three times daily
Atenolol	5 mg IV over 5 minutes, repeat in 10 minutes	25–100 mg once daily
Nadolol		20–120 mg once daily
Calcium-channel blockers		
Verapamil	5–20 mg in 5-mg increments IV every 30 minutes or 0.005 mg/kg/min infusion	120–360 mg daily in divided doses or in the slow-release form
Diltiazem	0.25–0.35 mg/kg IV followed by 5–15 mg/hour	120–360 mg daily as slow release
Cardiac glycoside		
Digoxin	0.75 mg–1.5 mg in 3–4 divided doses over 12–24 hours	0.125–0.5 mg daily

IV = intravenous

Table 15.4
Drug loading and maintenance doses for ventricular rate control in patients with atrial fibrillation

heart-rate control of chronic AF. Indeed, class Ia agents such as quinidine may even increase atrioventricular conduction due to their anticholinergic effects. Propafenone may control heart rate during paroxysms of AF, due to its effect on the atrioventricular node.

Prescribing for rate control in AF

As discussed above, there are various pharmacological possibilities to achieve heart rate control in AF (Table 15.4). Some drugs may be more appropriate for certain subgroups of patients with AF, for example beta-blockers or calcium antagonists in patients with hypertension. Nevertheless, digoxin is the most common drug prescribed as monotherapy for rate control in AF in the UK (Zarifis et al, 1997), despite its many limitations. By contrast, the beta-blockers and calcium antagonists are more commonly used in the USA.

In some patients, combination therapy will be required to achieve adequate control, such as digoxin plus beta-blocker or calcium antagonist. However, in some patients, rate control will still be problematic and a decision may be needed to proceed to non-pharmacological methods such as atrioventricular node modification or ablation with concomitant VVIR pacemaker implantation. Appropriate discussion with the patient and referral to the electrophysiologist will be useful.

References

Blevins RD, Kerin NZ, Benaderet D et al. Amiodarone in the management of refractory atrial fibrillation. *Arch Intern Med* 1987; **147:** 1401–4.

Botker HE, Toft P, Klitgaard NA, Simonsen EE. Influence of exercise on serum digoxin concentration and heart rate in patients with atrial fibrillation. *BMJ* 1991; **65:** 337–41.

Buys EM, van Hemel NM, Kelder JC et al. Exercise capacity after His bundle ablation and rate response ventricular pacing for drug refractory chronic atrial fibrillation. *Heart* 1997; **77:** 238–41.

CIBIS-II Investigators and Committees. The Cardiac Insufficiency Bisoprolol Study II: a randomised trial. *Lancet* 1999; **353:** 9–13.

Coumel P. Paroxysmal atrial fibrillation: a disorder of autonomic tone? *Eur Heart J* 1994; **15(suppl A):** 9–16.

Daoud EG, Knight BP, Weiss R et al. Effect of verapamil and procainamide on atrial fibrillation-induced electrical remodeling in humans. *Circulation* 1997; **96:** 1542–50.

David D, Segni ED, Klein HO, Kaplinsky E. Inefficacy of digitalis in the control of heart rate in patients with chronic atrial fibrillation: beneficial effect of an added beta-adrenergic blocking agent. *Am J Cardiol* 1979; **44:** 1378.

Lundstrom T, Ryden L. Ventricular rate control and exercise performance in chronic atrial fibrillation: effects of diltiazem and verapamil. *J Am Coll Cardiol* 1990; **16:** 86–90.

Farshi R, Kistner D, Sarma JSM et al. Ventricular rate control in chronic atrial fibrillation during daily activity and programmed exercise: a cross-over label study of five drug regimens. *J Am Coll Cardiol* 1999; **33:** 304–10.

Gallagher MM, Obel OA, Camm JA. Tachycardia-induced atrial myopathy: an important mechanism in the pathophysiology of atrial fibrillation. *J Cardiovasc Electrophysiol* 1997; **8:** 1065–74.

Galun E, Flugelman MY, Glickson M, Eliakim M. Failure of long-term digitalization to prevent rapid ventricular response in patients with paroxysmal atrial fibrillation. *Chest* 1991; **99:** 1038–40.

Galve E, Rius T, Ballester R et al. Intravenous amiodarone in treatment of recent-onset atrial fibrillation: results of a randomized, controlled study. *J Am Coll Cardiol* 1996; **27:** 1079–82.

Hsieh MH, Chen SA, Wen ZC et al. Effects of antiarrhythmic drugs on variability of ventricular rate and exercise performance in chronic atrial fibrillation complicated with ventricular arrhythmias. *Int J Cardiol* 1998; **64:** 37–45.

Klein H and Kaplinsky E. Verapamil and digoxin: their respective effects on atrial fibrillation and their interaction. *Am J Cardiol* 1982; **50:** 894–8.

Li Saw Hee FL, Lip GYH. Digoxin revisited. *Q J Med* 1998; **91:** 259–64.

Lundstrom T, Ryden L. Ventricular rate control and exercise performance in chronic and atrial fibrillation: effects of diltiazem and verapamil. *J Am Coll Cardiol.* 1990; **16:** 86–90.

MERIT-HF Investigators. Effect of metoprolol CR/XL in chronic heart failure: Metoprolol CR/XL Randomised Intervention Trial in Congestive Heart Failure (MERIT-HF). *Lancet* 1999; **353:** 2001–7.

Packer M, Bristow MR, Cohn J et al, for the US Carvedilol Heart Failure Study Group. The effect of carvedilol on morbidity and mortality in patients with chronic heart failure. *N Engl J Med* 1999; **334:** 1349–55.

Platia EV, Michelson EL, Porterfield JK, Das G. Esmolol versus verapamil in the acute treatment of atrial fibrillation or atrial flutter. *Am J Cardiol* 1989; **63:** 925–9.

Rawles JM, Metcalfe MJ, Jennings K. Time of occurrence, duration, and ventricular rate of paroxysmal atrial fibrillation: the effect of digoxin. *Br Heart J* 1990; **63:** 225–7.

RCPEdin. Final consensus statement of the Royal College of Physicians of Edinburgh Consensus Conference on atrial fibrillation in hospital and general practice, 3–4 September 1998. *Br J Haematol* 1999; **104:** 195–6.

Roth A, Kaluski E, Felner S et al. Clonidine for patients with rapid atrial fibrillation. *Ann Intern Med* 1992; **116:** 388–90.

Salerno DM, Dias VC, Kleiger RE et al. Efficacy and safety of intravenous diltiazem for treatment of atrial fibrillation and atrial flutter: The Diltiazem-Atrial Fibrillation/Flutter Study Group. *Am J Cardiol* 1989; **63:** 1046.

Scardi S, Humar F, Pandullo C, Poletti A. Oral clonidine for heart rate control in chronic atrial fibrillation. *Lancet* 1993; **341:** 1211–12.

Schwartz M, Michelson EL, Sawin HS, MacVaugh H 3rd. Esmolol: safety and efficacy in postoperative cardiothoracic patients with supraventricular tachyarrhythmias. *Chest* 1988; **93:** 705–11.

Shettigar UR, Toole JG, Appunn DO. Combined use of esmolol and digoxin in the acute treatment of atrial fibrillation or flutter. *Am Heart J* 1993; **126:** 368–74.

Tisdale JE, Padhi ID, Goldberg AD et al. A randomized, double-blind comparison of intravenous diltiazem and digoxin for atrial fibrillation after coronary artery bypass surgery. *Am Heart J* 1998; **135:** 739–47.

Tommaso C, McDonough T, Parker M, Talano JV. Atrial fibrillation and flutter. Immediate control and conversion with intravenously administered verapamil. *Arch Intern Med* 1983; **143:** 877.

Zarifis J, Beevers DG, Lip GYH. Acute admissions with atrial fibrillation in a British multiracial hospital population. *Br J Clin Pract* 1997; **51:** 91–6.

16

Antithrombotic therapy in atrial fibrillation

The high risks of stroke and thromboembolism in atrial fibrillation (AF) associated with valvular heart disease, especially mitral stenosis and prosthetic mitral valves, have long been appreciated. In the absence of rheumatic heart disease with mitral stenosis, however, AF had long been (erroneously) thought of as benign.

In recent years, non-valvular AF (NVAF) has gained much prominence, as this disorder has been identified as an important contributor to mortality and as one of the most powerful independent risk factors predisposing to stroke and thromboembolism, especially in the elderly (Flegel et al, 1987; Krahn et al, 1995; Onundarson et al, 1987; Feinberg et al, 1995; Benjamin et al, 1998). Importantly, recent large randomised trials have highlighted the value of antithrombotic prophylaxis against stroke and thromboembolism in non-valvular AF (AF Investigators, 1994; 1997). This has raised questions over the delivery of thromboprophylaxis for patients with AF in an efficient, effective, and safe manner. With an increasingly elderly general population, AF is also likely to become even more common, and the issues associated with thromboprophylaxis are likely to become an increasing public-health problem.

Valvular AF

In patients with thromboembolic cerebrovascular disease undergoing echocardiography, the most common abnormality (when present) is valvular heart disease (Hofmann et al, 1990; Nishide et al, 1983). Recurrent embolism occurs in 30%–75% of such patients — an annual rate of almost 10% (Sherman et al, 1990). The presence of mitral stenosis is a particular risk for thromboembolism, with systemic embolisation occurring in 9–20% of patients, of whom up to 75% have cerebral emboli (Cohen et al, 1993; Fleming et al, 1995; Sherman et al, 1990). When compared with someone with mitral stenosis in sinus rhythm, coexistent AF increases the risk of embolism by 3–7 times (Sherman et al, 1990). Indeed, 16% of 622 patients with mitral stenosis and AF had left atrial thrombi identified by echocardiography, compared with only 1% of 192 patients with mitral stenosis in sinus rhythm (Beppu et al, 1984) (Figure 16.1).

Valvular AF increases the risk of thrombogenesis by many mechanisms. For example, AF increases blood stasis within the left atrium in the presence of mitral stenosis, which is visualised as spontaneous echocontrast on transoesophageal echocardiography and detected by reduced left atrial appendage doppler velocities. Spontaneous echocontrast is a marker of previous thromboembolism in patients with non-valvular AF, mitral valve disease, or mitral valve replacement (Black et al, 1991) (Figure 16.2), and is highly specific (94%) and predictive for thromboembolic events (Tsai et al, 1992). Whilst uncorrected mitral stenosis com-

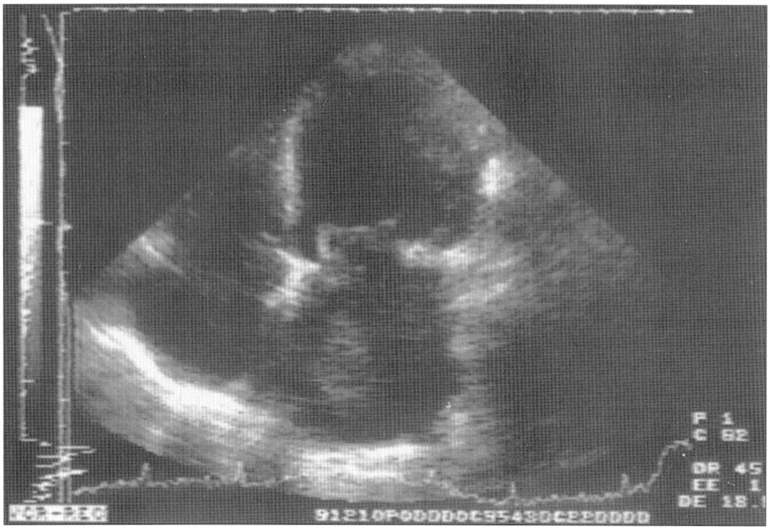

Figure 16.1
Two-dimensional echocardiogram (apical 4 chamber view) showing left atrial thrombus in patient with a prosthetic mitral valve.

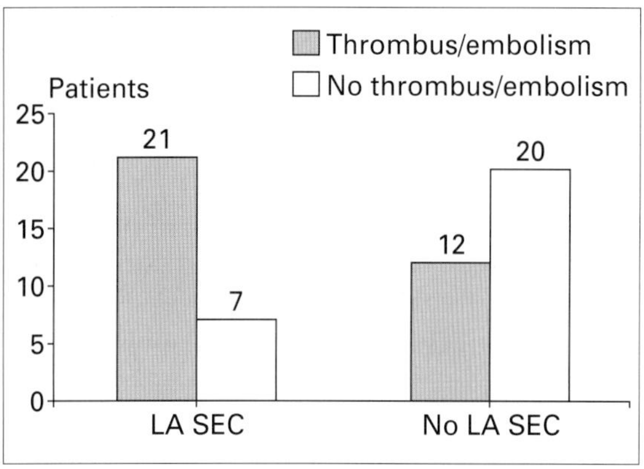

Figure 16.2
Association between left atrial spontaneous echo-contrast (LA SEC) and left atrial thrombus or suspected cardiogenic embolism (thrombus/embolism), or both, in 60 patients with non-valvular AF (p = 0.004). Reproduced with permission from Black et al (1991).

monly predisposes to the development of AF, a recent study suggests that anticoagulation is particularly indicated especially in the presence of aortic regurgitation, left atrial thrombus, or previous systemic thromboembolism, as these features are predictors of further systemic embolism even whilst in sinus rhythm (Chiang et al, 1998) (Table 16.1).

By contrast, in the absence of AF, aortic valve disease per se is a relatively uncommon cause of embolic stroke (Cohen et al, 1993; Kapila and Hart, 1986; Rancurel et al, 1989). Indeed, fibrin-platelet deposits (shown on disrupted valvular endothelium), and emboli from calcific aortic stenosis appear to be the principal pathological processes for the rare episodes of emboli associated with aortic stenosis. In later stages of aortic stenosis, however, when heart failure and AF occur, the risk of stroke and thromboembolism may substantially increase.

Thromboembolism in AF and its prevention using anticoagulation therapy

The size of the problem

NVAF carries a substantial risk of morbidity and mortality from stroke and thromboembolism (Wolf et al, 1991). It has been esti-

Variable	*Relative risk (95% CI)*	*p Value*
Patients in sinus rhythm (n = 132)		
Age	1.12 (1.04–1.21)	0.002
Mitral area	16.9 (1.53–187.0)	0.021
Left atrial thrombus	37.1 (2.82–487.8)	0.006
Significant aortic regurgitation	22.4 (2.72–184.8)	0.004
Patients in atrial fibrillation (n = 402)		
Percutaneous balloon mitral commissurotomy	0.37 (0.18–0.79)	0.010
Emboli	3.11 (1.66–5.85)	<0.001

*Only significant results are shown. Reproduced with permission from Chiang et al (1998)

Table 16.1
Cox regression analysis of predictors of systemic embolism in patients with mitral stenosis.*

mated that about 500 000 people in the USA suffer from stroke each year, and 15–20% of these strokes are thought to be attributable to cardiac emboli (Sherman et al, 1995) secondary to NVAF in the elderly. Silent cerebral infarction is also a common problem in chronic AF (Petersen et al, 1987). There is a distinct clustering of stroke events at the time of onset of the AF (Wolf et al, 1983) (Figure 16.3).

Patients with acute stroke and AF have a 1.5-fold to 3.0-fold higher mortality than that of stroke patients in sinus rhythm. For example, in a Glasgow study, patients admitted with acute severe stroke who also had AF (25%) had a significantly higher hospital mortality than patients in sinus rhythm (67% *vs* 44%) (Lowe et al, 1983). The Oxfordshire community stroke project reported that the 17% of patients with acute stroke and AF had a higher 30-day mortality (nearly threefold higher) than patients in sinus rhythm (Sandercock et al, 1992). Recent reports from the Copenhagen Stroke Study and the Framingham Study have suggested that patients with AF who develop a stroke have a higher mortality and more severe disability, a longer duration of in-hospital stay, and lower rate of

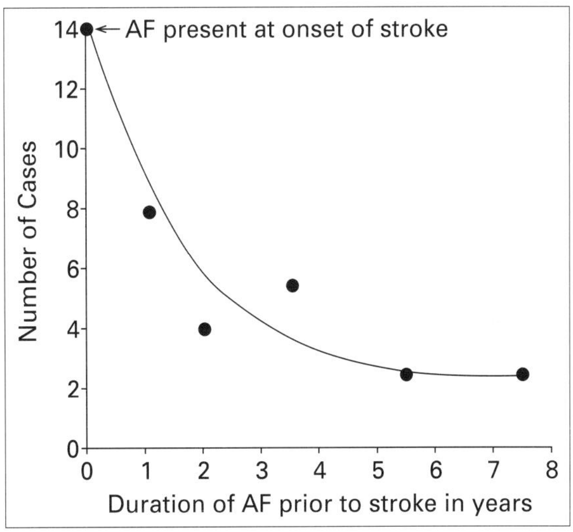

Figure 16.3
Temporal distribution of stroke events by duration of atrial fibrillation. Reproduced with permission from Wolf et al (1983).

discharge to their own homes (Jorgensen et al, 1997; Lin et al, 1996).

Until recently, the only evidence supporting the benefit of anticoagulation therapy in prophylaxis has been from retrospective studies. One example is the Montreal Heart Institute Study, which showed that the incidence of thromboembolic events was eight times more frequent during the period without anticoagulation therapy, whether or not mitral valve disease was present and irrespective of whether or not AF was chronic or paroxysmal (Roy et al, 1986). To fully address the issue of stroke and thromboembolism in NVAF, five large randomised primary prevention trials were initiated in the 1980s, in addition to one secondary prevention trial (Table 16.2). All five studies were terminated early by their data-monitoring boards in view of the marked benefit of warfarin therapy in the prevention of thromboembolic events, and all five primary prevention studies (most patients enrolled had no history of embolism) studies show consistent results.

Warfarin and aspirin for AF

Despite the limitations (which will be discussed further below), consideration of all trials together (as well as consideration of benefits and risks on antithrombotic treatment versus off treatment) allows the best current estimate of risks and benefits of warfarin and aspirin (Table 16.2).

Anticoagulation therapy

In the pooled meta-analysis by the Atrial Fibrillation Investigators of the five initial primary prevention trials, an annual rate of stroke of 4.5% was found in the control group and a rate of 1.4% in the warfarin group. This difference represents an overall risk reduction of 68% (95% CI 50%–79%) compared with the rate in untreated patients (AF Investigators, 1994). Warfarin prophylaxis also resulted in a similar risk reduction in stroke with residual deficit, a decrease in mortality by 33%, and a decrease in the combined adverse outcome (stroke, systemic embolism, or death) by 48%. Warfarin usage was particularly beneficial as secondary prevention in the EAFT study, in which the risk of stroke was reduced from 12% to 4% per year (Hazard Ratio 0.34 [95% CI 0.20–0.57]); (EAFT study, 1993). This was confirmed by the most recent meta-analysis of antithrombotic therapy in chronic AF, where the use of anticoagulation reduced the risk of stroke by 62% (95% CI 48%–72%) (Hart et al, 1999).

Despite these impressive figures, the optimal efficacy of warfarin prophylaxis is probably underestimated, because most strokes in patients randomised to warfarin occurred when the patients were not in fact taking warfarin or when they were significantly underanticoagulated.

Antiplatelet therapy

Aspirin has been evaluated as primary thromboprophylaxis against stroke and thromboembolism in AF in two randomised trials, compared with patients on no antithrombotic treatment (Petersen et al, 1989; SPAF, 1991), in one randomised trial against warfarin (SPAF2, 1992), one secondary prevention trial (EAFT, 1993) and in low risk patients (SPAF3, 1996); (Table 16.2). Doses of aspirin used daily ranged from 75 mg in the AFASAK study to 325 mg in the SPAF study. The SPAF-I data initially suggested that aspirin 325 mg daily may provide adequate thromboprophylaxis in patients aged below 75 years, but was not effective in preventing severe strokes (SPAF-I, 1991). In addition, 46% of patients in the placebo group of the BAATAF study were allowed to take aspirin 325 mg daily, with no beneficial effects found (Singer et al, 1992).

			Annual embolic event rate				Risk reduction in annual thromboembolic event rate	
1° prevention	*Mean follow-up (in years)*	*INR range*	*Aspirin*	*Warfarin*	*Placebo control*	*Low-dose warfarin and aspirin*	*With ASA*	*With adjusted warfarin*
SPAF I	1.3	2.0–3.5	3.6%	2.3%	6.3%–7.4%		42%	67%
SPAF II	2.3	2.0–4.5	<75y 1.9%	1.3%				>75y 33%*
			>75y 4.8%	3.6%				<75y 17%*
SPAF III	1.1	1.8–3.2		1.9%		7.9%		74%
		1.2–1.5						
CAFA	1.3	2.0–3.0		3.5%	5.2%			37%
BAATAF	2.2	1.5–2.7		0.41%	3%			86%
AFASAK	2	2.8–4.2	5.5%	2%	5.5%		14%	60%
AFASAK II+	3		3.6%	5.8% (1.25 mg)		7.2%		
		2.0–3.0		2.8%				
SPINAF	1.8	1.2–1.5		0.9%	4.3%			79%
2° prevention								
EAFT	2.3	2.5–4.0	10%	4%	12%		17%	66%

*The control group received aspirin at a dose of 325 mg once a day. +AFASAK II: warfarin 1.25 mg; warfarin 1.25 mg plus aspirin 300 mg; aspirin 300 mg once a day, versus adjusted dose-warfarin (INR 2.0–3.0). Comparison group was fixed, low-dose warfarin and aspirin.

SPAF = Stroke Prevention in Atrial Fibrillation; CAFA = Canadian Atrial Fibrillation Anticoagulation study; BAATAF = Boston Area Anticoagulation Trial in Atrial Fibrillation; AFASAK = Atrial Fibrillation, Aspirin, Anticoagulation Study from Copenhagen, Denmark; SPINAF = Veterans Affairs Stroke Prevention in Nonrheumatic Atrial Fibrillation Study; EAFT = European Atrial Fibrillation Trial; INR = International Normalized Ratio.

Table 16.2
Randomised trials for prevention of thromboembolic events in non-rheumatic AF.

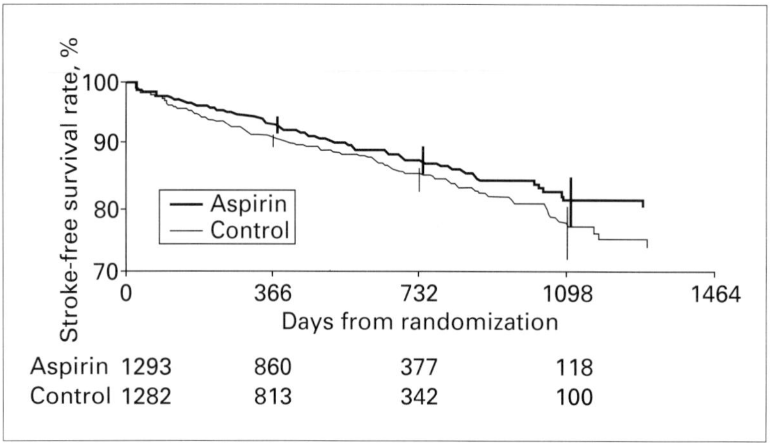

Figure 16.4
Cumulative stroke-free survival of all patients randomized to aspirin or placebo therapy. The vertical bars represent 95% confidence intervals. The log rank p value was 0.05. Aspirin and control indicate the number of patients at risk for stroke depending on their group assignment. Reproduced with permission from the Atrial Fibrillation Investigators (1997).

On-treatment analysis showed that aspirin was only about half as effective as warfarin. Importantly, aspirin has no significant effect on severe strokes or mortality, although in the pooled analysis, aspirin did reduce strokes by 21% (95% CI 0–37%, p = 0.05) and the combined outcome of stroke, embolism, or death by 28% (AF Investigators, 1997) (Figure 16.4; Table 16.3). In the EAFT study, aspirin was also less effective than warfarin when used as secondary prophylaxis in patients with previous stroke or transient ischaemic attack (warfarin *vs* aspirin hazard ratio 0.60 [95% CI 0.41–0.87]); (EAFT study, 1993). The most recent meta-analysis of antithrombotic therapy in chronic AF confirmed that the use of aspirin reduced the risk by 22% (CI 2%–38%) (Hart et al, 1999). A comparison of warfarin and aspirin suggests that warfarin was associated with a 45% risk reduction compared to aspirin (AF Investigators, 1994).

This reduction of stroke and thromboembolism with aspirin for AF is broadly similar to the 20% reduction found by the Antiplatelet Trialists (1994) in the meta-analysis of 144 trials of aspirin for the treatment and prevention of vascular disease.

Recently, the SIFA (Studio Italiano Fibrillazione Atriale); Morocutti et al, 1997) study showed in NVAF patients treated with indobufen, an antiplatelet agent, that indobufen may be similar in efficacy to warfarin. In this multicentre randomised secondary prevention trial, 916 patients with NVAF and recent (<15 days) minor stroke or transient ischaemic attack were treated with indobufen 200 mg twice daily or warfarin (INR 2.0–3.5), over a period of 12 months. The incidence of any vascular events was 10.6% in the indobufen group and 9.0% in the warfarin group (p = NS). The stroke rate was 5% in the indobufen arm and 4% in the warfarin arm. This study therefore implies that indobufen might be a valuable alternative in cases where anticoagulants are contraindicated and indobufen maybe more efficacious than aspirin.

The use of antiplatelet agents such as dipyridamole, clopidogrel, and ticlopidine in NVAF requires further assessment and clinical trials before their routine use can be recommended. In the European Stroke Prevention Study-2 (ESPS-2); (Diener et al, 1996), patients who had previous stroke or transient ischaemic attack were randomised to a trial of

Study group	SPAF 1	AFASAK	EAFT	All studies
		No. of Patients (Patient-Years of Exposure)		
Aspirin	552 (723)	336 (409)	404 (853)	1292 (1985)
Placebo	568 (734)	336 (398)	378 (734)	1282 (1867)
		No. of Strokes (Rate per Year, %)		
Aspirin	23 (3.2)	16 (3.9)	87 (10.2)	126 (6.3)
Placebo	42 (5.7)	19 (4.8)	90 (12.3)	151 (8.1)
Relative risk (95% CI)	0.56 (0.34–0.93; $p = .03$)	0.82 (0.42–1.60; $p = .57$)	0.85 (0.63–1.14; $p = .28$)	0.79 (0.62–1.0; $p = .05$)

*SPAF1 indicates Stroke Prevention in Atrial Fibrillation 1 Study; AFASAK, Atrial Fibrillation, Aspirin, Anticoagulation Study; EAFT, European Atrial Fibrillation Trial; and CI, confidence interval.

Table 16.3
Overall efficacy of aspirin therapy.*

low-dose (50 mg) aspirin alone sustained release dipyridamole (400 mg/day) alone, or a combination of the two agents, and results were compared with placebo over 24 months (Forbes, 1998). There was a significant benefit of combination therapy over aspirin or dipyridamole alone. A subgroup analysis of ESPS-2 showed a trend towards some benefit in secondary prevention from an aspirin-dipyridamole combination in patients with AF and previous cerebrovascular events.

Combined warfarin and aspirin therapy

The SPAF-III trial compared the use of low and fixed dose warfarin (INR of 1.2 to 1.5) plus aspirin (325 mg per day) with standard dose-adjusted warfarin therapy (INR 2–3) in 1044 patients with AF who were at high risk for stroke and thromboembolism (that is, women aged >75, systolic blood pressure >160 mm Hg, poor left ventricular function, or prior thromboembolic event). Compared with adjusted dose warfarin therapy, low and fixed dose warfarin plus aspirin was associated with significantly higher rates of ischemic stroke or systemic embolism (7.9% *vs* 1.9% per year, $p < 0.0001$), disabling stroke (5.6 *vs* 1.7%, $p = 0.0007$), and vascular death or a primary event (11.8 *vs* 6.4%, $p = 0.002$; SPAF-III, 1996). In the low risk patients ($n = 892$), a history of hypertension conferred a stroke risk of about 3.5-fold (approximately 3.5% per year [95% CI 2.5–5.2]) that of the remaining "low risk" cohort (1% per year [0.6–2.0]) despite aspirin 325 mg daily.

The second Copenhagen Atrial Fibrillation Aspirin Anticoagulation (AFASAK-2) trial compared daily treatment of warfarin 1.25 mg with warfarin 1.25 mg plus aspirin 300 mg, and with aspirin 300 mg versus adjusted dose warfarin (INR 2.0–3.0) in chronic AF (Gullov et al, 1998). After including 677 patients, the trial was terminated early following publication of SPAF-3, and the primary event rates at 3 years were 11.9%, 12.8%, 8.4%, and 8.3% ($p = 0.67$), suggesting a trend towards superiority of adjusted dose warfarin over low-intensity anticoagulation or aspirin-warfarin combination therapy.

A similar study by Pengo and colleagues (1998) of 303 patients randomised to low-intensity fixed mini-dose warfarin (INR < 1.5) or adjusted dose therapy (INR 2.0–3.0) reported an increased event rate in the fixed mini-dose warfarin group (11.1% *vs* 6.1%), suggesting that this regimen was not useful as thromboprophylaxis. The Primary prevention of Arterial Thromboembolism in patients with non-valvular Atrial Fibrillation in general practice (PATAF) study randomised 729 patients from 275 Dutch general practices to aspirin 150 mg, warfarin INR 2.5–3.5, or warfarin INR 1.1–1.6 (Hellemons et al, 1999). After a mean follow-up of 2.7 years, the primary event rate was similar (2% per year) in the three treatment groups, although in patients with contraindications to anticoagulation, the primary event rate was 10% per year in the aspirin group and the low dose warfarin group. However, the PATAF study excluded high-risk patients (age >78 years, heart failure, hypertension, valve disease, previous cerebrovascular event, or contraindications to aspirin or warfarin) and thus this trial could only confirm that aspirin was sufficient thromboprophylaxis in low-risk patients and that low-intensity or adjusted-dose warfarin did not confer further advantages.

The failure of low-intensity anticoagulation or fixed-dose aspirin-warfarin combinations comes as little surprise, since analyses of the optimal anticoagulation intensity for stroke prevention in AF showed that stroke risk appeared to be substantially increased at INR

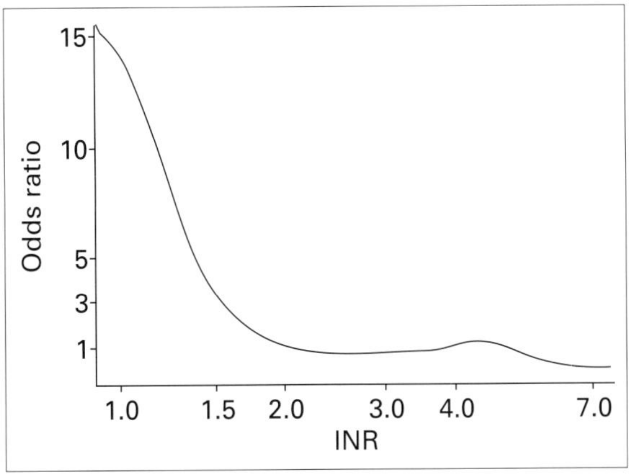

Figure 16.5
Odds ratio for stroke according to INR value. Hylek et al (1996).

INR	*Odds ratio (95% CI)**
1.0	17.6 (7.9–39.3)
1.1	11.9 (6.0–23.8)
1.2	8.3 (4.6–15.0)
1.3	6.0 (3.6–9.8)
1.4	4.4 (2.9–6.6)
1.5	3.3 (2.4–4.6)
1.6	2.5 (1.9–3.3)
1.7	2.0 (1.6–2.4)
1.8	1.5 (1.4–1.7)
1.9	1.2 (1.2–1.3)

*Odds ratios are the odds of ischemic stroke among patients with the INR in question as compared with the patients with an INR of 2.0. CI denotes confidence interval.

Table 16.4
Adjusted odds ratios for ischaemic stroke according to the INR. Hylek et al (1996).

levels below 2.0. In the case-controlled study by Hylek and colleagues (1996), the INR was a powerful and independent determinent of the risk of stroke. When compared with patients with an INR of 2.0, those with an INR of 1.7 had a two-fold increase in the risk of stroke (Hylek et al, 1996) (Figure 16.5; Table 16.4).

From trials to clinical practice

Despite convincing evidence for the effectiveness of warfarin prophylaxis, which appears to substantially outweigh the risk of intracranial bleeding, concern has been expressed that the efficacy of warfarin in clinical trials may not translate into effectiveness in practice. These trials have raised several important questions over its applicability to routine clinical practice.

These trials were also never designed to provide anything more than an estimate of treatment efficacy. Although widely interpreted as being studies of warfarin treatment, these trials have been described as "packages of care" that included drugs, monitoring, and follow-up. Patients in these trials were highly selected, especially for contraindications to warfarin, and on average fewer than 10% (range 3–40%) of eligible patients were randomised (Figure 16.6) For example, in the SPAF I study only 1330 (7.8%) patients of the 17 046 patients with AF who were screened were actually entered into the study. These trials had a relatively short-term follow-up, averaging 2 to 3 years, and despite this, the number of patients withdrawn from warfarin was relatively high, ranging from 10% in the BAATAF study (BAATAF, 1990) to 38% in the AFASAK study (Petersen et al, 1989). Very little information is available on patients who were withdrawn from therapy, and this number is likely to be sizeable in clinical practice. In addition, many patients were excluded after initial assessments for the absence of contraindications, and because of physicians' refusal

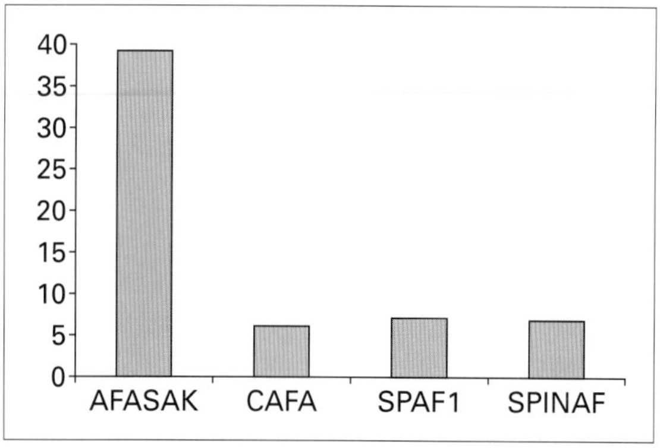

Figure 16.6
Percentage of patients enrolled in the primary prevention anticoagulation trials as a proportion of those screened.

to enter their patients into the study. Recruitment of these patients was therefore primarily from hospital practice, self-referral and referrals from interested physicians, suggesting that the populations were not representative of patients with AF in the community, or even of typical patients in our clinical practice. Furthermore, the frequent monitoring of warfarin therapy under trial conditions was probably more intense than that applied in usual clinical practice. For example, monitoring was done at least every 3 to 4 weeks in the trials that reported frequency, and between 0.6% and 15% of the tests showed the anticoagulant effect to be greater than intended. Hence, the ratio of antithrombotic benefit to bleeding risk may be lower in usual clinical practice than in published trials; and this may also reduce its cost-effectiveness.

A recent survey of patients with AF in a health-maintenance organisation in the USA showed a higher prevalence of concurrent illness, a less frequent monitoring interval, and a lower frequency of INR tests within the target therapeutic range, compared with patients in clinical trials (Gottlieb and Salem-Schatz, 1994). However, Caro and colleagues (1993) reported a study using decision-analysis techniques and concluded that the likely benefit of warfarin to all patients with AF was probably substantial in clinical practice. Since warfarin reduced the risk of stroke and thromboembolism by two thirds, but increased bleeding by 53% (or 0.5% per year), prophylaxis with warfarin should be given unless it is considered that the risk of bleeding is perceived to be over 6 times more detrimental than the risk of thromboembolism.

In addition, the five initial primary prevention trials used different target therapeutic ranges for the INR of the prothrombin time; these ranged between 1.5 and 4.5 (Table 16.3). However, the minimum risk of stroke appeared to occur in the INR range 2.0–3.0, which is now generally accepted as the optimum therapeutic range for anticoagulant prophylaxis of thromboembolism in all patient groups. Exceptions include those patients with older mechanical prosthetic heart valves, and those with recurrent thromboembolism (despite warfarin prophylaxis at INR 2.0–3.0, who require a higher intensity warfarin regimen (INR 3.0–4.5)). A target INR of 2.0–3.0 is therefore the recommended intensity of anticoagulation in the absence of the above indications for high intensity warfarinisation.

One critical appraisal and meta-analysis of the five published randomized controlled trials of primary stroke prevention with anticoagulation in chronic NVAF (Green et al, 1997) used the relatively objective endpoints of major strokes, fatal strokes, major bleeding, and fatal bleeding, in view of the lack of blinded assessment and documented low inter-rater reliability of soft neurological endpoints. The study showed that warfarin did not reduce the incidence of fatal strokes to a statistically significant extent, nor did the incidence of fatal bleeding increase significantly. Warfarin reduced the absolute annual incidence of major strokes in patients with chronic NVAF by 0.89%, but at the same time it increased the absolute annual risk of major bleeding incidents by 1.8%. This analysis concluded that on balance, the margin between expected benefit and harm for warfarin prophylaxis in patients with AF was uncomfortably thin.

Risk stratification for stroke and thromboembolism in patients with AF

Based upon clinical criteria from the pooled analysis of the AF Investigators, most patients with AF can be classified into high, moderate, and low risk patients (AF Investigators, 1994; Lip, 1999). The analysis by Ezekowitz and Levine (1999) of the prospective, randomized trials of patients with AF that evaluated warfarin, aspirin, or both, used MEDLINE from Jan 1, 1966, to Feb 23, 1999. The study identified five primary prevention placebo-controlled studies, which had been formally pooled. One study evaluated secondary prevention of stroke, one study compared warfarin with aspirin, and three studies assessed warfarin in combination with aspirin. They reported that the risk of developing stroke is heterogeneous and increased with each decade over 65 years, with history of high blood pressure, diabetes mellitus, previous transient ischemic attack, or stroke, with poor ventricular function, and in women older than 75 years. For patients younger than 65 years, without risk factors, and not receiving antithrombotic therapy, the risk of stroke is 1% per year; those without risk factors between the ages of 65 and 75 years have a risk of 1.1% per year if taking warfarin and 1.4% per year if taking aspirin. For all other patients, stroke risk per year is reduced from an untreated rate of between 4.3% and more than 12% to a rate of 1.2% to 4% with warfarin use. Thus, the researchers concluded that the protection afforded by warfarin was most pronounced in patients at the highest risk for stroke, who could be identified mainly from clinical risk factors, whilst aspirin treatment seemed adequate in low-risk populations.

Transthoracic echocardiographic features associated with a high risk of stroke in the SPAF-I study included left atrial dilatation (corrected for body surface area) and poor left ventricular function (SPAF, 1992b). However, in their recent overview of echocardiographic data from 1066 patients from three clinical trials, the AF Investigators (1998) reported that isolated left atrial enlargement per se was not an independent risk factor for stroke on multivariate analysis, although moderate to severe left ventricular systolic dysfunction on 2-dimensional echocardiography did appear to be a predictor (Figure 16.7; and Table 16.5). In the SPAF-III transoesophageal echocardiography substudy, features associated with a high risk of stroke included the presence of spontaneous echocontrast, thrombus in left atrial appendage, and complex aortic plaques (SPAF Committee on Echocardiography, 1998; Stollberger et al, 1998). Echocardiography therefore complements risk stratification on clinical grounds, and would be useful in the small study group of patients who have a low risk of stroke according to clinical risk factors. This is confirmed by the recent Newcastle survey, in which echocardiography was useful in deciding the need for warfarin in the small proportion of subjects with AF who did not have clinical risk factors (Sudlow et al, 1998).

Only rarely do clinicians need to proceed to TOE to assist risk stratification (Kulbertus, 1999), but in the SPAF-III TOE substudy, stroke and thromboembolism were correlated

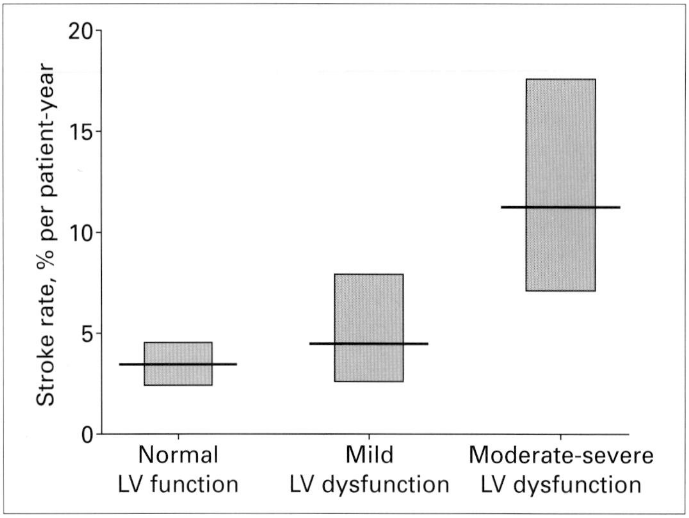

Figure 16.7
Atrial fibrillation echo analysis. CI = confidence interval; LV = left ventricle. Reproduced with permission from the Atrial Fibrillation Investigators (1998).

with dense spontaneous echocontrast, left atrial appendage thrombus, and complex aortic plaques (SPAF Committee on Echocardiography, 1998) (Table 16.6; Figure 16.8).

Reduced left atrial appendage velocity is also another risk factor (Kamp et al, 1999). In the study by Kamp and colleagues (1999), previous thromboembolism (odds ratio 5.3 [95% CI 1.9, 12.1], $p < 0.005$), history of hypertension (4.0 [1.4–10.4] $p < 0.01$), presence of left atrial spontaneous echocontrast (3.5 [1.2–10.0], $p < 0.025$), and presence of left atrial appendage peak velocity of 0.20 ms or less (4.1 [1.4, 11.6, $p < 0.01$) were significantly related to subsequent stroke and thromboembolic events in patients with AF (Figure 16.9).

The **highest risk** of stroke is observed in persons with previous transient ischaemic attack or stroke. In the pooled analysis, the annual risk of stroke was 12% in controls and 5% in warfarin groups (Table 16.3). In addition to a previous history of thromboembolism, independent risk factors for thromboembolism were increasing age, diabetes mellitus, and history of hypertension. The combination of age 75 years or over plus diabetes or hypertension also indicates a high-risk group, in whom warfarin prophylaxis appears highly effective (annual risk of stroke 8–12% in controls, and 1–2% on treatment with warfarin).

A **moderate risk** of stroke exists in people with non-rheumatic AF, without previous cerebrovascular events or thromboembolism; those who are aged under 65 years with a history of diabetes or hypertension; those who are aged 65–74 (with or without a history of diabetes or hypertension); and those aged 75 years or more with no history of diabetes or hypertension. In these patients, aspirin appears to be as effective as warfarin, with a reduction in the annual risk of stroke from 4% to 1–2%.

A **low risk** of stroke (annual risk 1%) exists in people with non-rheumatic AF who are aged under 65 years and who have no history of previous embolism, hypertension, or diabetes. Such patients include those with lone

	No risk factors†			≥1 Risk factor†		
Age, y	*Events per patients*	*Annual rate, %*	*95% CI for rate, %*	*Events per patients*	*Annual rate, %*	*95% CI for rate, %*
<65						
All patients	2/167	0.8	0.2–3.0	5/197	5.2	3.2–8.7
Normal LV‡	1/153	0.4	0.06–2.9	8/150	3.6	1.8–7.2
Abnormal LV§	1/10	9.3	1.3–66	5/36	9.7	4.0–23
65–75						
All patients	11/175	3.9	2.2–7.1	30/336	5.6	3.9–8.0
Normal LV	8/153	3.2	1.6–6.5	22/273	4.9	3.2–7.4
Abnormal LV	2/17	8.4	2.1–33	6/38	11.7	5.3–26
>75						
All patients	1/74	0.9	0.1–6.7	19/117	10.7	6.8–16.7
Normal LV	0/64	0.0	. . .	12/88	8.3	4.7–14.6
Abnormal LV	1/8	10.9	1.4–78	4/20	19.7	7.4–52

*The "all patients" includes some patients in whom information about LV function was not available. CI indicates confidence interval; ellipses, not applicable.
†Clinical risk factors (excluding age) are prior stroke or transient ischaemic attack, history of hypertension, or history of diabetes.
‡Includes patients with normal or mild LV dysfunction.
§Includes patients with moderate or severe LV dysfunction showed on echocardiography.

Table 16.5
Stroke rates by age and left ventricular (LV) function. Data from AF Investigators (1998).*

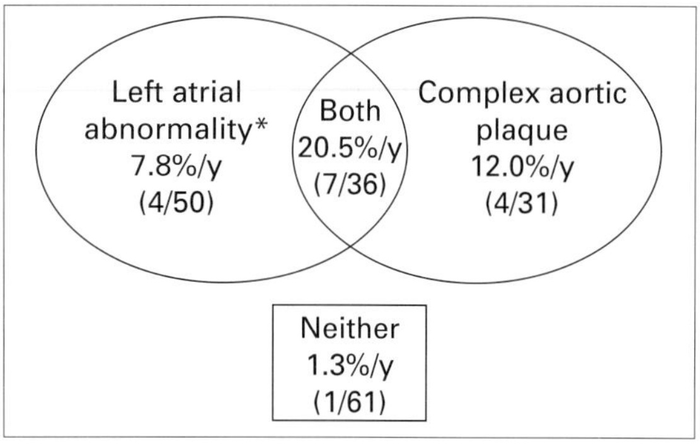

Figure 16.8
Event rates during combination therapy in subsets defined according to findings on transoesophageal echocardiography. Ratios in parentheses relate events to patients with the specified criteria.
** = Left atrial abnormality refers to thrombus of the left atrial appendage (14% of patients), dense spontaneous echocardiographic contrast (18% of patients) or peak antegrade (emptying) velocity of blood flow from the left atrial appendage less than 20 cm/s (35% of patients). The 95% CIs for the events are: left atrial abnormality, 2.9% to 21.0% per year; complex aortic plaque, 4.5% to 32.0% per year; both, 9.8% to 43% per year; and neither, 0.2% to 9.5% per year. SPAF Committee on Echocardiography (1998).*

AF, which is a diagnosis of exclusion after careful assessment has excluded any history, examination, ECG, or echocardiographic evidence of cardiovascular disease. In such people, antithrombotic prophylaxis with either aspirin or warfarin does not appear to be warranted unless some other indication or coexisting risk factor is present. Nevertheless, such patients are commonly prescribed aspirin in clinical practice.

Risk stratification may give a false sense of security for providing thromboprophylaxis in patients with chronic AF. However, many guidelines do exist (Table 16.7) such that a recent review by Thomson and colleagues (1998) concluded that the widespread nonsystemic production of guidelines could lead to wide variation in whether anticoagulation should be used in AF (range 13–100%). A survey by Lip and colleagues (1996) judged that the continued lack of consensus amongst consultant physicians over anticoagulation for AF and the varied perception of risk-benefit ratios

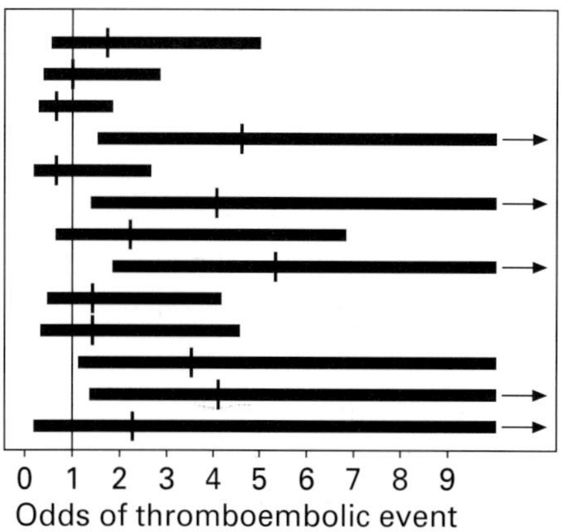

Adjusted OR	Variable	P value
1.6	Age>75 years	ns
1.0	Paroxysmal AF	ns
0.6	Duration AF<1 year	ns
4.5	Aspirin use	<0.010
0.6	OAC use	ns
4.0	History of hypertension	<0.010
2.2	History of heart failure	ns
5.3	Previous embolism	<0.005
1.4	LA area.20 cm^2	ns
1.4	LAA area>10 cm^2	ns
3.5	SEC	<0.025
4.1	LAA peak,20 cm s^{-1}	<0.010
2.3	Thrombus	ns

Figure 16.9
Odds ratio and 95% confidence intervals are presented to identify clinical and thromboembolic event predictors of a subsequent thromboembolic event in patients with atrial fibrillation. Reproduced with permission from Kamp et al (1999).

Feature	*RR*	*p*
LAA thrombi	2.5	0.04
Dense SEC	3.7	<0.001
LAA peak flow vel ≤ 20 cm/s	1.7	0.008
Complex aortic plaque	2.1	<0.001

n = 786
SPAF-III Investigators JACC 1998; 31: 1622–26.

Table 16.6
TOE correlates of thromboembolism in NVAF.

Atrial Fibrillation Investigators	*Stroke Prevention in Atrial Fibrillation Investigators*	*American College of Chest Physicians*
Previous stroke or TIA Moderate-severe LV dysfunction Previous hypertension Increasing age Diabetes	Previous stroke or TIA LV fractional shortening ≤25% or recent CHF Current SBP >160 mm Hg Women >75 y of age	Previous stroke or TIA Heart failure or coronary artery disease Previous hypertension Age >75 y Diabetes Mitral stenosis Prosthetic heart valves Thyrotoxicosis

*TIA indicates transient ischaemic attack; LV, left ventricular.

Table 16.7
Risk stratification schemes for patients with atrial fibrillation and increased stroke risk.*

in this survey suggests that much work is still needed for adequate risk stratification and provision of suitable thromboprophylaxis for patients with chronic NVAF. Equally, prescription of warfarin to low-risk patients who do not need it increases the risk of bleeding in those patients, and imposes the inconvenience of regular attendance at anticoagulant clinics for monitoring.

For now, a strategy of careful clinical assessment and risk stratification for AF, where the highest risk groups for stroke and thromboembolism are targeted for anticoagulation, whilst low risk subjects could be adequately treated with aspirin, is probably the way forward (Figure 16.10). A practical guide

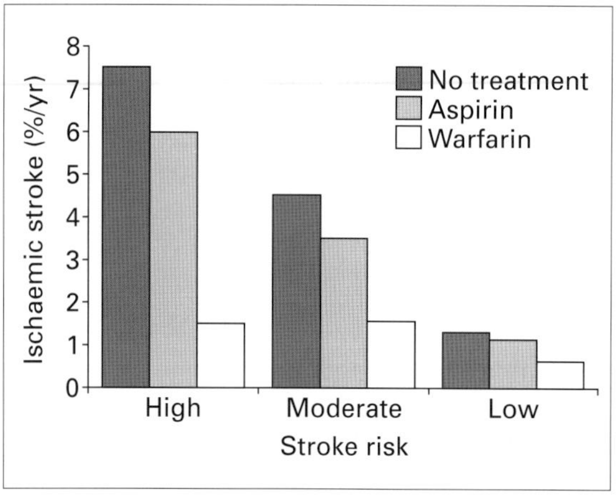

Figure 16.10
Absolute reduction in ischaemic stroke by aspirin and warfarin according to intrinsic stroke rate in patients with atrial fibrillation.

to risk stratification in patients with AF is provided in Table 16.8 which has been adopted locally and nationally.

Risk stratification for patients with AF

Paroxysmal AF

Epidemiological studies suggest that paroxysmal AF (PAF) confers an intermediate risk of stroke compared with chronic AF and sinus rhythm (Petersen and Godtfredsen, 1986). By contrast, data from the SPAF and BAATAF trials suggest that stroke rates in PAF and chronic AF are similar (BAATAF, 1990; SPAF, 1991). Both the SPAF II study and the European Atrial Fibrillation Trial also enrolled patients with chronic AF and PAF, though specific results are not available for those patients with PAF. Nevertheless there are no trials specifically examining the value of antithrombotic therapy in patients with PAF per se.

However, the risks of stroke and thromboembolism with PAF are likely to be significant. Patients with PAF show abnormalities of haemostasis (Lip, 1997), which appear to be related to the duration of paroxysms of AF and to whether the patient was in AF at the time of blood sampling (Sohara et al, 1997) PAF has also been associated with abnormalities of atrial function, as evident by the appearance of spontaneous echocontrast on transoesophageal echocardiography (Obarski et al, 1990). Patients who are started on anticoagulation or cardioverted from AF to sinus rhythm (Lip et al, 1995) show significant changes in markers of haemostasis, suggesting a reduction in the hypercoagulable state. However, a large percentage (50%) of patients with PAF have no underlying structural heart disease or have "lone" PAF (Suttorp et al, 1993; Clementy et al, 1992); this is in contrast to the small percentage of chronic AF patients who can be confidently diagnosed as "lone" chronic AF (Godtfredsen et al, 1982).

A recent analysis from the SPAF investigators reported that the annual rate of stroke was similar in paroxysmal (3.2%) and sustained (3.3%) AF (Hart et al, 2000). Independent predictors of stroke in PAF were age (relative risk RR 2.1 per decade), hypertension (RR 3.4) and prior stroke (RR 4.1), with a stroke rate of 7.8/yr (95% CI 4.5–14) in "high risk" subjects.

Our recommendation, therefore, is to use warfarin in patients with PAF unless they can be clearly classified as having lone AF or there is contraindication to the use of anticoagulation. As with NVAF, it appears that individuals with PAF but no underlying heart disease are at a low risk of thromboembolism and do not require anticoagulation. Aspirin therapy may suffice in such patients.

ASSESS RISK:

1. High Risk **(annual risk of CVA = 8–12%)**

- All patients with NVAF and previous TIA or CVA
- All patients aged 75 and over with NVAF and diabetes and/or hypertension
- All patients with NVAF and clinical evidence of valve disease, heart failure, thyroid disease and/or impaired LV function on echocardiography.*

2. Moderate Risk **(annual risk of CVA = 4%)**

- All patients under 65 with NVAF and clinical risk factors: diabetes, hypertension, peripheral arterial disease, ischaemic heart disease.
- All patients over 65 with NVAF who have not been identified in High Risk group.

3. Low Risk **(annual risk of CVA = 1%)**

- All other patients under 65 with NVAF with no history of embolism, hypertension, diabetes or other clinical risk factors.

*ECHOCARDIOGRAM – not needed for routine risk assessment but refines clinical risk stratification in case of impaired LV function and valve disease (see 1 above). A large Left Atrium per se is not an independent risk factor on multivariate analysis.

REASSESS RISK FACTORS AT REGULAR INTERVALS

TREATMENT:

- **High Risk:** use WARFARIN (target INR 2.0–3.0) if no contraindications and possible in practice.
- **Moderate Risk:** Either WARFARIN or ASPIRIN. In view of insufficient clearcut evidence, treatment may be decided on individual cases. Referral and ECHOCARDIOGRAPHY may help.
- **Low Risk:** use ASPIRIN 75–300 mg daily

Table 16.8
Risk stratification and anticoagulation in non-valvular atrial fibrillation (NVAF) – a practical guide for clinicians. Adapted with permission from Lip GYH (1999).

	Aspirin	*No aspirin*	
With atrial fibrillation			
Cast	99/680	111/692	
IST	322/1622	308/1547	
Total	421/2302	419/2239	χ^2=0.136; d.f =1; p=NS
Without atrial fibrillation			
Cast	441/9552	500/9514	
IST	776/8097	898/8167	
Total	1217/17649	1398/17681	χ^2=13.178; d.f =1; p=0.0003

Table 16.9
Effect of aspirin in patients with atrial fibrillation and acute stroke. Adapted from Lip and Beevers (1997).

Patients with AF and a recent stroke

In the acute management of stroke, the use of subcutaneous heparin in the International Stroke Trial (1997) and the Chinese Acute Stroke Trial (1997) reduced recurrent ischaemic stroke, but this was offset by an increase in haemorrhagic transformation, leading to a neutral effect on outcomes. The use of aspirin in both trials led to a marginal benefit in mortality, but this appeared to be less so among patients with AF at time of presentation (Lip and Beevers, 1997) (Table 16.9). Low molecular weight heparin is not any superior to aspirin in acute ischaemic stroke and AF (Berge et al, 2000).

When, and whether or not to start anticoagulation after an acute cardioembolic stroke poses another problem, as there is a small risk of haemorrhagic transformation of the cerebral infarct by bleeding into the infarcted, softened brain.

In cases of established thromboembolic strokes, intravenous heparin followed by warfarin (target INR 2–3) could be commenced in non-hypertensive patients with small to moderate strokes after computed tomography or magnetic resonance imaging (MRI) done 48 h or more after symptom onset confirms the absence of intracranial haemorrhage (Sherman et al, 1995). Anticoagulation should, however, be postponed for 1–2 weeks in patients with large thromboembolic strokes due to the potential risk of haemorrhagic transformation (Laupacis et al, 1995). In patients with AF as the presumed cause of thromboembolism, initiation of warfarin therapy (after CT at 48 h) without initial heparin therapy is reasonable in view of the relatively low risk of early recurrent thromboembolism.

Anticoagulation intensity, stroke, and bleeding risk

It is important to balance the risks (especially bleeding) and benefits in the individual patients before starting antithrombotic prophylaxis with warfarin or aspirin. Current evidence favours a target INR of 2.0–3.0, although some physicians target a lower range of INR (1.5–2.5) in patients at increased risk of bleeding. To minimise the risk of intracranial bleeding on prophylactic warfarin, hypertension should be adequately controlled and closely monitored. The risks and benefits of warfarin should also be reviewed annually, especially in patients aged over 80 years. Intracranial haemorrhage should be excluded in patients with acute stroke and AF, before commencing warfarin. This is an important consideration since 11% of patients with haemorrhagic stroke have AF, compared with the frequency of 18% in stroke due to cerebral infarction (Sandercock et al, 1992).

In the BAATAF study, no significant differences between warfarin-treated patients and controls were found for quality of life as shown by measures of functional status, well-being, and health perceptions, unless complicated by a bleeding episode. Surprisingly, the quality-of-life assessment of patients in the BAATAF study showed that 76% did not mind regular blood tests (Lancaster, 1991). Patients on warfarin who sustain a bleeding complication show a significant decrease in health perceptions. It should be noted that primary prophylaxis with anticoagulant therapy in AF is cost-effective if the rate of intracranial bleeding during such therapy is only 0.3%, as in the major published trials (Gustafsson et al, 1992). However, if this rate increases to 2% per year, warfarin therapy is no longer cost-effective. This "cost" has to be balanced against the reduction of the annual risk of stroke and the associated morbidity and mortality "costs", which are likely to be large. This emphasises the importance of careful selection of patients for warfarin prophylaxis, regular monitoring and control, and regular review of the balance of risks and benefits. Thus, in high-risk patients in whom warfarin is judged to be contraindicated, aspirin prophylaxis may be appropriate. Whatever prophylaxis is given, however, risk factors should be reviewed annually because they change: for example, the risk of stroke increases with age (Figure 16.1).

Gastrointestinal tract
Potentiating drugs – Antacids (magnesium salts); cimetidine; liquid paraffin and other laxatives.
Antagonistic drugs – Cholestyramine; colestipol
Cardiovascular system
Potentiating drugs – Amiodarone; clofibrate; dextrothyroxine; diazoxide; dipyridamole; ethacrynic acid; quinidine; sulphinpyrazone
Antagonistic drugs – Cholestyramine; colestipol; spironolactone
Respiratory system
Antagonistic drugs –Antihistamines
Central nervous system
Potentiating drugs – Chloral hydrate and related compounds; chlorpromazine; dextropropoxyphene; dichloralphenazone (initial); diflunisal; mefenamic acid; monoamine oxidase inhibitors; triclofos sodium; tricyclic antidepressants
Antagonistic drugs – Barbiturates; carbamazepine; dichloralphenazone – late; haloperidol; phenytoin; primidone
Infections
Potentiating drugs – Aminoglycosides; ampicillin (oral); cephalosporins; chloramphenicol; co-trimoxazole; cycloserine; erythromycin; isoniazid; ketoconazole; metronidazole; miconazole; nalidixic acid; penicillin G (large doses) – intravenous; quinine salts; streptotriad; sulphonamides (long acting); tetracycline
Antagonistic drugs – Griseofulvin; rifampicin
Endocrine system
Potentiating drugs – Anabolic steroids; chlorpropamide; corticosteroids; danazol; glucagon; metoclopramide; propylthiouracil; sulphonyl urea; thyroxine; tolbutamide
Antagonistic drugs – Oral contraceptives
Malignant disease and immunosuppression
Potentiating drugs – Cyclophosphamide; metcaptopurine; methotrexate; immunosuppressant drugs; tamoxifen
Musculoskeletal and joint disease
Potentiating drugs – Allopurinol; aspirin and the salicylates; azapropazone; diflunisal; fenclofenac; fenoprofen; febrazone; flufenamic acid; flubiprofen; indomethacin; ketoprofen; mefenamic acid; naproxen; paracetamol (high daily doses (with dextropropoxyphene distalgesic/coproxamol)); piroxicam; sulindac; sulphinpyrazone
Nutrition and blood
Potentiating drugs – Alcohol (dose dependent potentiator)
Antagonistic drugs – Vitamin K; alcohol
Ear, nose and oesophagus
Antagonistic drugs – Antihistamines; phenazone
Skin
Antagonistic drugs – Antihistamines
Alcoholism
Potentiating drugs – Disulfiram (antabuse)

Table 16.10
Drugs that may interact with oral anticoagulants.

Bleeding risk and anticoagulation intensity

The most devastating complication associated with warfarin prophylaxis is the risk of intracranial haemorrhage. This is a particular problem in the elderly, in whom frailty, poor mobility, forgetfulness or poor compliance with medication, concomitant medications (resulting in drug interactions), and frequent falls may jeopardise the benefits from warfarin (Table 16.10).

The intensity of anticoagulation may be an important factor in the prevention of stroke in NVAF, and in the risk of bleeding, which occurs in up to 2–3% of patients per year on warfarin. In the pooled analysis of five primary prevention trials, the annual rate of major haemorrhage (defined as an intracranial haemorrhage, a haemorrhage requiring at least two units of blood, or an event requiring hospital admission) was 1% in control patients and 1.3% in warfarin-treated patients (AF Investigators, 1994). The overall risk of bleeding associated with the usage of warfarin was therefore 2–3% of patients per year.

The annual risks of intracranial haemorrhage increased from 0.1% in control to 0.3% in warfarin groups in the pooled analysis, which represents an excess of two intracranial bleeds per annum per 1000 patients treated. The risk is increased as much as threefold in patients who have bled previously, and both bleeding and haemorrhagic stroke may be more common in patients aged over 75 years. The risk of death from a major bleed ranged from 13–33% and the risk of morbidity in those who survive a major bleed is as high as 15%.

Possible factors which may increase the risk of bleeding whilst on warfarin include the following: age, uncontrolled hypertension (defined as systolic blood pressure >180 mm Hg or diastolic blood pressure >100 mm Hg), alcohol excess, liver disease, poor drug or clinic compliance, and bleeding lesions (especially gastrointestinal blood loss, for example, peptic ulcer disease; or previous cerebral haemorrhage) or bleeding tendency (including coagulation defects and thrombocytopenia). Concomitant use of aspirin with oral anticoagulants may also increase the risk of bleeding.

In the SPAF-II study, the benefits of warfarin were nearly counteracted by an increased risk of intracranial haemorrhage in the warfarin group, which was unexpectedly high in patients older than 75 years (1.8% per year); however, the rate of intracranial haemorrhage in this group was substantially higher than that reported in the original five trials (on average 0.3% per year), which may reflect the higher intensity of anticoagulation in the SPAF-II study (INR up to 4.5) (Figure 16.11). For patients 75 years or younger, the annual rate of intracranial haemorrhage in the SPAF-II study was 0.2% on aspirin and 0.5% on warfarin. For those older than 75 years, the annual rate of intracranial haemorrhage was higher (0.8% on aspirin, 1.8% on warfarin). By contrast, the pooled data from five initial primary prevention trials (AF Investigators, 1994) showed only one intracranial haemorrhage in 223 patients aged older than 75 years who were receiving warfarin. Even low-dose aspirin increases the risk of major haemorrhage by two-fold (0.5% per year in elderly people).

What is the risk of bleeding associated with antithrombotic therapy in the "real world"? Petty and colleagues (1999) reported a population-based study of complication rates of medical therapy for secondary stroke prevention in the general population. They found that 20 aspirin-associated complications (one fatal) during an average 1.7 years of treatment, eight warfarin-associated complications

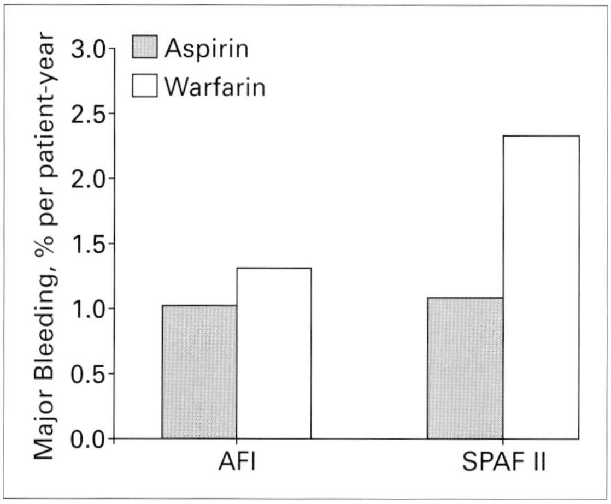

Figure 16.11
Rates of major bleeding events among patients receiving warfarin sodium compared with aspirin from the pooled analysis of 5 trials performed by the Atrial Fibrillation Investigators and the Stroke Prevention in Atrial Fibrillation II (SPAF II) study. In the AFI analysis, major haemorrhage was defined as intracranial bleeding or a bleeding event that required hospitalization or 2 U blood. In the SPAF trial, major bleeding was defined as a haemorrhagic event that involved the central nervous system; required hospitalization, blood transfusion, and/or surgical intervention; or resulted in permanent functional impairment to any degree.

occurred during an average of 0.7 years of treatment, and three heparin-associated complications (one fatal) occurred during an average 5.1 days of treatment. Complication rates were 3.5 per 100 person-years (95% CI 2.1–5.4) for aspirin, 7.9 per 100 person-years (3.4–15.6) for warfarin, and 0.30 (0.06–0.86) per 100 person-days for heparin. Rates of fatal complications were 0.2 per 100 person-years (0–1.0) for aspirin, 0 per 100 person-years (0–3.6) for warfarin, and 0.10 per 100 person-days (0–0.55) for heparin. Interestingly, the complication rates for warfarin and intravenous heparin given as therapy for secondary stroke prevention in this study from Rochester were much lower than rates reported from earlier trials and observational studies. However, complication rates for warfarin were higher than in more recent referral-based studies and multicentre randomised trials. One prospective cohort study to determine if trial efficacy of warfarin for stroke prevention in AF translated into clinical effectiveness reported that the rate of stroke (2% per year, 95% CI 0.7–4.4) were comparable to patients in the pooled studies (1.4%/year); similarly, major bleeding rates (1.7% versus 1.6%) were comparable (Kalra et al, 2000).

What is the right INR range?

In the multicentre trials most strokes occurred in patients assigned to warfarin therapy with INR values under 2.0 (Hylek et al, 1996). At the other end of the spectrum, the bleeding risk is higher in patients with INR values over 3.0. Whilst some studies have suggested that the risk of bleeding with anticoagulation increases with age (Coon and Willis, 1974; Wintzen et al, 1984), this has not been confirmed by others (Forfar et al, 1979; Gurwitz et al, 1988; Enrichete et al, 1985). In the AFASAK-2 study (Gullov et al, 1999), fixed mini-dose warfarin and aspirin alone or in combination were associated with both minor and major bleeding; after 3 years of treatment with mini-dose warfarin, warfarin plus aspirin, aspirin, and adjusted-dose warfarin, the cumulative rate of any bleeding was 24.7%, 24.4%, 30.0%, and 41.1% ($p = 0.003$), respectively. Increasing INR value ($p < 0.001$) and prior myocardial infarction ($p = 0.001$) were independent risk factors for bleeding, whereas (importantly)

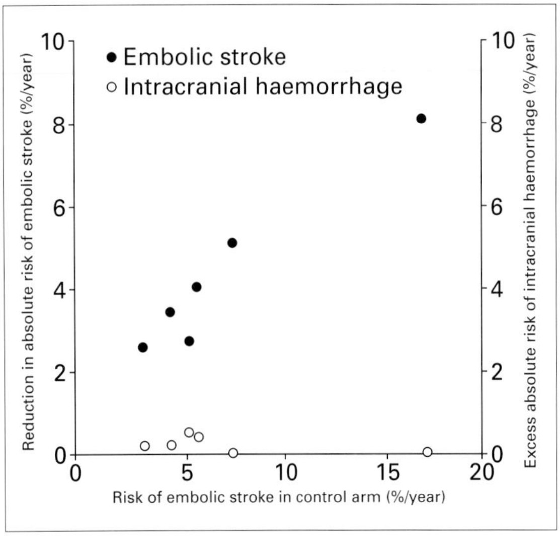

Figure 16.12
Trials of warfarin in non-valvular AF show that benefit (reduction in absolute risk of stroke) increases with increasing risk of stroke but that harm (intracranial haemorrhage) seems to be constant. Reproduced with permission from Glaszion and Irwig (1995).

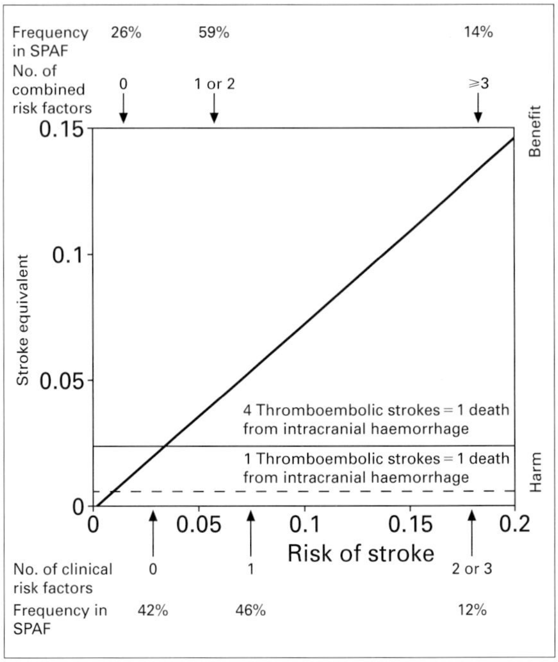

Figure 16.13
Benefit compared with harm for warfarin on basis of six trials. If one death from an intracranial haemorrhage is equivalent to four thromboembolic strokes, threshold is about 2% per year. This may be predicted from three clinical risk factors (previous embolism, recent cardiac failure, and hypertension; bottom axis) or three clinical plus two echocardiographic risk factors (clinical risk factors plus atrial size and left ventricular dysfunction; bottom axis).
SPAF = stroke prevention in AF trial. Reproduced with permission from Glaszion and Irwig (1995).

increasing age was not. The finding that the small number of major bleeding events in patients receiving adjusted-dose warfarin therapy (INR 2–3) compared with those receiving less intensive antithrombotic treatment, and the finding of no significant influence of age on the risk for bleeding, suggests that even elderly patients with AF should be able to tolerate adjusted-dose warfarin therapy.

The target INR for anticoagulation in NVAF should therefore be 2.0–3.0, providing maximal thromboprophylaxis with minimal bleeding risk (Glaszion and Irwig, 1995) (Figures 16.12 and 16.13). Maintenance of INR values between 2.0 and 3.0 is much more difficult than it seems, however (Table 16.11). In the SPAF III study (SPAF III, 1996b), only 61% of INR values had an INR between 2 and 3, despite the fact that a nurse carefully followed monthly prothrombin times and adjusted warfarin doses with physician assistance and the use of a warfarin nomogram developed by the investigators. In the Italian group (Pengo et al, 1998), the warfarin dose-adjusted group spent only 70% of their time in the optimal INR

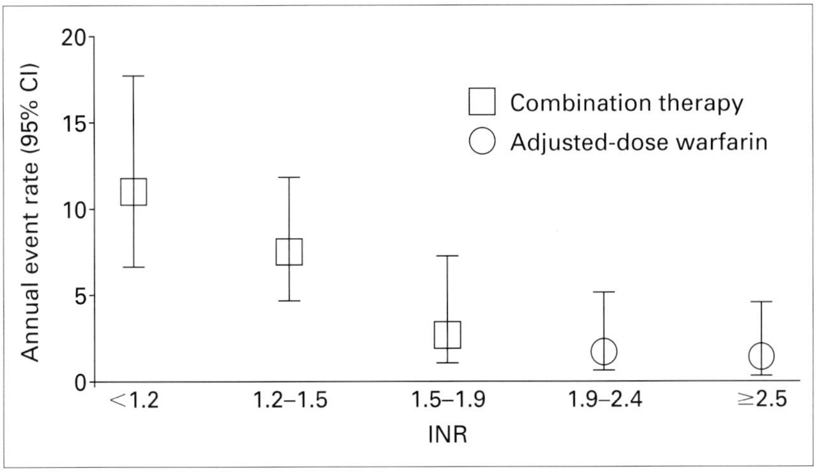

Figure 16.14
Event ratios for ischaemic stroke or systemic embolism in the SPAF III Study. Reproduced with permission of Stroke Prevention in Atrial Fibrillation Investigators (1996a).

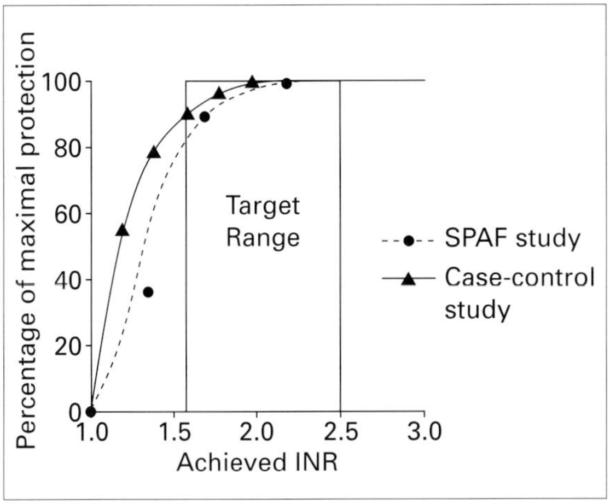

Figure 16.15
Relative efficacy of target international normalized ratios (INRs) of 1.6 to 2.5. SPAF = Stroke Prevention in Atrial Fibrillation. Hylek et al (1996).

therapeutic range of 2.0–3.0 and had an excessive anticoagulation intensity (INR > 3.0) for 12% of the time. As discussed previously, the safety and tolerability of long-term anticoagulation titrated to conventional levels is less clear in the very elderly (age >75 years), which is the age group encompassing perhaps half of AF-associated stroke patients. It has been suggested that INR 1.6–2.5 can provide substantial, if partial efficacy (estimated to be nearly 90% of the highest intensities; SPAF III, 1996b; Hylek et al, 1996) (Figure 16.14). Given the uncertainty about safety of INRs above 3.0, particularly for elderly AF patients, a target INR of 2.0 (range 1.6–2.5) may be a reasonable compromise between toxicity and efficacy for this age group, pending further data about the safety of higher intensities (Figure 16.15). Indeed, this was suggested in a small trial where low intensity warfarin (INR 1.5–2.1) was safer, with less bleeding, than conventional warfarin (Yamaguchi, 2000).

Overall, oral anticoagulation therapy does appear to be a relatively safe therapeutic stratagem and should therefore be standard therapy for most patients with AF, in the absence of contraindications. However, patients on warfarin need regular instructions, and the effect of warfarin must be regularly monitored (and the dose adjusted). General practitioners looking after such patients also need to be aware of potential drug interactions and risks in such patients (Lip et al, 1996). Patients who are anticoagulated long-term also require regular follow-up in anticoagulant clinics to optimise anticoagulant control, thus imposing

Study	Mode of monitoring	Anticoagulation below range	Estimated INR range	Estimated average INR	Anticoagulation above range
AFASAK	INR	58%	2.8–4.2	Not given	0–6%
SPAF-I	PTR	23%	2.0–4.5	~2.5	5%
BAATAF	PTR	8%	1.5–2.7	Not given	9%
CAFA	INR	40%	2.0–3.0	2.4	17%
SPINAF	PTR	29%	1.4–2.8	Not given	15%
EAFT	INR	32%	2.5–4.0	2.9	9%
SPAF-II	PTR/INR	20%/22%	2.0–4.5	2.7/2.6	5%/6%
<75 years/>75 years					

INR = International normalized ratio.
PTR = Prothrombin time ratio.
For other abbreviations see Table 16.2.

Table 16.11
Adequacy of anticoagulant control in studies of atrial fibrillation

some restrictions on their lives. There have been concerns that service provision for the use of anticoagulants in AF may be insufficient, particularly with the need for caution in interpreting the results of the large studies and extrapolating these results to the UK population (Sudlow et al, 1995).

Current practice with anticoagulation for AF

Despite the compelling evidence of the benefits of stroke reduction in patients with AF, antithrombotic therapy continues to be underused. Many studies have consistently shown that the usage of antithrombotic therapy in the community remains low, with only 44% of patients with AF aged 65 to 74 years, and only 11% of patients over 75 years with AF being treated with warfarin (Sudlow et al, 1995; Lip et al, 1997). Our survey of AF in two general practices in West Birmingham (Lip et al, 1997) broadly agrees with these findings, with warfarin being prescribed to only 36% of 111 patients with AF. A low rate of anticoagulation was particularly seen in the elderly patients (over the age of 75 years) in whom the benefits of antithrombotic therapy might be expected to be greatest. Physician surveys have consistently cited patient age as a deterrent to the use of warfarin in AF (McCroy et al, 1995; Kutner et al, 1991). In a survey of UK consultant physicians, there was also significant difference in the management of AF, with more cardiologists than non-cardiologists considering cardioversion or antithrombotic therapy (Lip et al, 1996). Furthermore, other risk factors, such as poor compliance, recurrent falls, cognitive impairment, and the risk of interaction with multiple drug therapies are also cited as deterrents to the use of warfarin in AF, especially in the elderly (Kutner et al, 1991).

The problems and uncertainties about anticoagulation in the elderly are clearly illustrated by a cross-sectional analysis of a subgroup of elderly (aged >70 years) participants in the Cardiovascular Health Study (White et al, 1999), in which 4.1% had AF and 37% used warfarin. Of the 109 participants not reporting warfarin use, 84% had at least one of the clinical risk factors (aside from age) associated with stroke in patients with AF. Of the participants not taking warfarin, 47% were taking aspirin. Factors that were independently associated with warfarin use included age (odds ratio of less than 0.6 per 5-year increment [95% CI 0.5–0.9]), a modified mini-mental examination score of less than 85 points (0.3 [0.1–0.9]), and, among patients without prior stroke, female sex (0.5 [0.2–1.0]). Thus, despite widely publicised practice guidelines to treat patients who have AF with warfarin, most participants who had AF were at high risk for stroke but were not treated with warfarin. Elderly patients in rural areas with AF also seemed to be receiving antithrombotic therapy less frequently than urban patients, despite having a similar high-risk profile and fewer relative contraindications (Flaker et al, 1999). One reason for this may be that primary-care physicians prescribed antithrombotic therapy less often than cardiologists (69% *vs* 52%).

One reason frequently cited as an influence on the choice of antithrombotic therapy in elderly patients with AF is the risk of falling (with a possible increased chance of intracranial haemorrage). Man-Son-Hing and colleagues (1999) reported a Markov decision analytic model used to determine the preferred treatment strategy (no antithrombotic therapy, long-term aspirin use, or long-term warfarin use) for patients with AF who are 65 years of age and older, are at risk for falling, and have no other contraindications to antithrombotic therapy. They showed that for patients with average risks of stroke and falling, warfarin therapy was associated with 12.90 quality-adjusted life-years per patient. Aspirin therapy was associated with 11.17 quality-adjusted life-years, and no antithrombotic therapy gave 10.15 quality-adjusted life-years. Sensitivity analysis showed that, irrespective of the patients' age or baseline risk of stroke, the risk of falling was not an important factor in determining their optimal antithrombotic therapy.

Thus, as discussed in this chapter, for elderly patients with AF the choice of optimal therapy to prevent stroke depends on many clinical factors, especially their baseline risk of stroke. The patients' propensity to fall is not an important factor in this decision. Furthermore, the patient's perspective may be just as important. The same investigators (Man-Son-Hing et al, 1996) interviewed patients with AF and found that 52% of the patients would take warfarin for an absolute decrease in stroke risk of 1% over 2 years. Nevertheless, AF patients generally showed poor knowledge of their stroke risk.

In a recent analysis of Medicare beneficiaries, only 55% were prescribed antithrombotic therapy (34% warfarin, 21% aspirin). Advanced age, female gender and rural residency predicted underuse of antithrombotic therapy (Gage et al, 2000).

One option to improve anticoagulation management of these patients with AF may be to increase involvement by general practitioners. There is clear evidence that many general practitioners can monitor anticoagulation intensity more efficiently than hospital anticoagulant clinics (Pell et al, 1993), and many patients prefer to attend their local general practitioner rather than busy hospital clinics that may be far away. This issue requires further clarification, and possible solutions, such as decision support for dosing and self-monitoring, need further evaluation. A recent survey of hospital consultants and general practitioners broadly concluded that general practitioners could perform this role satisfactorily (Rogers et al, 1997). However, general practitioners vary in their willingness to undertake anticoagulation monitoring, and some practices do not even offer this service (Taylor et al, 1993). If better, safer, and increasing use of anticoagulation in patients with AF is intended, increasing provision of general practitioner-based anticoagulation monitoring aided by computerised support systems and near-patient testing may become a necessary step (Rogers et al, 1997; Fitzmaurice et al, 1998).

Conclusion

AF is very common, and consideration of appropriate antithrombotic strategies remains a major public-health problem, in view of the potential avoidance of mortality and morbidity from stroke and thromboembolism. Until we can develop more effective, efficient, and safe methods to provide adequate thromboprophylaxis, efforts at careful risk stratification with clinical risk factors (with some refinement from echocardiography) are needed. This would allow the highest risk patients with AF to be identified and treated with warfarin, with lower risk individuals prescribed aspirin. Concurrent comorbidity, especially in the elderly, needs to be carefully evaluated and considered in any treatment strategy.

References

Antiplatelet Trialists' Collaboration. Collaborative overview of randomized trials of antiplatelet therapy. I. Prevention of death, myocardial infarction, and stroke by prolonged antiplatelet therapy in various categories of patients. *BMJ* 1994; **308:** 81–106.

Atrial Fibrillation Investigators. Echocardiographic predictors of stroke in patients with atrial fibrillation: a prospective study of 1066 patients from three clinical trials. *Arch Intern Med* 1998; **158:** 1316–20.

Atrial Fibrillation Investigators. Risk factors for stroke and efficacy of antithrombotic therapy in atrial fibrillation: analysis of pooled data from five randomized controlled trials. *Arch Intern Med* 1994; **154:** 1449–57.

Atrial Fibrillation Investigators. The efficacy of aspirin in patients with atrial fibrillation. Analysis of pooled data from 3 randomized trials. *Arch Intern Med* 1997; **157:** 1237–40.

Benjamin EJ, Levy D, Varizi SM et al. Independent risk factors for atrial fibrillation in a population-based cohort. *JAMA* 1994; **271:** 840–4.

Benjamin EJ, Wolf PA, D'Agostino RB et al. Impact of atrial fibrillation on risk of death. The Framingham Heart Study. *Circulation* 1998; **98:** 946–52.

Beppu S, Park YD, Sakakibara H et al. Clinical features of intracardiac thrombosis based on echocardiographic observation. *Jpn Circ J* 1984; **48:** 75–82.

Berge E, Abdelnoor M, Nakstad PH, Sandset PM. Low molecular weight heparin versus aspirin in patients with acute ischaemic stroke and atrial fibrillation: a double blind randomised study. *Lancet* 2000; **355:** 1205–10.

Black IW, Hopkins AP, Lee LC et al. Left atrial spontaneous echo contrast: a clinical and echocardiographic analysis. *J Am Coll Cardiol* 1991; **18:** 398–404.

The Boston Area Anticoagulation Trial for Atrial Fibrillation Investigators. The effect of low-dose warfarin on the risk of stroke in patients with nonrheumatic atrial fibrillation. *N Engl J Med* 1990; **323:** 1505–11.

Caro JJ, Groome PA, Flegel KM. Atrial fibrillation and anticoagulation: from randomised trials to practice. *Lancet* 1993; **341:** 1381–4.

Chiang CW, Lo SK, Ko YS et al. Predictors of systemic embolism in patients with mitral stenosis. *Ann Intern Med* 1998; **128:** 885–9.

Chinese Acute Stroke Trial (CAST) Collaborative Group. CAST: randomised placebo-controlled trial of early aspirin use in 20,000 patients with acute ischaemic stroke. *Lancet* 1997; **349:** 1641–9.

Clementy J, Dulhoste MN, Laiter C et al. Fleclainide acetate in the prevention of paroxysmal atrial fibrillation: a nine-month follow-up of more than 500 patients. *Am J Cardiol* 1992; **70(suppl):** 44A–49A.

Cohen BA, Hilderbrand F, Biller J. Cardioembolic Stroke: part I – clinical patterns and associated cardiac conditions. *ACC Current Journal Review* 1993; **2:** 51–2.

Connolly SJ, Laupacis A, Gent M et al. Canadian Atrial Fibrillation Anticoagulation (CAFA) Study. *J Am Coll Cardiol* 1991; **18:** 349–55.

Coon WW, Willis PW III. Hemorrhage complications of anticoagulant therapy. *Arch Intern Med* 1974; **133:** 386–92.

Diener HC, Cunha L, Forbes C et al. European Stroke Prevention Study. 2. Dipyridamole and acetylsalicylic acid in the secondary prevention of stroke. *J Neurol Sci* 1996; **143:** 1–13.

EAFT (European Atrial Fibrillation Trial) Study Group. Secondary prevention in non-rheumatic atrial fibrillation after transient ischaemic attack or minor stroke. *Lancet* 1993; **342:** 1255–62.

Enrichete AM, Holden A, Ansell J. Management of oral anticoagulant therapy: experience with an anticoagulant clinic. *Arch Intern Med* 1985; **144:** 1966–8.

Ezekowitz MD, Bridgers SL, James KE et al, for the Veterans Affairs Stroke Prevention in Nonrheumatic Atrial Fibrillation Investigators. Warfarin in the prevention of stroke associated with nonrheumatic atrial fibrillation. *N Engl J Med* 1992; **327:** 1406–12.

Ezekowitz MD, Levine JA. Preventing stroke in patients with atrial fibrillation. *JAMA* 1999; **281:** 1830–5.

Feinberg WM, Blackshear JL, Laupacis A et al. Prevalence, age distribution, and gender of patients with atrial fibrillation: analysis and implications. *Arch Intern Med* 1995; **155:** 469–73.

Fitzmaurice DA, Hobbs FD, Murray ET. Primary care anticoagulant clinic management using computerized decision support and near patient International Normalized Ratio (INR) testing: routine data from a practice nurse-led clinic. *Fam Pract* 1998; **15:** 144–6.

Flaker GC, McGowan DJ, Boechler M et al. Underutilization of antithrombotic therapy in elderly rural patients with atrial fibrillation. *Am Heart J* 1999; **137:** 307–12.

Flegel KM, Shipley MJ, Rose G. Risk of stroke in non-rheumatic atrial fibrillation. *Lancet* 1987; **1:** 526–9.

Fleming HA, Bailey SM. Mitral valve disease, systemic embolism and anticoagulants. *Postgrad Med J* 1995; **47:** 599–604.

Forbes CD. Secondary stroke prevention with low-dose aspirin, sustained release dipyridamole alone and in combination. ESPS Investigators. European Stroke Prevention Study. *Thromb Res* 1998; **92(suppl 1):** S1–6.

Forfar JC. A 7-year analysis of haemorrhage in patients on long term anticoagulant treatment. *Br Heart J* 1979; **42:** 128–32.

Gage BF, Boechler M, Doggette AL et al. Adverse outcomes and predictors of underuse of antithrombotic therapy in medicare beneficiaries with chronic atrial fibrillation. *Stroke* 2000; **31:** 822–87.

Glaszion PP, Irwig LM. An evidence-based approach to individualizing treatment. *BMJ* 1995; **311:** 1356–9.

Godtfredsen J. Atrial fibrillation, etiology, course, and prognosis: a follow-up of 1212 cases. In: Kulbertus HE, Olsson SB, Schlepper M, eds. *Atrial Fibrillation.* Molndal: AB Hassle, 1982; 134–45.

Gottlieb LK, Salem-Schatz S. Anticoagulation in atrial fibrillation. Does efficacy in clinical trials translate into effectiveness in practice? *Arch Intern Med* 1994; **154:** 1945–53.

Green CJ, Hadorn DC, Bassett K, Kazanjian A. Anticoagulation in chronic nonvalvular atrial fibrillation: a critical appraisal and meta-analysis. *Can J Cardiol* 1997; **13:** 811–15.

Gullov AL, Koefoed BG, Petersen P et al. Fixed minidose warfarin and aspirin alone and in combination vs adjusted-dose warfarin for stroke prevention in atrial fibrillation: Second Copenhagen AFASAK Study. *Arch Intern Med* 1998; **158:** 1513–21.

Gullov AL, Koefoed BG, Petersen P. Bleeding during warfarin and aspirin therapy in patients with atrial fibrillation: the AFASAK 2 Study. *Arch Intern Med* 1999; **159:** 1322–8.

Gurwitz JH, Goldberg RJ, Holden A et al. Age-related risks of long term oral anticoagulant therapy. *Arch Intern Med* 1988; **148:** 1733–6.

Gustafsson C, Asplund K, Britton M et al. Cost-effectiveness of primary stroke prevention in atrial fibrillation: Swedish national perspective. *BMJ* 1992; **305:** 1457–60.

Hart RG, Benavente O, McBride R, Pearce LA. Antithrombotic therapy to prevent stroke in patients with atrial fibrillation: A meta-analysis. *Ann Intern Med* 1999; **131:** 492–501.

Hart RG, Pearce LA. Rothbart RM et al. Stroke with intermittent atrial fibrillation: incidence and predictors during aspirin therapy. SPAF investigators. *J Am Coll Cardiol* 2000; **35:** 183–7.

Hellemons BSP, Langenberg M, Lodder J et al. Primary prevention of arterial thromboembolism in non-rheumatic atrial fibrillation in primary care: randomised controlled trial comparing two intensities of conmarin with aspirin. *BMJ* 1999; **319:** 958–64.

Hofmann T, Kasper W, Meinertz T, et al. Echocardiographic evaluation of patients with clinically suspected arterial thrombi. *Lancet* 1990; **336:** 1421–4.

Hylek EM, Skates SJ, Sheehan MA, Singer DE. An analysis of the lowest effective intensity of prophylactic anticoagulation for patients with non-rheumatic atrial fibrillation. *N Engl J Med* 1996; **335:** 540–6.

International Stroke Trial (IST): a randomised trial of aspirin, subcutaneous heparin, both, or neither among 19 435 patients with acute ischaemic stroke. International Stroke Trial

Collaborative Group. *Lancet* 1997; **349:** 1569–81.

Jorgensen HS, Nakayama H, Reith J et al. Stroke recurrence: predictors, severity, and prognosis. The Copenhagen Stroke Study. *Neurology* 1997; **48:** 891–5.

Kalra L, Yu G, Perez I et al. Prospective cohort study to determine if trial efficacy of anticoagulation for stroke prevention on atrial fibrillation translates into clinical effectiveness. *BMJ* 2000; **320:** 1236–9.

Kamp O, Verhorst PM, Welling RC, Visser CA. Importance of left atrial appendage flow as a predictor of thromboembolic events in patients with atrial fibrillation. *Eur Heart J* 1999; **20:** 979–85.

Kapila A, Hart R. Calcific cerebral emboli and aortic stenosis: detection of computed tomography. *Stroke* 1986; **17:** 619–21.

Krahn AD, Manfreda J, Tate RB et al. The natural history of atrial fibrillation: incidence, risk factors and prognosis in the Manitoba Follow-Up Study. *Am J Med* 1995; **98:** 476–84.

Kulbertus H. Assessment of risk of thromboembolism in atrial fibrillation: which patients should we anticoagulate? *Eur Heart J* 1999; **20:** 923–4.

Kutner M, Nixon G, Silverstone F. Physicians' attitudes towards oral anticoagulants and antiplatelet agents for stroke prevention in elderly patients with atrial fibrillation. *Arch Intern Med* 1991; **151:** 1950–3.

Lancaster TR, Singer DE, Sheehan MA et al. The impact of long-term warfarin therapy on quality of life. Evidence from a randomized trial. Boston Area Anticoagulation Trial for Atrial Fibrillation Investigators. *Arch Intern Med* 1991; **1:** 1944–9.

Laupacis A, Albers G, Dalen J et al. Antithrombotic therapy in atrial fibrillation. *Chest* 1995; **168:** 3525–95.

Lin HJ, Wolf PA, Kelly-Hayes M et al. Stroke severity in atrial fibrillation. The Framingham Study. *Stroke* 1996; **27:** 1760–4.

Lip GYH, Beevers DG. Interpretation of IST and CAST stroke trials. International Stroke Trial. Chinese Acute Stroke Trial. *Lancet* 1997; **350:** 443–4.

Lip GYH, Golding D, Nazir M et al. A survey of atrial fibrillation in general practice: the West Birmingham Atrial Fibrillation Project. *Br J Gen Pract* 1997; **47:** 285–9.

Lip GYH, Rumley A, Dunn FG, Lowe GD. Plasma fibrinogen and fibrin D-dimer levels in atrial fibrillation: effect of cardioversion to sinus rhythm. *Int J Cardiol* 1995; **51:** 245–53.

Lip GYH, Zarifis J, Watson RD, Beevers DG. Physician variation in the management of patients with atrial fibrillation. *Heart* 1996; **75:** 200–5.

Lip GYH. Does paroxysmal atrial fibrillation confer a paroxysmal thromboembolic risk? *Lancet* 1997; **349:** 1565–6.

Lip GYH. Thromboprophylaxis for atrial fibrillation. *Lancet* 1999; **353:** 4–6.

Lowe GD, Jaap AJ, Forbes CD. Relation of atrial fibrillation and high haematocrit to mortality in acute stroke. *Lancet* 1983; **1:** 784–6.

Man-Son-Hing M, Laupacis A, O'Connor A et al. Warfarin for atrial fibrillation. The patient's perspective. *Arch Intern Med* 1996; **156:** 1841–8.

Man-Son-Hing M, Nichol G, Lau A, Laupacis A. Choosing antithrombotic therapy for elderly patients with atrial fibrillation who are at risk for falls. *Arch Intern Med* 1999; **159:** 677–85.

McCrory DC, Matchar DB, Smasa G et al. Physician attitudes about anticoagulation for nonvalvular atrial fibrillation in the elderly. *Arch Intern Med* 1995; **155:** 277–81.

Morocutti C, Amabile G, Fattapposta F et al, for the SIFA (Studio Italiano Fibrillazione Atrial) Investigators. Indobufen versus warfarin in the secondary prevention of major vascular events in nonrheumatic atrial fibrillation. *Stroke* 1997; **28:** 1015–21.

Nishide M, Irino T, Gotoh M et al. Cardiac abnormalities in ischaemic cerebrovascular disease studied by two-dimensional echocardiography. *Stroke* 1983; **14:** 541–5.

Obarski TP, Salcedo EE, Castle LW, Stewart WJ. Spontaneous echo contrast in the left atrium during paroxysmal atrial fibrillation. *Am Heart J* 1990; **120:** 988.

Onundarson PT, Thorgeirsson G, Jonmundsson E et al. Chronic atrial fibrillation – epidemiologic features and 14 year followup: a case control study. *Eur Heart J* 1987; **3:** 521–7.

Pell JP, McIver B, Stuart P et al. Comparison of anticoagulant control among patients attending general practice and a hospital anticoagulant clinic. *Br J Gen Prac* 1993; **43:** 152–4.

Pengo V, Zasso A, Barbero F et al. Effectiveness of fixed minidose warfarin in the prevention of thromboembolism and vascular death in nonrheumatic atrial fibrillation. *Am J Cardiol* 1998; **82:** 433–7.

Petersen P, Boysen G, Godtfredsen J et al. Placebo-controlled, randomised trial of warfarin and aspirin for prevention of thromboembolic complications in chronic atrial fibrillation: the Copenhagen AFASAK Study. *Lancet* 1989; **1:** 175–9.

Petersen P, Godtfredsen J. Embolic complications in paroxysmal atrial fibrillation. *Stroke* 1986; **17:** 622–5.

Petersen P, Madsen EB, Brun B et al. Silent cerebral infarction in chronic atrial fibrillation. *Stroke* 1987; **18:** 1098–100.

Petty GW, Brown RD Jr, Whisnant JP et al. Frequency of major complications of aspirin, warfarin, and intravenous heparin for secondary stroke prevention. A population-based study. *Ann Intern Med* 1999; **130:** 14–22.

Rancurel G, Marelle L, Vincent C et al. Spontaneous calcific cerebral embolus from a cardiac aortic stenosis in a middle cerebral artery infarct. *Stroke* 1989; **20:** 691–3.

Rogers H, Sudlow M, Dobson R et al. Warfarin anticoagulation in primary care: a regional survey of present practice and clinicians' views. *Br J Gen Pract* 1997; **47:** 309–10.

Roy D, Marchand E, Gagné P et al. Usefulness of anticoagulant therapy in the prevention of embolic complications of atrial fibrillation. *Am Heart J* 1986; **112:** 1039–43.

Sandercock P, Bamford J, Dennis M et al. Atrial fibrillation and stroke: prevalence in different types of stroke and influence on early and long term prognosis (Oxfordshire Community Stroke Project). *BMJ* 1992; **305:** 1460–5.

Shaper AG, Pocock SJ, Walker M et al. British Regional Heart Study: cardiovascular risk factors in middle-aged men in 24 towns. *BMJ* 1981; **283:** 179–86.

Sherman DG, Dyken ML Jr, Gent M et al. Antithrombotic therapy for cerebrovascular disorders: an update. *Chest* 1995; **108:** 444s–56s.

Sherman DG, Dyken ML, Fisher M et al. Antithrombotic therapy for cerebrovascular disorders. *Chest* 1990; **95(suppl):** 140S–55S.

Shimomura K, Ohe T, Uehara S et al. Significance of atrial fibrillation as a precursor of embolism. *Am J Cardiol* 1989; **63:** 1405–7.

Singer DE, Hughes RA, Gress DR et al, for the BAATAF Investigators. The effect of aspirin on the risk of stroke in patients with nonrheumatic atrial fibrillation: the BAATAF study. *Am Heart J* 1992; **124:** 1567–73.

Sohara H, Amitani S, Kurose M, Miyahara K. Atrial fibrillation activates platelets and coagulation in a time-dependent manner: a study in patients with paroxysmal atrial fibrillation. *J Am Coll Cardiol* 1997; **29:** 106–12.

Stollberger C, Chnupa P, Kronik G et al. Transesophageal echocardiography to assess embolic risk in patients with atrial fibrillation. *Ann Int Med* 1998; **128:** 630–8.

Stroke Prevention in Atrial Fibrillation Committee on Echocardiography. Transesophageal echocardiographic correlates of thromboembolism in high-risk patients with atrial fibrillation. *Ann Intern Med* 1998; **128:** 639–47.

The Stroke Prevention in Atrial Fibrillation Investigators. Bleeding during antithrombotic therapy in patients with atrial fibrillation. *Arch Intern Med* 1996a; **156:** 409–16.

Stroke Prevention in Atrial Fibrillation Investigators. Predictors of thromboembolism in atrial fibrillation: II. Echocardiographic features of patients at risk. *Ann Intern Med* 1992b; **116:** 6–12.

Stroke Prevention in Atrial Fibrillation Investigators. Stroke prevention in atrial fibrillation study: Final results. *Circulation* 1991; **84:** 527–39.

Stroke Prevention in Atrial Fibrillation Investigators. Adjusted-dose warfarin versus low-intensity, fixed-dose warfarin plus aspirin for high risk patients with atrial fibrillation: Stroke Prevention in Atrial Fibrillation III randomized clinical trial. *Lancet* 1996b; **348:** 633–8.

Stroke Prevention in Atrial Fibrillation Investigators. Predictors of thromboembolism in atrial fibrillation: I. Clinical features of patients at risk. *Ann Intern Med* 1992a; **116:** 1–5.

Stroke Prevention in Atrial Fibrillation Investigators. Warfarin versus aspirin for prevention of thromboembolism in atrial fibrillation: Stroke

Prevention in Atrial Fibrillation II Study. *Lancet* 1994; **343:** 687–91.

Sudlow CM, Rodgers H, Kenny RA, Thomson RG. Service provision and use of anticoagulants in atrial fibrillation. *BMJ* 1995; **311:** 558–61.

Sudlow M, Thomson R, Thwaites B et al. Prevalence of atrial fibrillation and eligibility for anticoagulants in the community. *Lancet* 1998; **325:** 1167–71.

Suttorp MJ, Kingma JH, Koomen EM et al. Recurrence of paroxysmal atrial fibrillation or flutter after successful cardioversion in patients with normal left ventricular function. *Am J Cardiol* 1993; **71:** 710–13.

Taylor F, Ramsay M, Voke J, Cohen H. Anticoagulation in patients with atrial fibrillation: GPs not prepared for monitoring anticoagulation. *BMJ* 1993; **307:** 1493.

Thomson R, McElroy H, Sudlow M. Guidelines on anticoagulant treatment in atrial fibrillation in Great Britain: variation in content and implications for treatment. *BMJ* 1998; **316:** 509–13.

Tsai LM, Chen JH, Fang CJ et al. Clinical implications of left atrial spontaneous echo contrast in nonrheumatic atrial fibrillation. *Am J Cardiol* 1992; **70:** 327–31.

White RH, McBurnie MA, Manolio T et al. Oral anticoagulation in patients with atrial fibrillation: adherence with guidelines in an elderly cohort. *Am J Med* 1999; **106:** 165–71.

Wintzen AR, de Jonge H, Loeliger EA, Bots GT. The risk of intracerebral hemorrhage during oral anticoagulation treatment: a population study. *Ann Neurol* 1984; **16:** 553–8.

Wolf PA, Abbot RD, Kannel WB. Atrial fibrillation as an independent risk factor for stroke. The Framingham Study. *Stroke* 1991; **22:** 983.

Wolf PA, Kannel WB, McGee et al. Duration of atrial fibrillation and imminence of stroke. The Framingham Study. *Stroke* 1983; **14:** 664.

Yamaguchi T, for Japanese nonvalvalone atrial fibrillation – Embolism Secondary Prevention Cooperative Study Group. Optimal intensity of warfarin therapy for secondary prevention of stroke in patients with nonvalvular atrial fibrillation. *Stroke* 2000; **31:** 817–21.

Index